A NOTEBOOK OF DERMATOPATHOLOGY

A NOTEBOOK OF DERMATOPATHOLOGY

Mastering the Basics, Pattern Recognition, and Key Pathologic Findings

Edited by

Mariya Miteva, MD

Department of Dermatology and Cutaneous Surgery
University of Miami Miller School of Medicine
Miami, FL
USA

With contributions from

Jacquelyn Dosal, MD, and Andrew Miner, MD

Department of Dermatology and Cutaneous Surgery
University of Miami Miller School of Medicine, Miami, FL, USA

CRC Press
Taylor & Francis Group
Boca Raton London New York

CRC Press is an imprint of the
Taylor & Francis Group, an **informa** business

CRC Press
Taylor & Francis Group
6000 Broken Sound Parkway NW, Suite 300
Boca Raton, FL 33487-2742

Printed on acid-free paper

International Standard Book Number-13: 978-1-138-70408-4 (Hardback)

Visit the Taylor & Francis Web site at
http://www.taylorandfrancis.com

and the CRC Press Web site at
http://www.crcpress.com

Contents

Preface

The great Albert Einstein said: "Logic will get you from A to B. Imagination will take you everywhere." Love for morphology and the imagination inspired this book; I am convinced that studying skin pathology can be entertaining.

This book is dedicated to the dermatology residents at the University of Miami, who motivated me to simplify dermatopathology by using easy-to-memorize images (photomnemonics). Encouraged by the positive response to these over the years, I have put together this book in order to introduce residents, fellows, and students, as well as anyone interested in skin, to the basics of skin pathology. I hope readers will find the book useful and will benefit from it, but, most importantly, I hope they will enjoy it.

This book would not have happened without the help of my colleagues and dear friends Paolo Romanelli, MD, and Clara Milikowski, MD, who generously provided me with many pathologic slides from their collections. Other individual contributions are credited in the captions of the illustrations.

My colleague and dear friend Antonella Tosti, MD, deserves special recognition for encouraging and helping me to accomplish this project. I am also indebted to Robert Peden from Taylor & Francis for his great help and patience. Last but not least, I am grateful to Jackie Dosal, MD and Andrew Miner, MD for sharing my enthusiasm and contributing to the preparation of the book.

Mariya Miteva, MD
Miami, March 2016

Acknowledgments

In preparing this book various sources have helped with some of the text and inspired some of the figures, including but not limited to the following:

Barnhill RL, ed., *Textbook of Dermatopathology,* 1st edn, McGraw-Hill, 1998.

Brinster NK, Liu V, Diwan H, McKee PH, *Dermatopathology,* 1st edn, Elsevier Inc., 2011.

Cerroni C, Gatter K, Kerl H, *An Illustrated Guide to Skin Lymphoma*, 2nd edn, Blackwell, 2004.

Elder DE, Elentsias R, Johnson BL, Murphy GF, Xu X, *Lever's Histopathology of the Skin,* 10th edn, Lippincott-Williams & Wilkins, 2009.

Hood AF, Kwan TH, Mihm MC, Horn TD, *Primer of Dermatopathology*, 2nd edn, Little, Brown and Company, 1993.

Kazakov D, Michal M, Kacerovska D, McKee PH, *Cutaneous Adnexal Tumors,* 1st edn, Lippincott-Williams & Wilkins, 2012.

LeBoit PE, Burg G, Weedon D, Sarasin A, *Pathology and Genetics of Tumours of the Skin (IARC WHO Classification of Tumours)*, 1st edn, IARC Press, 2006.

McKee PH, Calonje E, Granter S, *Pathology of the Skin with Clinical Correlations*, 3rd edn, Elsevier, 2005.

Nasemann T, Jänner M, Schűtte B, *Histopathologie der Hautkrankheiten fűr Studenten der Medizin und Wissentschaftliche Assistenten Orientiert am Gegenstandskatalog der Dermatovenerologie,* Springer, 1982.

Rapini R, *Practical Dermatopathology,* 1st edn, Elsevier, 2005.

Weedon D, *Skin Pathology,* 3rd edn, Elsevier, 2013.

I also owe a general debt to the main references in the field:

American Journal of Dermatopathology, Wolters Kluwer
Journal of Cutaneous Pathology, John Wiley & Sons, Inc.
Journal of the American Academy of Dermatology, Elsevier
www.pathologyoutlines.com

Finally, many of the photomnemonic images are used as free images from www.pixabay.com and some are used under license from www.shutterstock.com.

SECTION I: THE BASICS OF DERMATOPATHOLOGY

1 Characteristics of the cells at low power and close-up view

Mariya Miteva and Jacquelyn Dosal

EPIDERMIS

Definition: The superficial layer of the skin made of stratified, squamous epithelium of different thickness; consists primarily of keratinocytes in progressive stages of differentiation; contains no blood vessels.

(Photomnemonic 1.1)

Keratinocytes

Description: The main cells of the epidermis, organized in the following layers from the bottom to the top:

- Stratum basale (blue): cuboidal or columnar
- Stratum spinosum (pink): angulated with spines between cells
- Stratum granulosum (purple): prominent granules with the cells beginning to flatten
- Stratum lucidum: hypochromatic thin layer only on palms and soles
- Stratum corneum (pink): flattened, anucleated cells appearing as "basket weave"

(Photomnemonic 1.2, Figure 1.1)

Immunohistochemistry: Cytokeratin, p63

Anatomical variations:

- Flat rete ridges on the face
- Thick stratum corneum and stratum granulosum on acral skin
- No stratum corneum or stratum granulosum on mucosal epithelium (stratum granulosum is present only on the tongue and hard palate)
- No stratum granulosum on the nail matrix or nail bed

(Figure 1.2, Table 1.1)

Table 1.1 Granular layer variations

Prominent	Absent
Acral skin	Mucosa (*present on tongue)
	Nail matrix
	Nail bed

Langerhans cells (LC)

Description: Bone-marrow derived dendritic cells which reside in the epidermis. They have a kidney-shaped nucleus with pale blue cytoplasm and Birbeck granules (like tennis rackets on electron microscopy)

Location: Middle layers of the epidermis

Immunohistochemistry: Langerhans cells stain with CD1a, S100 and Langerin, CD207 (specific for LC)

(Figure 1.3, Figure 1.4)

Melanocytes

Description: Pigment-producing cells of the epidermis. They have dendrites, via which they deliver melanin to keratinocytes. Melanocyte to keratinocyte ratio is 1:10 on body sites, 1:4 on the face, and up to 1:1 in sun-damaged skin (with larger melanosomes as in dark skin)

Location: Basal layer of the epidermis

NB Keratinocytes have ample cytoplasm and are connected via desmosomes; melanocytes have a nucleus surrounded by a clear halo as the cytoplasm shrinks during tissue processing.

Immunohistochemistry: S-100, Melan-A (MART-1), MITF, HMB-45

(Figure 1.5, Figure 1.6, Photomnemonic 1.3)

DERMOEPIDERMAL JUNCTION (DEJ)

Definition: A basement membrane that adheres the epidermis to the dermis; composed of two layers: the lamina lucida and the lamina densa.

- **The lamina lucida** is thinner and connects through hemidesmosomes directly with the basal layer of the epidermis.
- **The lamina densa** is thicker and is in direct contact with the underlying dermis through type VII collagen and anchoring fibrils.

The junction is significant in a number of disorders:
- It harbors the antigens for subepidermal immunobullous disorders.
- It is the target area in lichenoid and interface dermatitis.

DERMIS

DERMAL STROMA

Definition: Composed of collagen, elastic fibers, and ground substance which together with the stromal cells (fibroblasts, histiocytes, mast cells), vessels, adnexal structures, and nerve endings form the middle layer of the skin, the dermis.

(Table 1.2)

Table 1.2 Dermal stroma components

Cells: • spindle cells • histiocytes (dendritic cells, macrophages) • lymphocytes • mast cells • plasma cells • neutrophils • eosinophils • plasmacytoid dendritic cells • smooth muscle cells	Collagen fibers Elastic fibers Vessels Nerves Adnexal structures: • hair follicles • sweat glands • sebaceous glands

- The papillary (superficial) dermis has loose, fine collagen, elastic fibers, and capillaries organized in fingerlike projections (dermal papillae) oriented perpendicular to the skin surface. They are surrounded by similar projections of the epidermis (rete ridges) and create an undulating surface.

NB The face has flat rete ridges and the nail bed has parallel longitudinal grooves.

- The reticular (mid and lower) dermis has coarse and large parallel collagen fibers, closely interlaced elastic fibers, and larger blood vessels.

(Figure 1.7)

Collagen bundles

- Dermal collagen: type I (type III in the papillary dermis)
- Human collagen polarizes under polarized light; bovine collagen does not
- Specimens from the back show thick collagen bundles

NB Infants have small collagen bundles and many fibroblasts. Adults have the opposite: thick bundles and few fibroblasts.

(Photomnemonic 1.4)

Elastic fibers

- Normal elastic fibers are not visible to the naked eye; abnormal elastic tissue in solar elastosis is visible as conglomerates of blue–purple fragmented fibers in the upper dermis.
- Stains: Verhoeff–Van Gieson (VVG), orcein

(Figure 1.8)

Ground substance (extrafibrillar matrix)

- Amorphous gel-like substance surrounding the cells
- Primarily composed of water, glycosaminoglycans (hyaluronic acid, proteoglycans, and glycoproteins)
- Stains: Alcian blue and colloidal iron (highlight increased mucin)

DERMAL CELLS

Fibroblasts

Description: The active form of fibrocytes; bipolar elongated (plump) spindle to stellate cells with ovoid nuclei; surrounded by collagen; they synthesize collagen, elastic tissue, and ground substance
Location: Dermis
Immunohistochemistry: CD10, CD68, factor XIIIa, vimentin
(Figure 1.9, Figure 1.10, Photomnemonic 1.5)

Myofibroblasts

Description: Appear as fibroblasts but act as smooth muscle cells (important for contracting the wound edges); have elongated nuclei, vesicular cytoplasm, and blunt ends

Location: Dermis
Immunohistochemistry: Desmin+/–, SMA (smooth muscle actin)
(Figure 1.11)

Smooth muscle

Description: Elongated, cigar-shaped nuclei with blunt ends
Location: Dermis
Immunohistochemistry: Desmin, SMA (smooth muscle actin), H-caldesmon
(Figure 1.12, Photomnemonic 1.6, Figure 1.13, Table 1.3)

Table 1.3 Staining pattern of fibroblasts, myofibroblasts, and smooth muscle cells

	Fibroblasts	Myofibroblasts	Smooth muscle
Morphology	Elongated spindle	Plump vesicular	Vesicular blunt ends
Factor XIII	Yes	No	No
SMA	No	Yes	Yes
Desmin	No	Yes/No	Yes
H-caldesmon	No	No	Yes

Histiocytes

Description: Dermal dendritic cells (APC, antigen presenting cells) and macrophages (professional phagocytes): oval light blue (pale) cells with ample cytoplasm and large vesicular nuclei with clearly delineated nuclear membrane; the cells form syncitia (multinucleated mass of connecting cytoplasms that cannot be separated into individual cells). Histiocytes are involved in: fibrohistiocytic tumors (soft tissue tumors), cutaneous histiocytic disorders (histiocytoses) and granulomatous disorders.
(Figure 1.4, Figure 1.14, Photomnemonic 1.7, Figure 1.15)
Location: Dermis
Immunohistochemistry: Factor XIIIa (APC); CD68 (phagocytes)
Macrophages fuse to form giant cells in granulomatous disorders.
(Figure 1.16, Table 1.4)

Table 1.4 Types of macrophages and their derivative giant cells

Macrophages	Giant cells
Foamy	Touton (xanthogranuloma)
Stellate	Foreign body
Oncocytic	Ground glass (reticulohystiocytoma)

Lymphocytes

Description: Small to medium-sized blue cells with minimal visible cytoplasm. The size of lymphocytes is typically used as the baseline standard (i.e. "large cells" are larger than lymphocytes).
(Figure 1.17, Photomnemonic 1.8)

NB Lymphocytes and histiocytes are mononuclear cells, often present together around vessels forming lymphohistiocytic infiltrate (mononuclear cell infiltrate), which is the most common infiltrate in inflammatory skin disorders. Polymorphonuclear cells have segmented nuclei (neutrophils and eosinophils).

(Figure 1.18)

- **T-cells** (T-thymus derived) are most lymphocytes found in the skin; they are epidermotropic (like the epidermis) and change its architecture while moving through it (spongiosis, acanthosis); malignant T-cells are passive and do not change the epidermis.
- **B-cells** (bone-marrow derived) are minimally presented in skin; they are epidermophobic (dislike the epidermis) and stay in the dermis.

NB In nodular infiltrates B-cells are separated by a Grenz zone (a clear band of papillary dermis spared by the inflammatory or neoplastic collections in the dermis).

Location: Circulate in the dermis; usually found around vessels
Immunohistochemistry: CD3, CD4 (Th – helper), CD8 (Tc – cytotoxic), FoxP3 (Treg – regulatory); CD20 (B-cells), CD79a (B-cells); CD3-C20-CD56+ (NK cells – natural killer)
(Table 1.5)

Table 1.5 Immunohistochemistry of T- and B-cells

T-cells	B-cells	Natural killer cells (10% of the circulating lymphocytes)
CD3+	CD20+	CD3–
CD4+ (TH, helper T-cells)	CD79a+	CD20–
CD4+FoxP3+ (Treg, regulatory T-cells)		CD56+
CD8+ (Tc, cytotoxic T-cells)		
Lymphocytes (T- and B-cells) are indistinguishable by light microscopy. Most lymphocytes circulating in the skin are found in the dermis perivascularly.		

Mast cells

Description: Dark blue cells with prominent cytoplasmic granules and central, round nucleus. The cut-off value for increased number of mast cells is not well defined but it is considered to range from 6 to 10 per high power field. They usually hang out with eosinophils around dilated blood vessels (telangiectasia) and love dermal edema and mucin.
(Photomnemonic 1.9, Figure 1.19)
Location: Often perivascular in the dermis
Immunohistochemistry: C-kit (CD117), tryptase; special stains: Giemsa, toluidine blue, Leder stain (chloroacetate esterase) for the granules
(Figure 1.20)

Plasma cells

Description: Large purple cells with eccentric nucleus with a clock-face arrangement. They are tissue cells derived from activated B-lymphocytes and are not present in peripheral circulation. In infiltrates with numerous plasma cells (syphilis) Russell bodies (compact pink cytoplasmic accumulation of immunoglobulin) are found.
(Photomnemonic 1.10, Figure 1.21)
Location: Mucosal sites; in the dermis as part of a perivascular infiltrate
Immunohistochemistry: CD19, CD20, CD79a, CD138
(Table 1.6)

Table 1.6 Skin conditions with plasma cells

Normal mucosal skin	Zoon's balanitis
Morphea profunda	Plasmacytoma
Infectious dermatoses:	Necrobiosis lipoidica
• syphilis	Kaposi's sarcoma
• granuloma inguinale	Syringocystadenoma papilliferum
• rhinoscleroma	
• leishmaniasis	
• Lyme disease	

Plasmacytoid dendritic cells (PDC)

Description: Mononuclear cells which circulate in the peripheral blood and are occasionally found in the skin. They have overlapping characteristics of lymphocytes and dendritic cells, and play a crucial role in the initiation of immune responses and activation of T-cells and B-cells.
Derivation: Controversial: lymphoid or myeloid progenitors
Immunohistochemistry: CD4+, CD56+, CD123+
Implicated conditions: Pseudolymphoma, CD4+/CD56+ hematodermic neoplasm (also known as plasmacytoid dendritic cell tumor), psoriasis (Koebner phenomenon is thought to arise due to PDC), systemic lupus erythematosus, dermatomyositis, contact dermatitis
(Table 1.7)

Table 1.7 Skin conditions with plasmacytoid dendritic cells

Koebner phenomenon
Lymphoid hyperplasia of the skin
Psoriasis
Systemic lupus erythematosus
Dermatomyositis
Contact dermatitis
CD4+/CD56+ hematodermic neoplasm (plasmacytoid dendritic cell tumor)

Neutrophils

Description: White blood cells of medium size with bright eosinophilic cytoplasm due to red granules (containing myeloperoxidase, hydrolases, collagenase, elastase, and lysozymes) and multilobulated blue nuclei of at least three connected segments. Fragmentation of the nuclei is known as karyorrhexis (nuclear dust, leukocytoclasia) and characterizes leukocytoclastic vasculitis.
Location: Dermis, around blood vessels, epidermis (including stratum corneum)

> NB IgA deposits (dermatitis herpetiformis, linear IgA disease), ulcerations, and necrosis attract neutrophils.

(Photomnemonic 1.11, Figure 1.22, Table 1.8, Figure 1.23, Photomnemonic 1.12)

Table 1.8 Skin conditions with neutrophils (according to site)

Stratum corneum	Papillary dermis	Dermis
Psoriasis	Bullous lupus erythematosus	Neutrophilic dermatoses (Sweet's syndrome, pyoderma gangrenosum)
PLEVA (busy stratum corneum)	Dermatitis herpetiformis	Folliculitis
Clear cell acanthoma		Palisaded neutrophilic granulomatous dermatitis
Tinea		Leukocytoclastic vasculitis
		Fibrinoid necrosis (rheumatoid nodule, chronic ulcers)

Eosinophils

Description: White blood cells with bright eosinophilic cytoplasm due to red granules (containing major basic protein) and a blue, bilobed nucleus (only two connected segments)
Location: In the dermis perivascular; interstitial

- Eosinophils can phagocytize: 1) antigen–antibody complexes in atopic dermatitis/dermal hypersensitivity reactions, autoimmune bullous disorders, and granuloma faciale; 2) mast cell granules in mast cell disorders and anaphylactoid conditions

- Flame figures: bright red aggregates of smudged necrobiotic material in the dermis from decomposed eosinophilic granules, nuclear debris and collagen (eosinophilic cellulitis / Wells' syndrome, arthropod bite reaction)

(Photomnemonic 1.13, Figure 1.24, Table 1.9)

Table 1.9 Skin conditions with eosinophils in the epidermis (eosinophilic spongiosis)

Allergic contact dermatitis
Bullous disease
Arthropod bite reaction
Incontinentia pigmenti
Erythema multiforme

OTHER DERMAL STRUCTURES

BLOOD VESSELS

Definition: Horizontally arranged superficial and deep plexuses which are interconnected via communicating vessels oriented perpendicular to the skin surface.

- Upper horizontal plexus (in the papillary dermis): loops of capillaries, venules, and arterioles, most pronounced around adnexal structures (adventitial dermis)
- Lower horizontal plexus (at the border of the dermis and subdermis): larger vessels: small arteries and veins

NB Any vessel visible at 2× magnification is of a large caliber.

Endothelial cells

Line the inner layer of blood vessels and lymphatic vessels

- Often cannot be appreciated unless very swollen
- Immunohistochemistry: CD31, CD34, factor VIII-related antigen, and *Ulex europaeus*-1 lectin
- Interact with pericytes (vascular smooth muscle cells which envelop the surface of the vascular tube, provide scaffold for the vessels, and regulate their luminal opening), with which they share a basement membrane **(Figure 1.25)**

Capillaries

Microscopic vessels in the upper dermis; vessel wall made of only one layer of endothelial cells and an incomplete layer of pericytes

(Figure 1.26)

Arteries and arterioles (small arteries)

Organized in three "onion-like" layers from inside out: 1) intima: endothelial cells and elastic lamina; 2) media: two or three layers of muscle cells (but only one layer in arterioles); 3) adventitia: connective tissue **(Photomnemonic 1.14, Figure 1.27)**

Veins

Three-layered walls but thinner than arteries due to fewer muscular layers.

Three layers: 1) intima with endothelial cells, 2) media (muscle layers), 3) adventitia (usually thicker than the media)

(Figure 1.28, Table 1.10)

Table 1.10 Comparison of veins and arteries (Modified from: Sanchez EY, et al. *Am J Dermatopathol* 2012; 34(2): 229.)

	Veins	Arteries
Muscular layer	Thick	Thicker
Inner elastic lamina	Thinner, discontinuous	Thick, distinct, and undulated
Valves	Always seen at step sections	Never seen

Venules

Larger than capillaries but smaller than veins (vary from 40–100 μm diameter); resemble capillaries as they consist of 1) endothelial cells, 2) basement membrane and 3) pericytes

NB The endothelial cells of the venules are the primary site of adhesive interactions for antigen–antibody complexes leading to diapedesis of white blood cells and vasculitis.

Lymphatics

Blind-ended lymphatic capillaries arise within the interstitial spaces of the papillary dermis; invisible in normal skin due to poorly developed walls but visible when dilated (as seen in urticaria)

- Angulated shape compared to round blood vessels **(Figure 1.29)**

- NB Structure: flat endothelial cells; no basement membrane, no pericytes

- Immunohistochemistry: D2-40

(Figure 1.30, Figure 1.31)

CUTANEOUS NEURAL NETWORK

Definition: Sensory (myelinated) and autonomic (unmyelinated, from the sympathetic nervous system) nerves follow the blood vessels to the skin and form a network of interconnected branches throughout the dermis.

NB Only larger myelinated nerve fibers are visible on hematoxylin and eosin (H&E) stain.

Dermatome

Skin area mainly supplied by a single spinal nerve

Autonomic nerves

Supply the blood vessels and the adnexal structures

NB Sebaceous glands do not have autonomic innervations: they function through endocrine stimuli.

Free neural endings/encapsulated receptors

Free neural endings are found in the epidermis and encapsulated receptors are found in the dermis; specialized to detect various stimuli:

- Merkel cells in the epidermis (invisible on light microscopy) and Meissner corpuscles in the papillary dermis detect light touch.
- Pacini corpuscles (flat, modified Schwann cells) in the deep dermis and subdermis detect pressure.

(Figure 1.32)

Sensory myelinated nerves

Cordlike structures that contain closely packed nerve fibers (axons)

- **Axons (neuroaxons)** – long, slender projections of the neurons; stain with silver stains
- **Endoneurium** – a mucinous fibrous matrix with fibroblasts, capillaries, and mast cells which surrounds each axon; stains with colloidal iron and focally with CD34 (fibroblasts)
- **Perineurium** – surrounds fascicles (bundles of grouped axons); perineural cells stain positive with EMA
- **Epineurium** – a layer of connective tissue that wraps up the entire nerve

Schwann cells

Wrap around axons forming the myelinated sheaths; stain with S100, neuron-specific enolase (NSE), and CD57 (Leu-7)

NB The normal ratio of axons to Schwann cells is 1:1.

(Photomnemonic 1.15, Figure 1.33, Figure 1.34)

SWEAT GLANDS

Definition: Tubular structures in the skin which produce and excrete sweat. There are two types of sweat glands: eccrine and apocrine.

Eccrine glands

Produce sweat to cool the skin surface

NB Sweat glands are present everywhere on the skin except on the vermillion border of the lip, the external ear canal, the labia minora, the glans penis, and the nail bed.

They consist of three segments:

- **Eccrine coils** – secretory portion of convoluted tubules in the subdermis and lower dermis, made of one layer of clear and dark cells and an outer thin layer of myoepithelial cells (stellate cells above the basement membrane and beneath the epithelial cells which stain with SMA, calponin, p63, and S100); there is a myxoid change in the stroma around sweat glands, especially in acral skin
- **Intradermal duct** – two layers of small basophilic cuboidal cells
- **Acrosyringium** – a single layer of inner cells, two or three layers of outer cells, and eosinophilic cuticle (lines the lumen prior to keratinization)

Eccrine glands stain with S100 and CEA.
(Figure 1.35, Figure 1.36, Figure 1.37, Figure 1.38, Figure 1.39)

Apocrine glands

In human skin are found only in the axillae, the anogenital region, and, as modified glands, in the external ear canal (ceruminous glands), the eyelid (Moll's glands); consist of the same three segments with the following differences:

- The secretory coil has larger lumina and contains only pale cells (glycogen).
- The intradermal duct is the same.
- The intraepidermal portion opens in the infundibulum of a hair follicle, above the entrance of the sebaceous duct.

(Figure 1.40)

NB Eccrine and apocrine glands are often indistinguishable. Look for decapitation secretion (detachment of the apical portion of the secretory cells into the lumina) as a clue to apocrine differentiation.

SEBACEOUS GLANDS

Definition: Exocrine glands which secrete sebum to lubricate the skin.

- Absent from palms and soles; densest on scalp and face
- Fordyce spots: ectopic sebaceous glands found on the lips, inner cheeks or gums; present at birth (due to maternal hormones) but after that undergo involution and develop in puberty

Structure:

- Several lobules of sebocytes (pale cells with vacuolated fenestrated cytoplasm which contains lipids and stellate central nuclei)
- Basaloid (blue) cuboidal cells at the periphery of the lobule (contain no lipids)

- A common duct (sebaceous duct) drains the lobules in the hair canal (lined by stratified squamous epithelium and crenulated pink lining)

(Figure 1.41, Table 1.11)

Table 1.11 Glands at a glance

	Eccrine	Apocrine	Sebaceous
Mechanism of secretion	Exocytosis	Decapitation: the apical portion of the cell is pinched off and released in the lumen	The membrane ruptures and releases the lipids into the lumen
EMA, CEA	+	+	+
S100	+	–	–
GCDFP	–	+	–
Androgen receptor	–	–	+

HAIR FOLLICLE

Definition: A sac-like epithelial structure which produces the hair shaft (keratinized non-viable structure) through phases of growth and involution: 1) anagen (growing hairs, more than 85% of all hairs); 2) catagen (transitional hairs to rest, less than 1% of all hairs); 3) telogen (resting hairs, up to 15% of all hairs).

Based on the diameter of the hair shaft, the follicles are also divided into:

- Terminal (thicker than 0.06 mm)
- Intermediate (between 0.03–0.06 mm)
- Vellus (thinner than 0.03 mm)

There are recognizable levels along the follicular length:

- **Bulbar level** – the anagen follicles have bulbs (hair matrix cells and melanocytes) which surround the dermal papilla (fibroblasts and blood vessels) and are situated in the subdermis (terminal anagen follicles) or the dermis (vellus follicles)
- **Isthmus** – the attachment site of the sebaceous duct and the arrector pilar muscle (smooth muscle bundle which attaches the follicular unit to the dermis)
- **Infundibulum** – the follicle opens to the surface

(Figure 1.42, Figure 1.43)

Anagen follicle

This has a concentric arrangement of the follicular epithelial layers around the hair shaft in the center: 1) inner root sheath (pink and compact; supports the hair shaft and keratinizes and disappears at the isthmus); 2) outer root sheath (layers of pale cells due to glycogen); 3) connective tissue sheath (loose collagen, vessels, and fibroblasts).

(Figure 1.44, Photomnemonic 1.16)

Catagen and telogen follicle

These have a shrunken outer root sheath (with/without apoptotic cells), no hair shaft or, if still present, look like "a flame" (bright and degenerated serrated keratin mass).

(Figure 1.45, Photomnemonic 1.17, Photomnemonic 1.18, Photomnemonic 1.19)

Vellus follicle

This has a very thin hair shaft; it also goes through phases of growth and involution.

(Photomnemonic 1.20)

NAIL

Definition: Hard envelope made of keratin covering the dorsal aspect of the terminal phalanges. Composed of: 1) the nail plate, 2) the nail matrix, 3) the nail bed, and 4) the grooves surrounding the nail bed (proximal, lateral, and distal nail fold)

(Figure 1.46)

Nail plate

Acellular layered structure of thick compact "hard" keratin.

Nail matrix

The nail root which produces the nail plate; consists of 1) proximal part below the proximal nail fold which produces the dorsal nail plate, and 2) distal part (below the lunula) which produces the ventral nail plate; the matrix is composed of several layers of germinative basaloid cells (compared to one in the epidermis) and upper keratogenous zone (angulated flat keratinocytes with resin-like nuclei but no granular layer) which transitions into the acellular nail plate.

Nail bed

Adheres the nail plate to the dermis and periosteum; distal from the lunula to the hyponychium (the distal attachment of the nail plate); consists of flat, thinner than the matrix epithelium, with less prominent basal layer, no melanocytes, and no granular layer.

NB Melanocytes are present in the distal matrix but not in the nail bed.

SUBDERMIS

Definition: The lowest layer of the skin composed of mature fat (also called subcutaneous fat); consists of compartmentalized lobules of adipocytes separated by fibrous septae.

(Figure 1.47)

Adipocytes

Description: Large, uniform cells with eccentric nucleus displaced to the side due to the accumulation of lipids in the cytoplasm

- The lipid in the cytoplasm is not visible as it is removed during processing (stain with Sudan black).
- The nucleus has a vacuole and looks as if it has been perforated by a hole (*lochkern* in German).

(Figure 1.48, Figure 1.49)

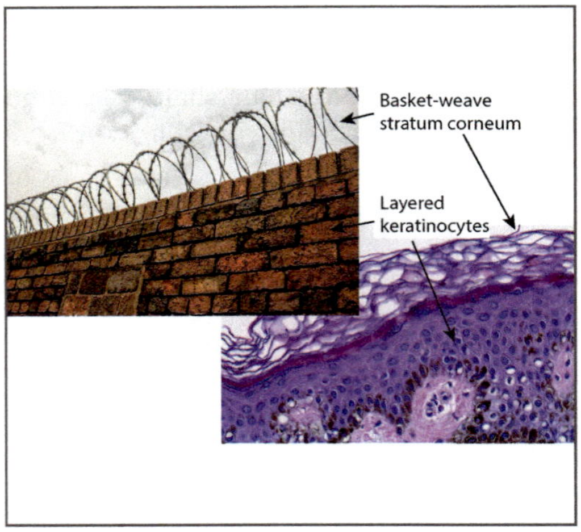

Photomnemonic 1.1 The epidermis is reminiscent of a brick wall with barbed wire on top (stratum corneum).

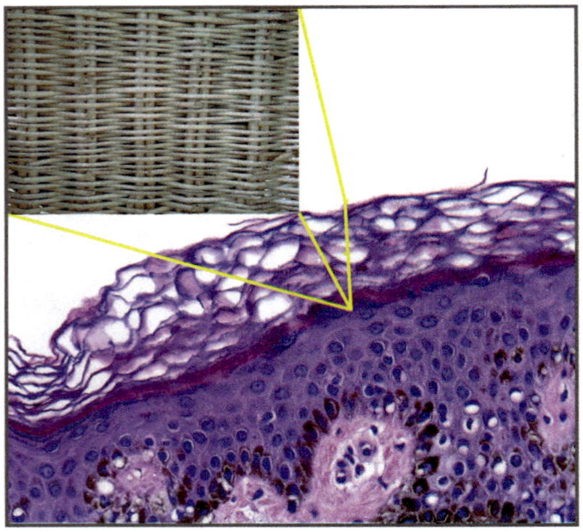

Photomnemonic 1.2 Stratum corneum – composed of anucleated cells woven in a flat "basket-weave" pattern.

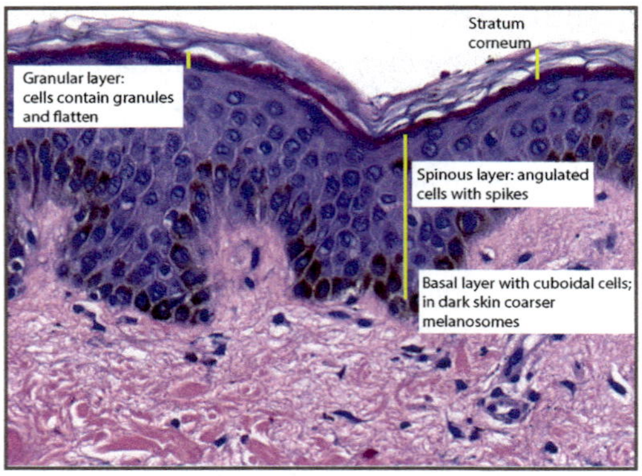

Figure 1.1 Layers of the epidermis.

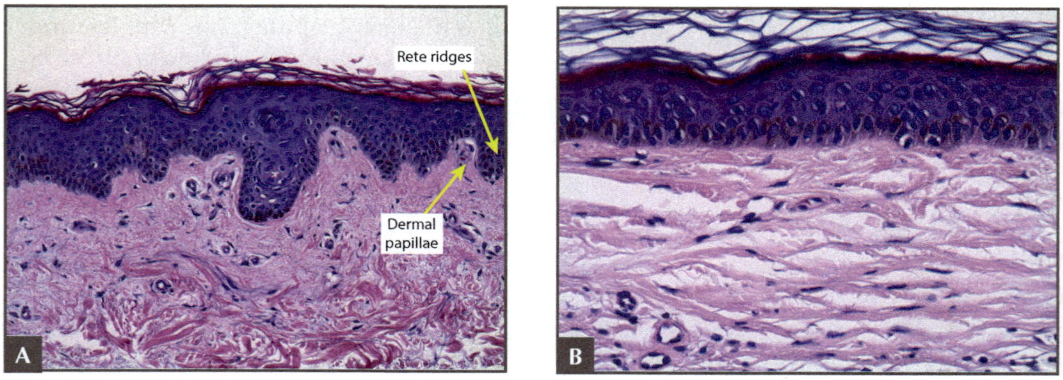

Figure 1.2 Epidermis. **A** The uppermost part of the skin derived from the ectoderm, illustrating basket-weave stratum corneum, rete ridges, and dermal papillae. **B** Epidermis on the face with flat rete ridges.

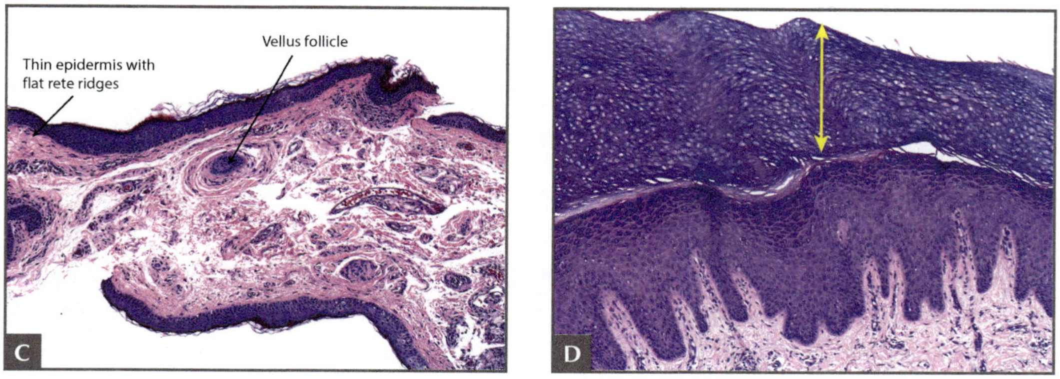

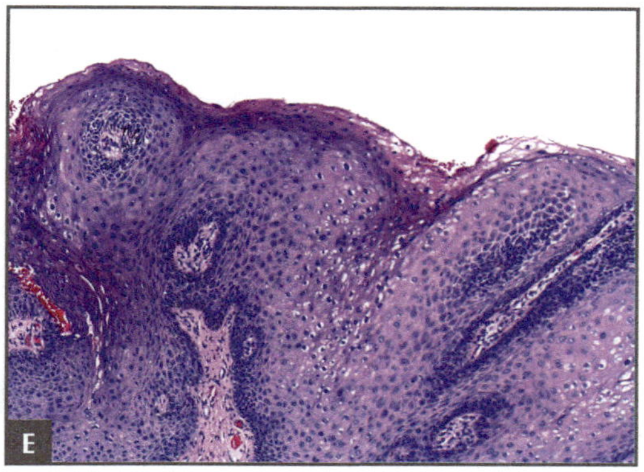

Figure 1.2 Epidermis. **C** Flat rete ridges, thin epidermis, minimal stratum corneum, and vellus hairs seen in eyelid skin. **D** Acral epidermis with thick stratum corneum. **E** Mucosa without stratum corneum.

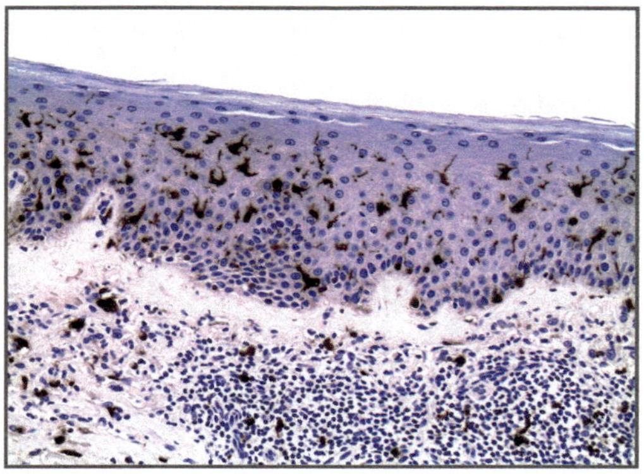

Figure 1.3 Langerhans cells stained with S100.

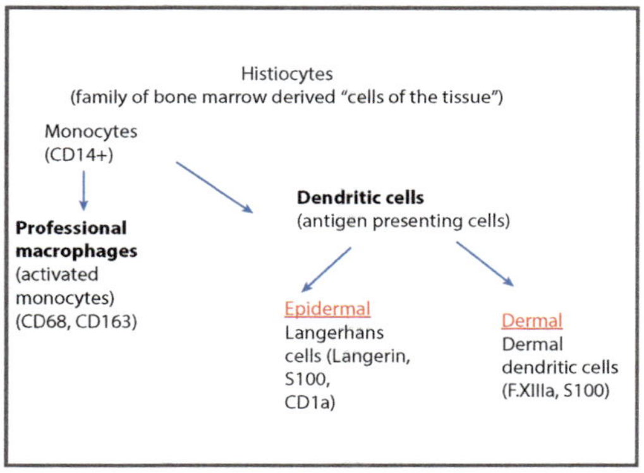

Figure 1.4 Lineage of histiocytes (family of bone-marrow derived "cells of the tissue").

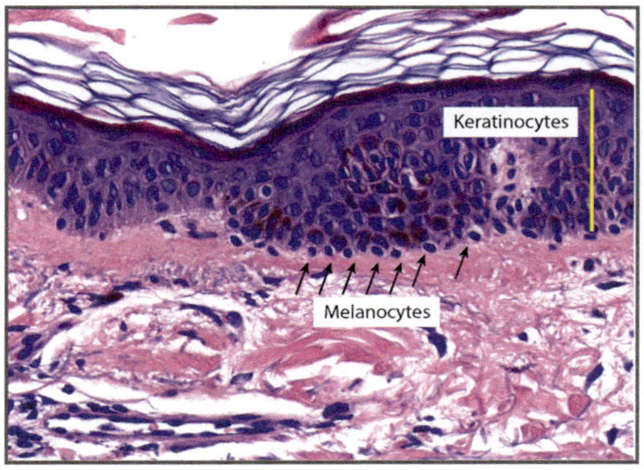

Figure 1.5 Melanocytes in the basal layer of black skin.

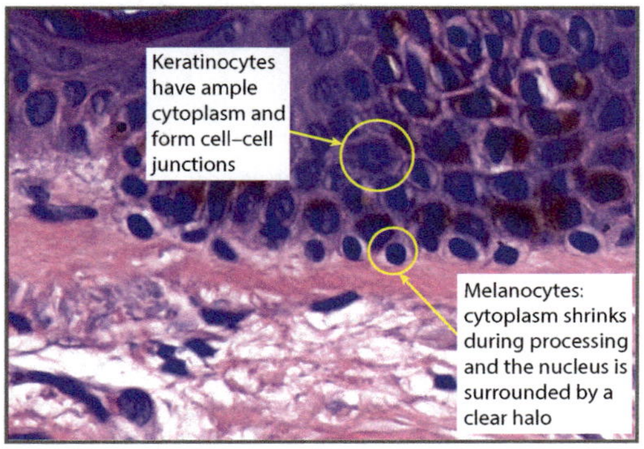

Figure 1.6 Close-up view of the cellular differences between keratinocytes and melanocytes.

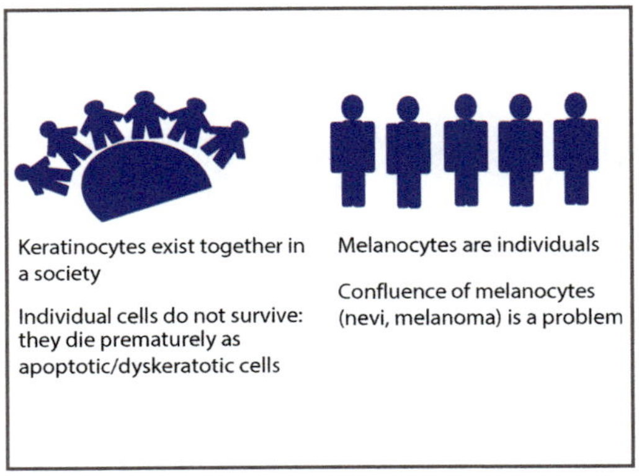

Photomnemonic 1.3 Keratinocytes are collectivists – if they dare detach, they die as apoptotic cells; melanocytes are individualists.

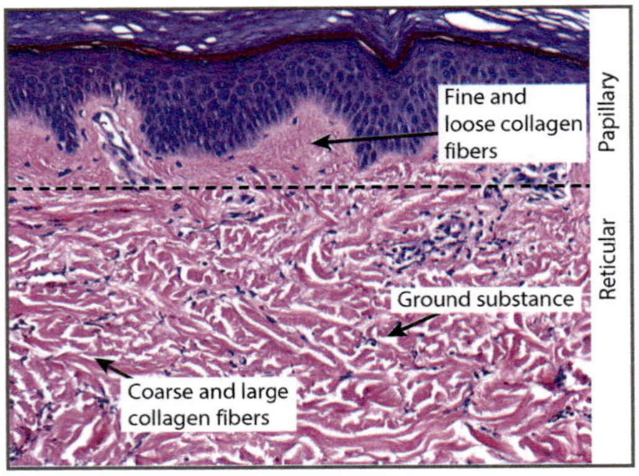

Figure 1.7 Dermis: collagen and elastic bundles in the papillary and reticular dermis.

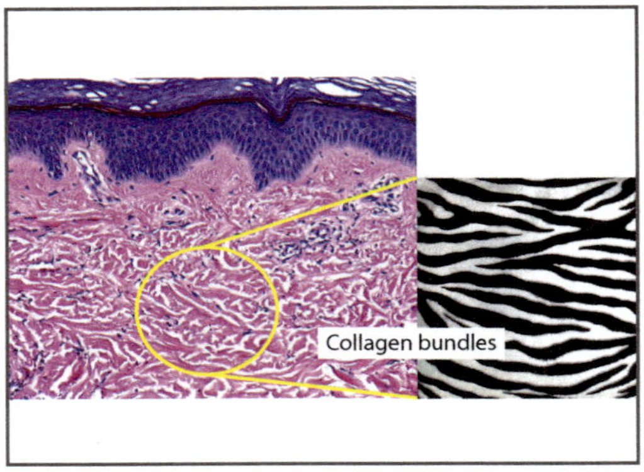

Photomnemonic 1.4 Due to the way collagen bundles are cut in processing, they appear wavy, resembling the skin pattern of zebras.

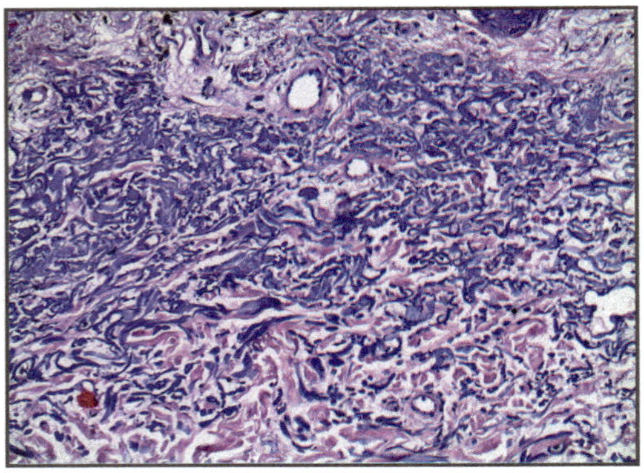

Figure 1.8 Solar elastosis: abnormal elastic fibers due to excessive sun exposure.

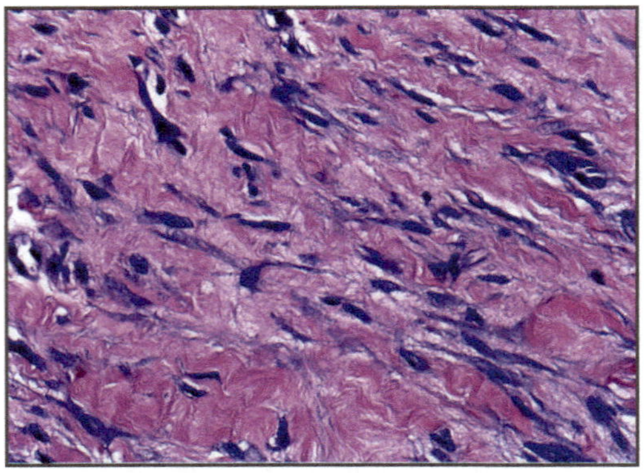

Figure 1.9 Fibroblasts in a pink collagenous stroma.

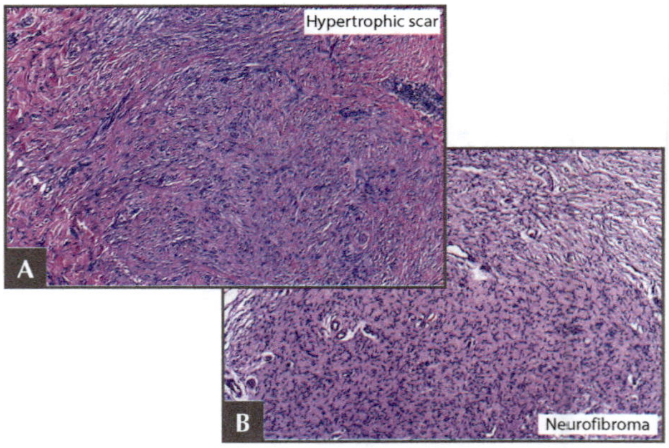

Figure 1.10 Fibroblasts. **A** Dermal fibroblasts in a hypertrophic scar. **B** Neural fibroblasts in a neurofibroma.

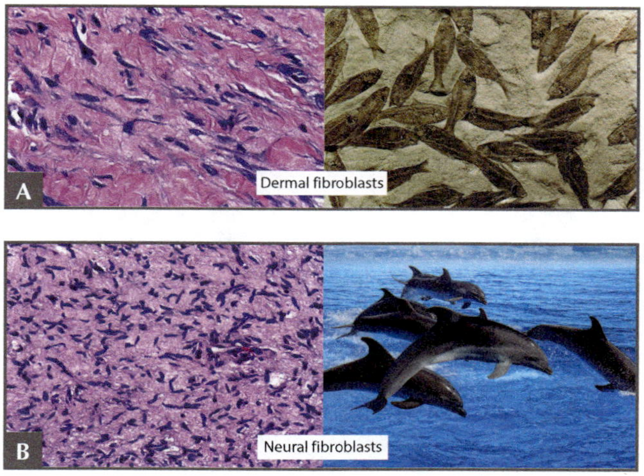

Photomnemonic 1.5 Fibroblasts. **A** Dermal fibroblasts are embedded among dermal collagen and are immobile, similar to a fish fossil. **B** Neural fibroblasts float within a mucinous "delicate stroma" and are wavy and light, similar to dancing dolphins.

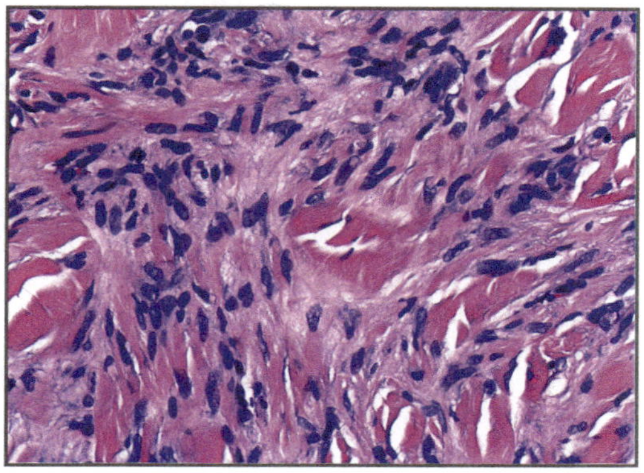

Figure 1.11 Myofibroblasts are an intermediate between fibroblasts and smooth muscle cells. Myofibroblasts have elongated nuclei, vesicular cytoplasm, and blunt ends. Distinction between fibroblasts and smooth muscle cells may be impossible on H&E.

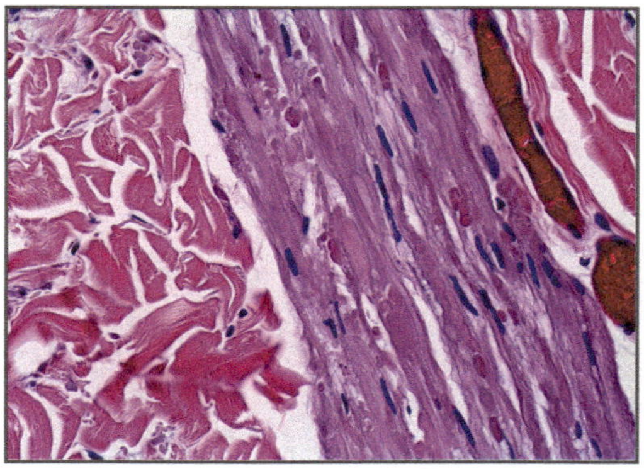

Figure 1.12 Arrector pili muscle from a follicular unit.

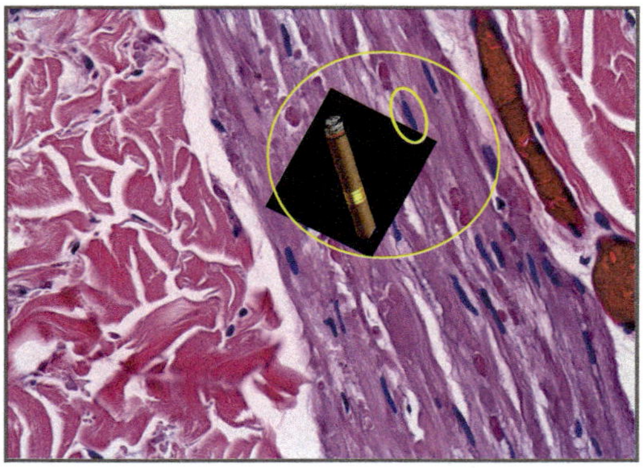

Photomnemonic 1.6 Smooth muscle cells show cigar-shaped nuclei with blunt (rounded) edges.

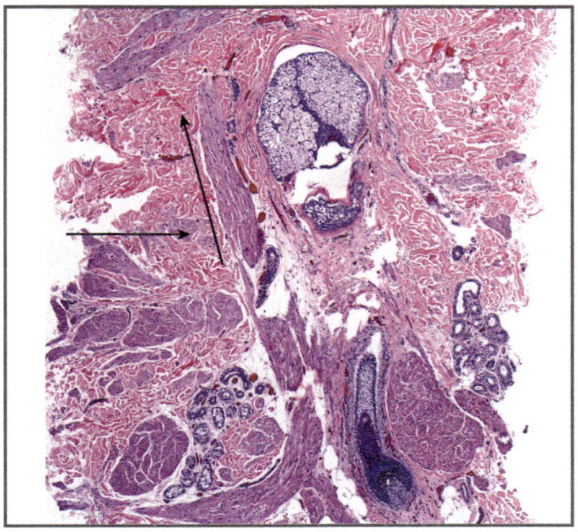

Figure 1.13 Smooth muscle hamartoma – increased number of "independent" smooth muscle bundles attached to a hair follicle that do not intermingle. The arrows show the vertical and parallel arrangement of the smooth muscle bundles.

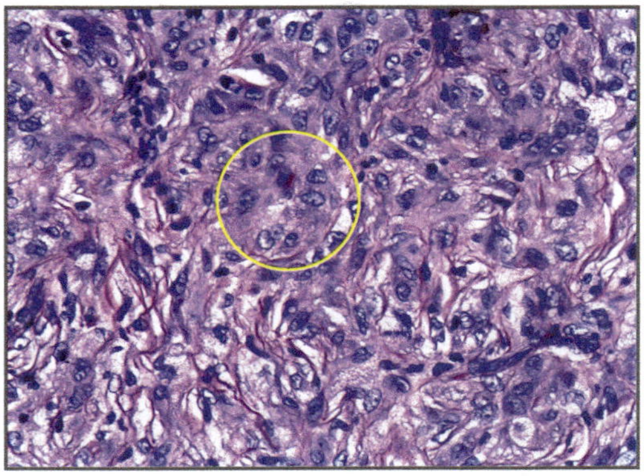

Figure 1.14 Histiocytic infiltrate in the dermis.

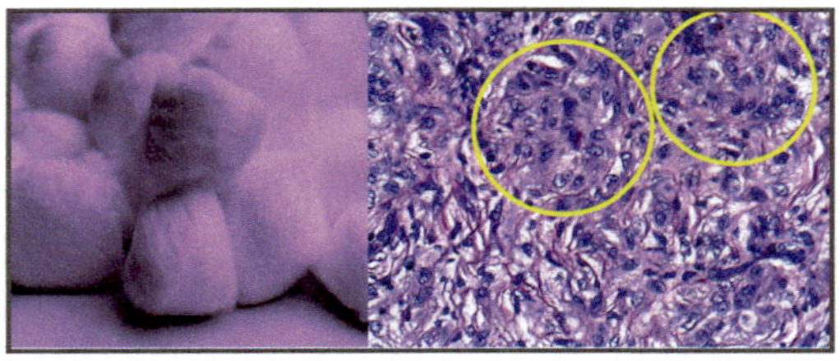

Photomnemonic 1.7 Round histiocytes resemble light blue/purple cotton balls in the dermis; they have ample pale cytoplasm and lie close to each other, forming syncytia in which the cell membranes are not well delineated.

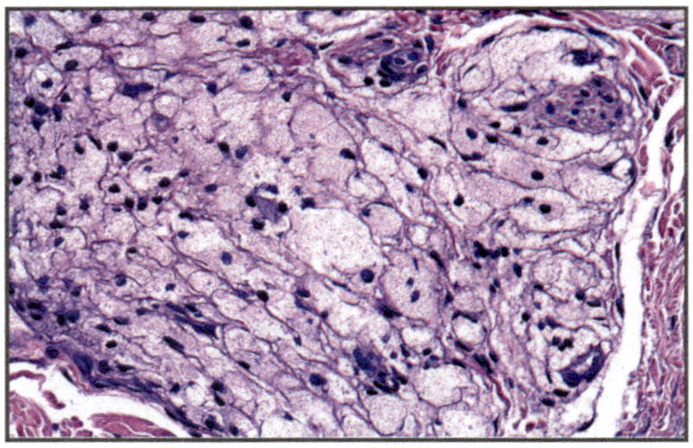

Figure 1.15 Foamy histiocytes in xanthelasma. The cytoplasm of the cells is clear and foamy.

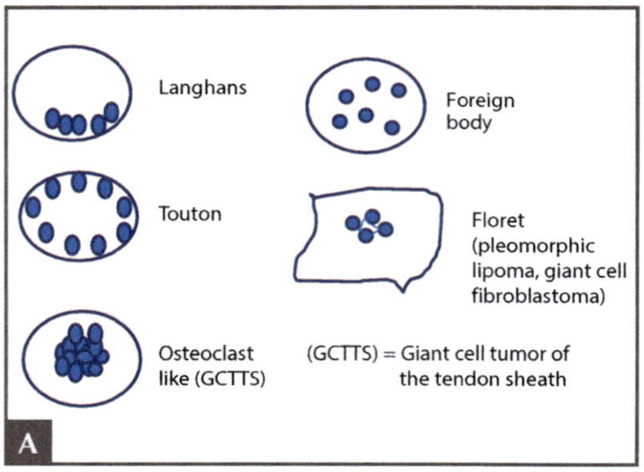

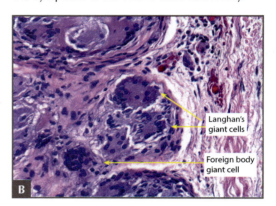

Figure 1.16 Giant cells. **A** Types of giant cell. **B** Examples of giant cells.

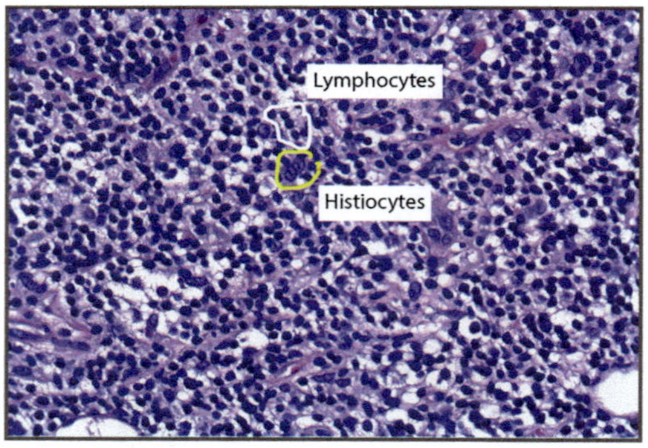

Figure 1.17 Lymphocytes and histiocytes.

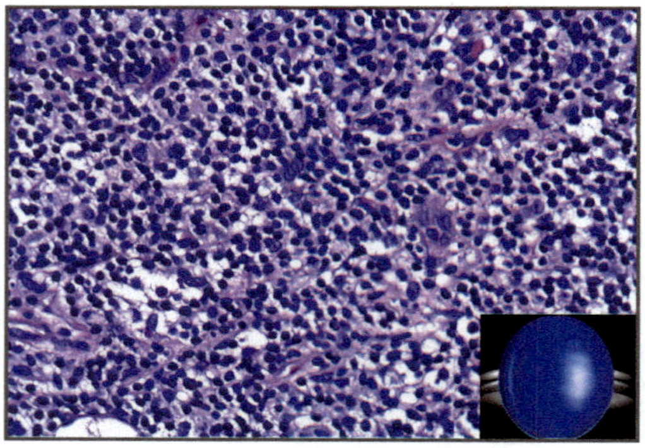

Photomnemonic 1.8 Lymphocytes resemble the head-on view of an oval blue ring.

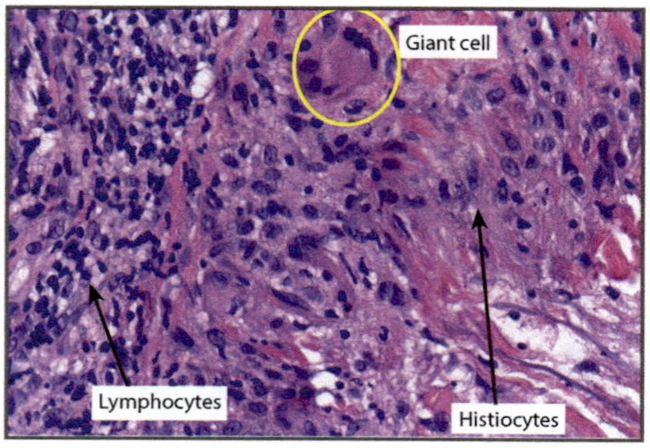

Figure 1.18 Lymphohistiocytic infiltrate: lymphocytes are small individual, blue cells with no visible cytoplasm; histiocytes are larger pale, oval cells with ample cytoplasm, forming pale masses (syncitia).

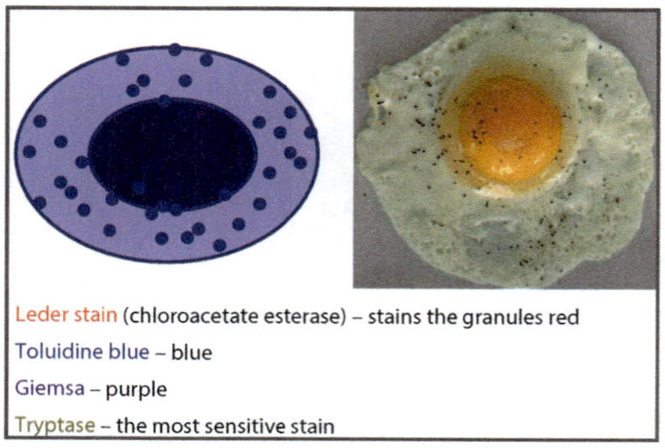

Photomnemonic 1.9 Mast cells resemble a fried egg with dots of black pepper. They are dark blue cells with prominent granules and a central round nucleus.

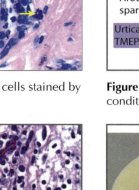

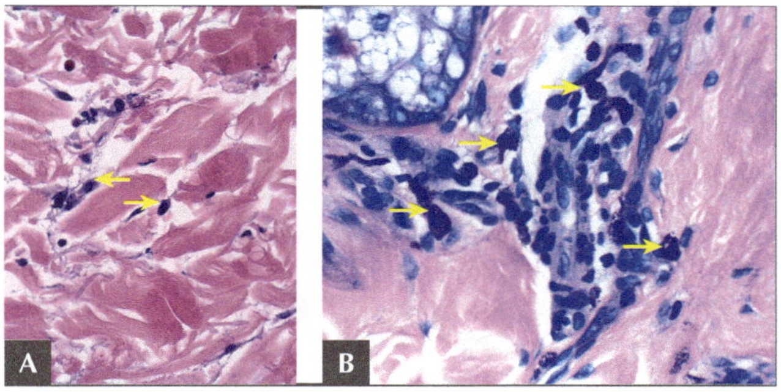

Figure 1.19 A Mast cells. **B** Perivascular mast cells stained by Giemsa in purple.

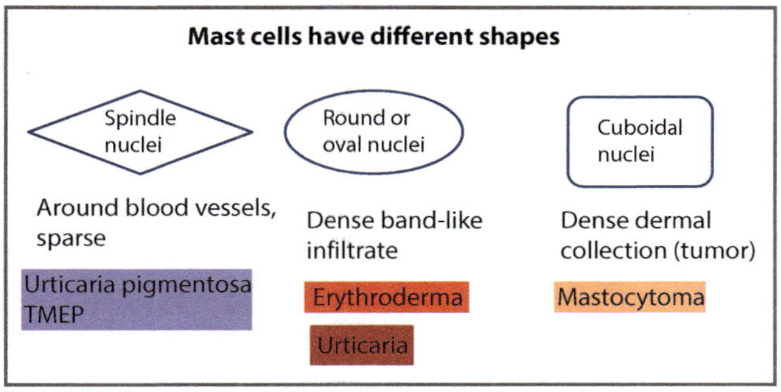

Figure 1.20 Mast cells have different shapes depending on the condition. TMEP = telangiectasia macularis eruptiva perstans.

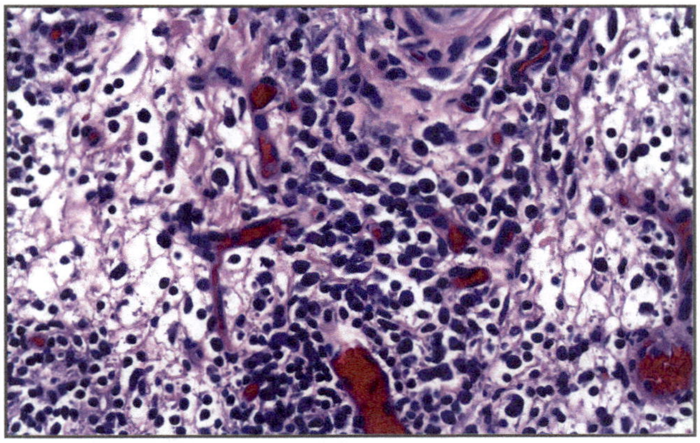

Figure 1.21 Perivascular plasma cell-rich infiltrate with a close-up view of plasma cells.

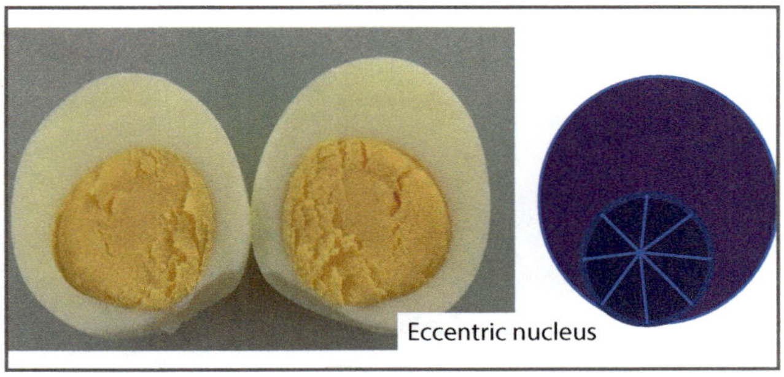

Photomnemonic 1.10 The eccentric nucleus of a plasma cell can resemble that of a hard-boiled egg (as opposed to the fried egg for mast cells).

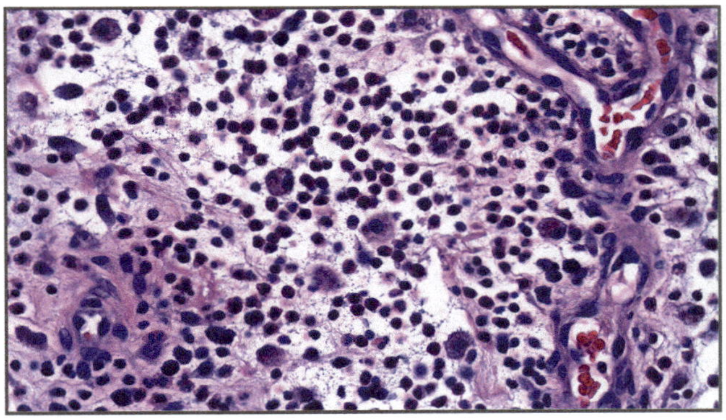

Figure 1.22 Polymorphonuclear cell infiltrate.

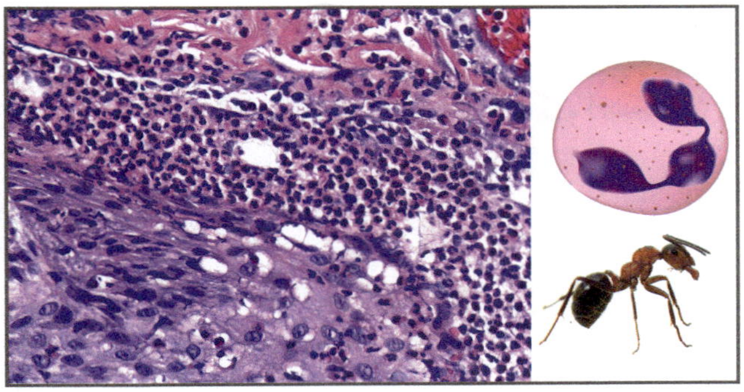

Photomnemonic 1.11 The segmented nucleus of a neutrophil resembles the body of an ant.

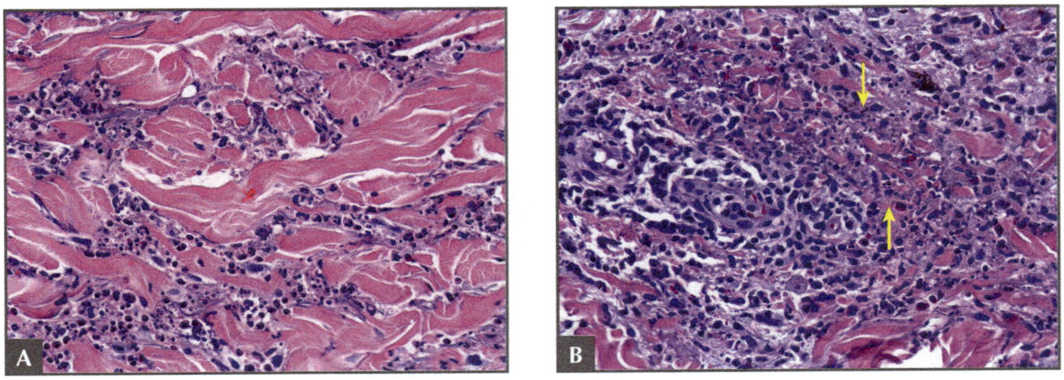

Figure 1.23 Leukocytoclastic vasculitis. **A** Nuclear dust in the dermis (karyorrhexis) can be found in leukocytoclastic vasculitis, folliculitis or necrosis (eschar). **B** Karyorrhexis in leukocytoclastic vasculitis.

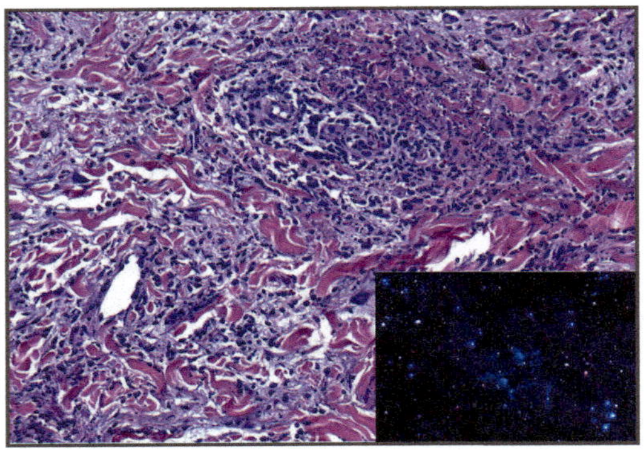

Photomnemonic 1.12 Leukocytoclastic vasculitis exhibiting karryorhexis/nuclear dust, which resembles a starry sky.

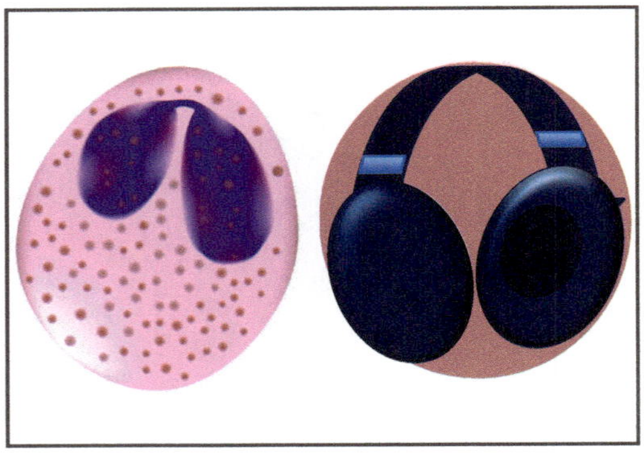

Photomnemonic 1.13 Eosinophils – the nucleus resembles dark blue headphones.

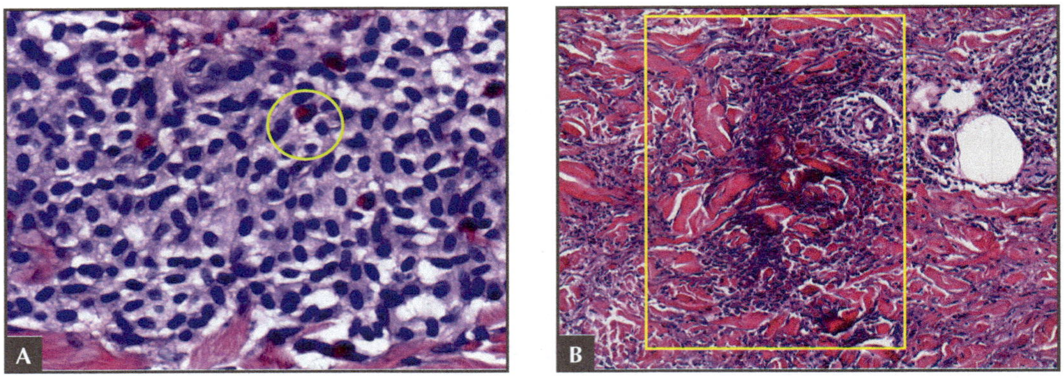

Figure 1.24 A Eosinophils. **B** Flame figure.

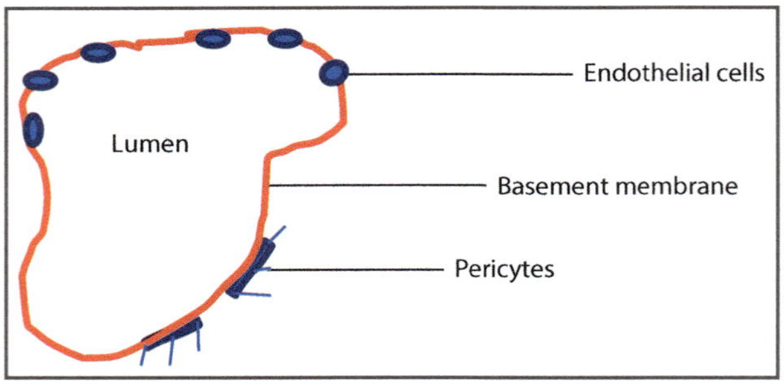

Figure 1.25 Blood vessel showing the endothelial lining and the pericytes separated by a basement membrane.

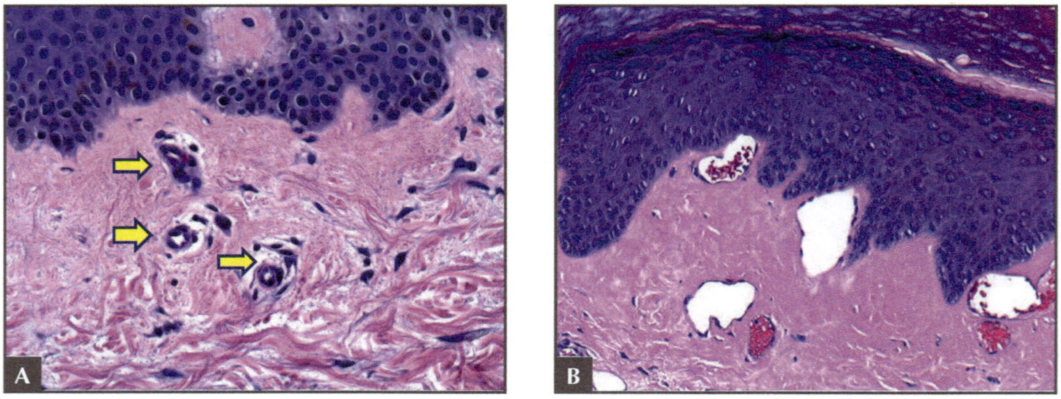

Figure 1.26 Capillaries. **A** Capillaries in papillary dermis with only one cell layer of endothelial cells. **B** Dilated capillaries in the papillary dermis.

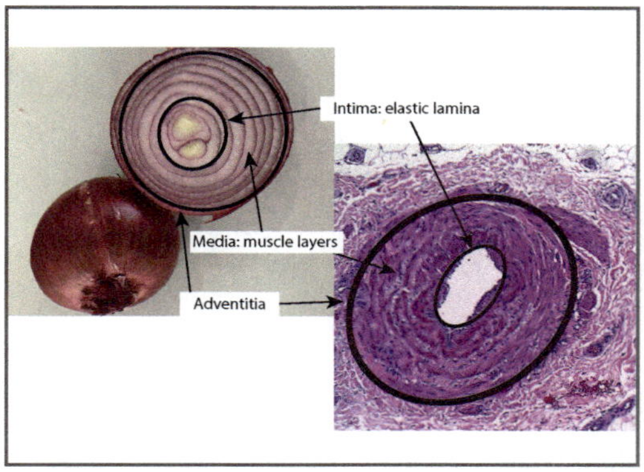

Photomnemonic 1.14 The layers of arteries and arterioles mimic a transversally cut red onion. The wall has three layers: 1) intima, which consists of endothelial cells and elastic lamina; 2) media, two or more layers of muscle cells (*only one layer in arterioles); and 3) adventitia, which contains mostly collagen.

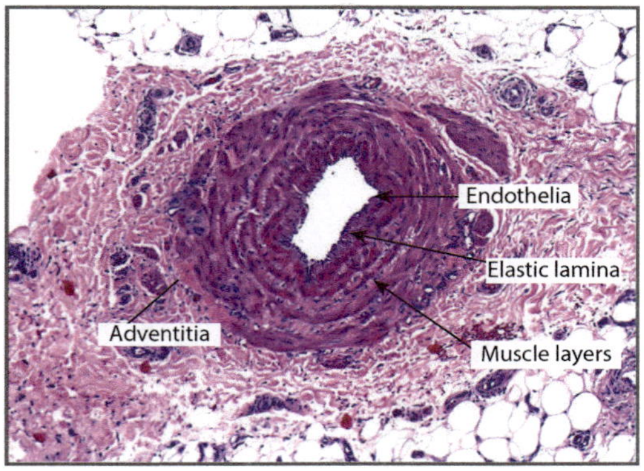

Figure 1.27 High-power view of an arteriole in the lower dermis.

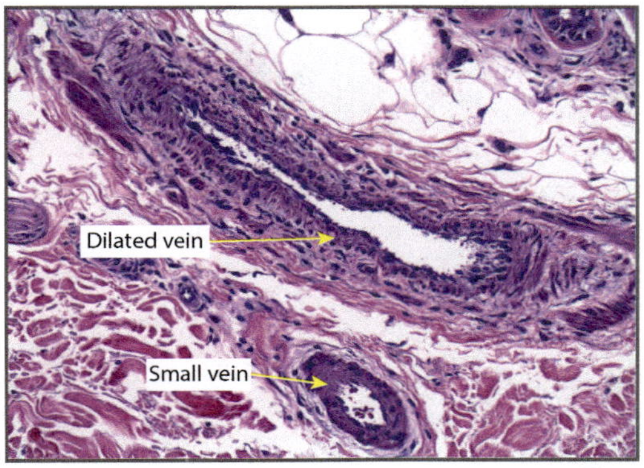

Figure 1.28 A dilated vein in the lower dermis.

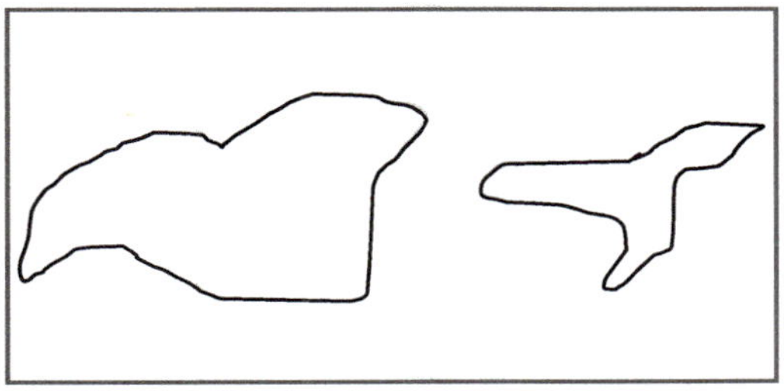

Figure 1.29 Drawing of lymphatics. Lymphatics have a more angulated contour compared to round blood vessels. The lumen of lymphatics is lined by flat endothelial cells. Lymphatics do not have a basement membrane or pericytes.

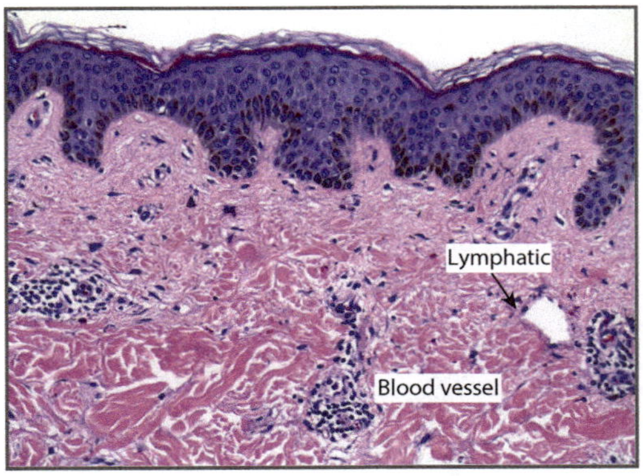

Figure 1.30 Lymphatics look like angulated holes through the dermis.

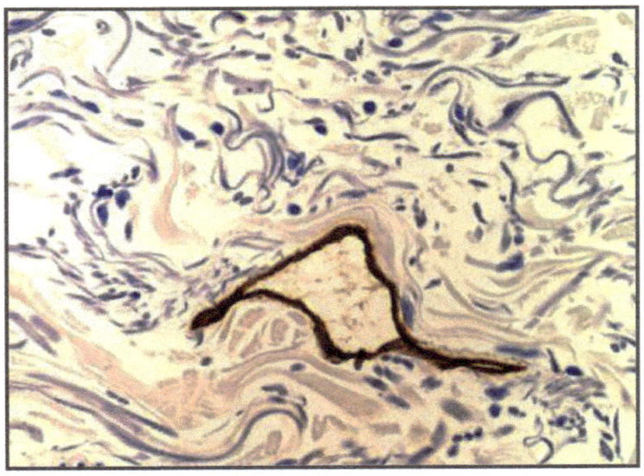

Figure 1.31 Angulated dilated lymphatic vessel stained by D2-40.

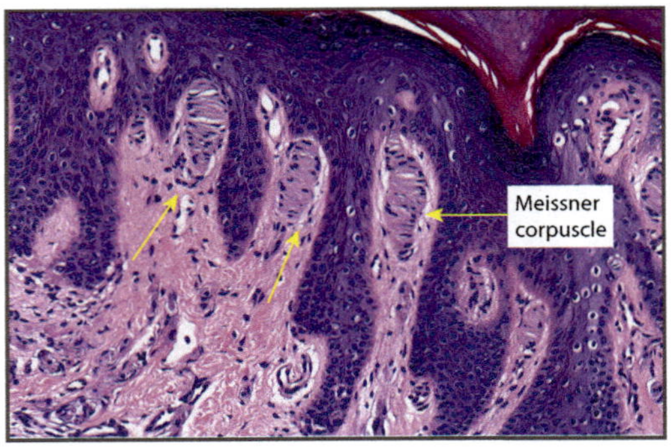

Figure 1.32 Meissner corpuscles in the dermal papillae.

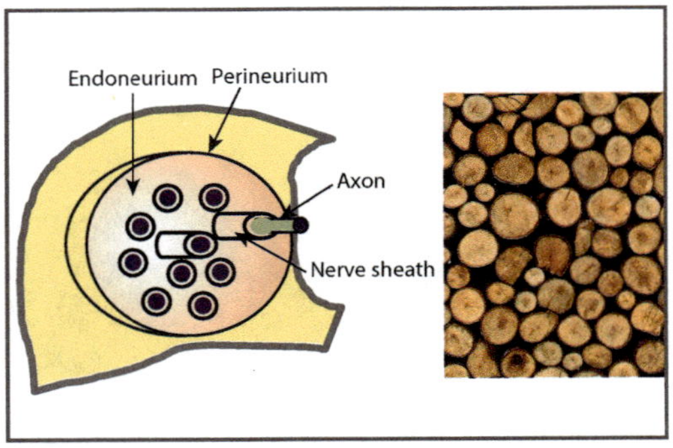

Photomnemonic 1.15 The nerve resembles the cross section of a stack of firewood.

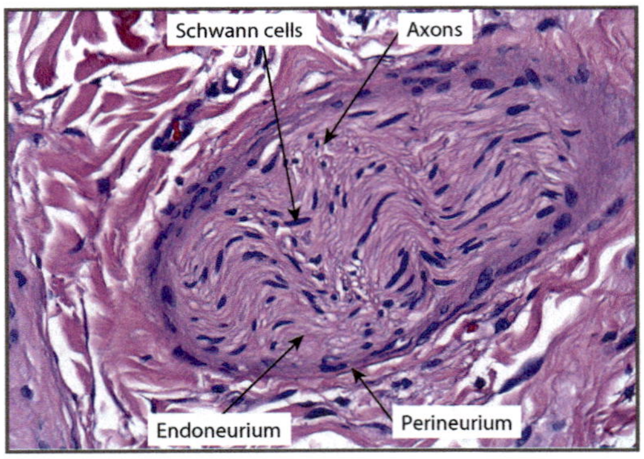

Figure 1.33 Cross section of a nerve, exhibiting axons, Schwann cells, endoneurium, and perineurium.

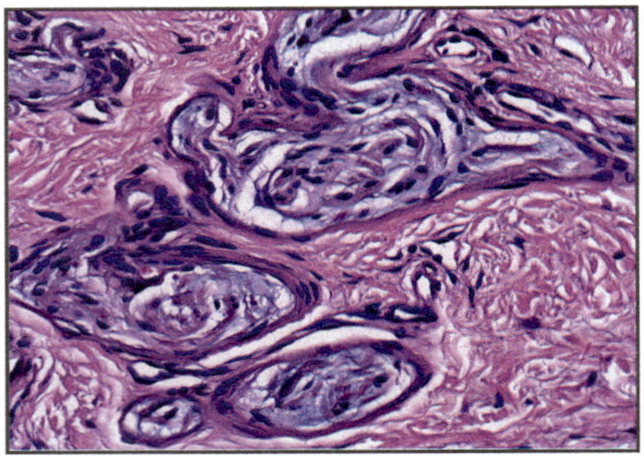

Figure 1.34 Hyperplasia of axons and Schwann cells (neuroma) in a rudimentary digit.

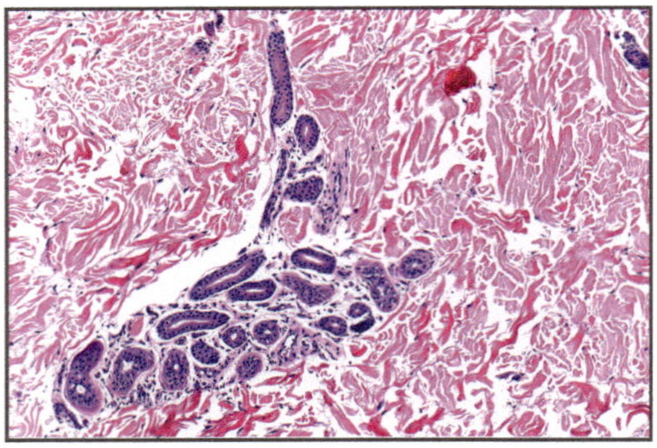

Figure 1.35 Secretory portion of sweat glands.

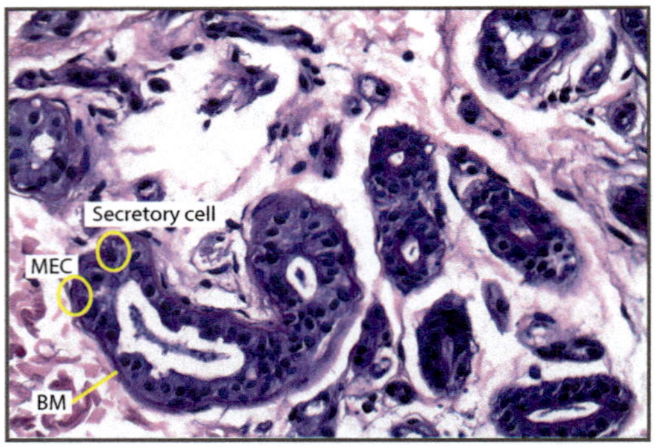

Figure 1.36 Cell layers in eccrine coils. MEC = myoepithelial cells (contract to deliver sweat to the surface); BM = hyaline basement membrane.

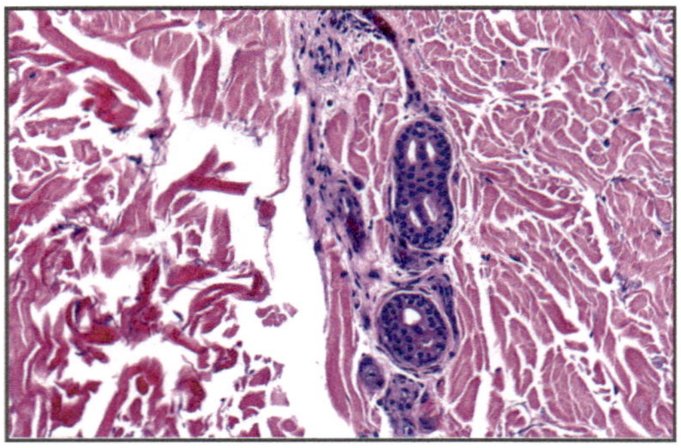

Figure 1.37 Intradermal duct of eccrine gland: two layers of small basophilic cuboidal cells.

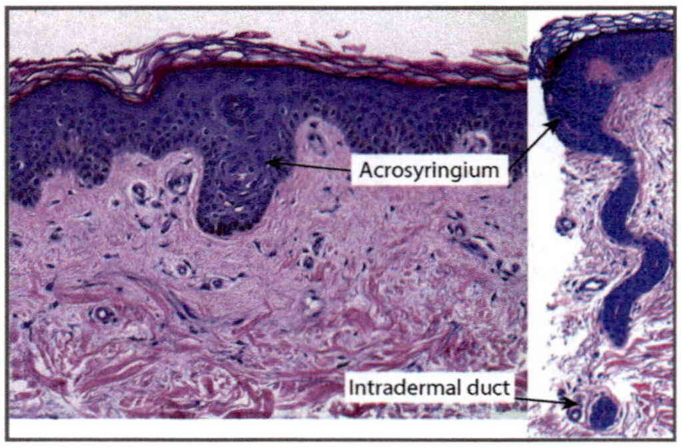

Figure 1.38 Acrosyringium of eccrine gland.

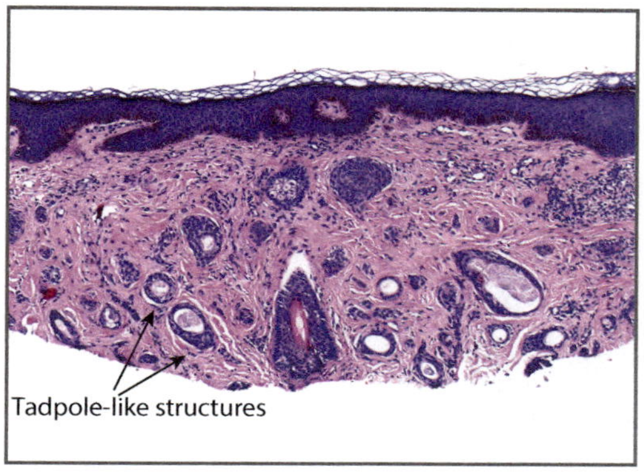

Figure 1.39 Syringoma is a tumor forming from the acrosyringium. Note the presence of tadpole-like structures.

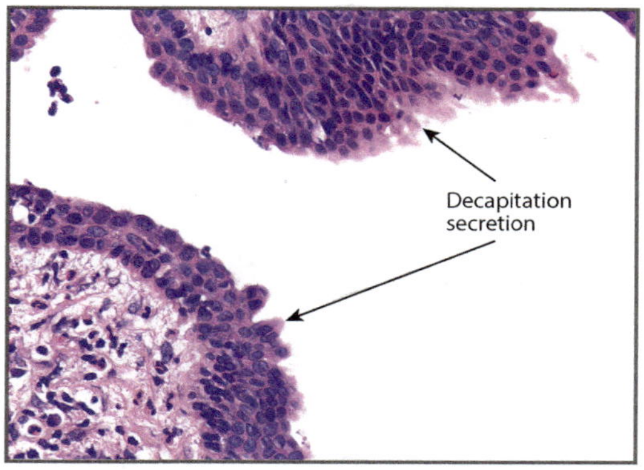

Figure 1.40 Decapitation secretion in an apocrine gland in Syringocystadenoma papilliferum.

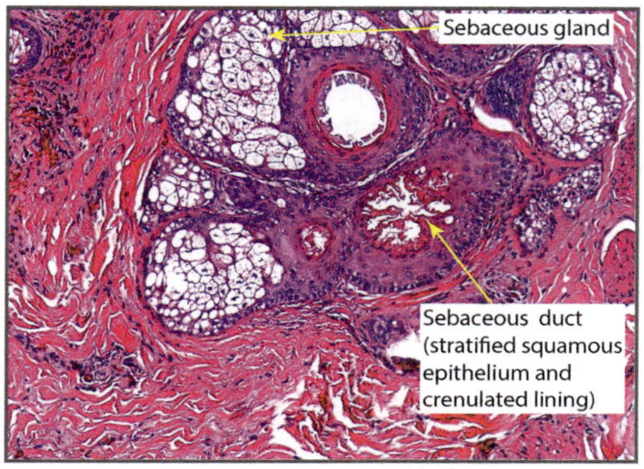

Figure 1.41 Follicular unit with the sebaceous glands. Note the dilated sebaceous duct with crenulated eosinophilic lining. Sebocytes have a stellate, centrally located nucleus with vacuolated cytoplasm, outlined by basaloid cells.

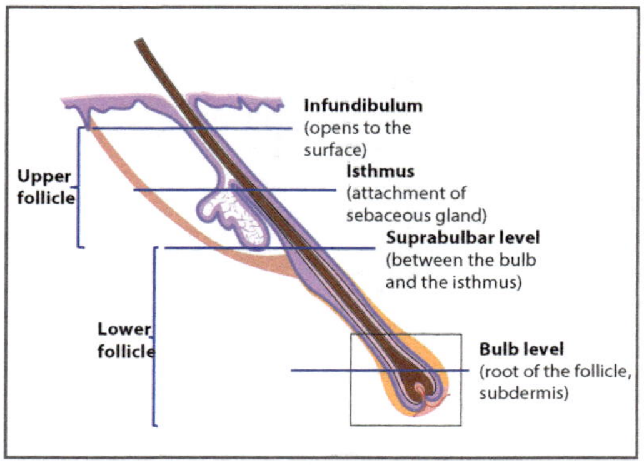

Figure 1.42 Longitudinal view of a hair follicle showing the segments along its length.

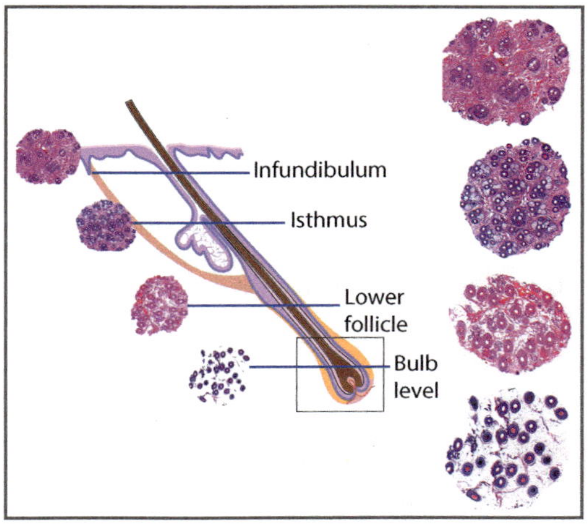

Figure 1.43 Transverse (horizontal) sections of a hair follicle throughout its length.

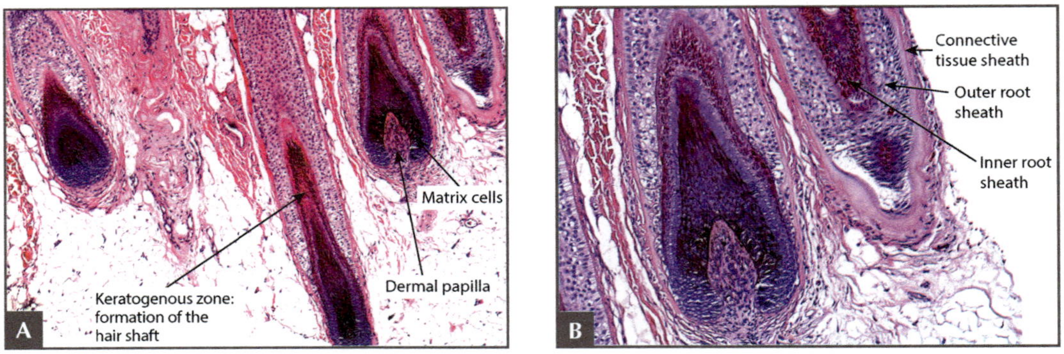

Figure 1.44 Anagen hair follicles. **A** Bulbs of terminal anagen follicles. The bulbs are embedded in the subdermis. Matrical cells (keratinocytes and melanocytes) enclose the dermal papillae (fibroblasts and blood vessels). **B** Close-up view of the bulbs of anagen follicles. Note the inner root sheath, outer root sheath, and connective tissue sheath.

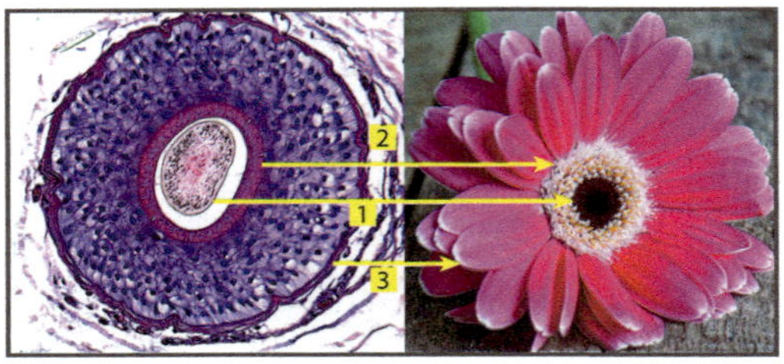

Photomnemonic 1.16 Cross-section view of an anagen follicle resembles the *Gerbera* flower.
1 = Hair shaft (thicker than the inner root sheath).
2 = Thinner inner root sheath (the inner root sheath disappears at the isthmus. 3 = Outer root sheath.

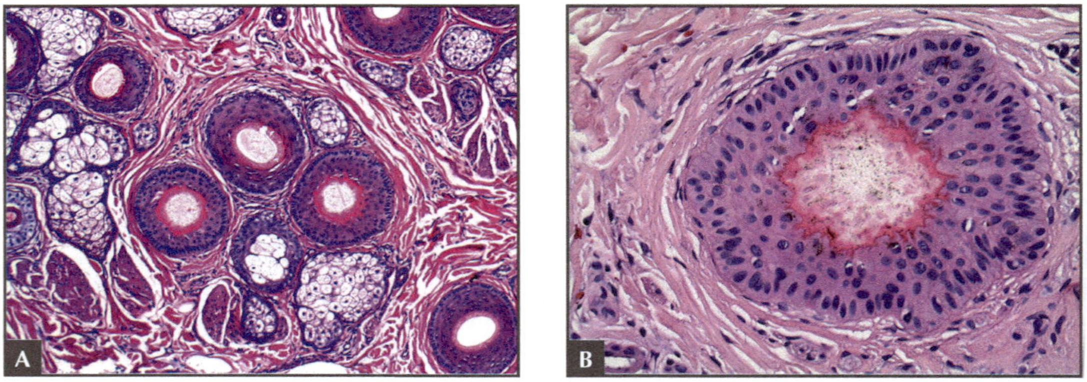

Figure 1.45 Telogen hair follicles. **A** Transverse section of telogen hair follicles. **B** Close-up transverse section of a telogen follicle: the normal layered structure of the hair shaft with the surrounding inner root sheath is absent and instead is replaced by trichilemmal keratin in the middle with red serrated borders.

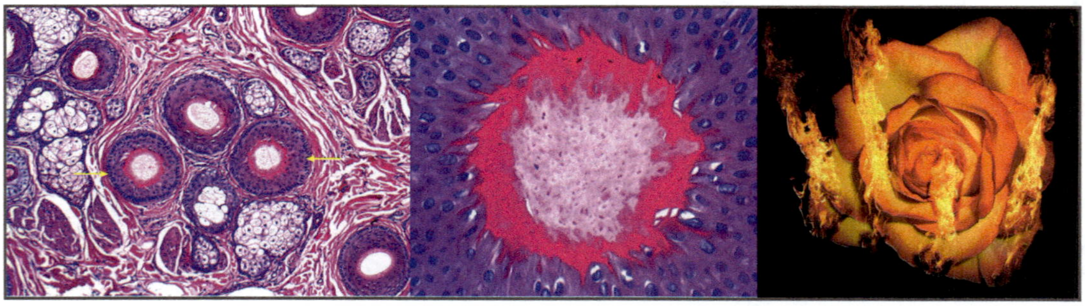

Photomnemonic 1.17 A telogen follicle in cross section resembles a burning flower.

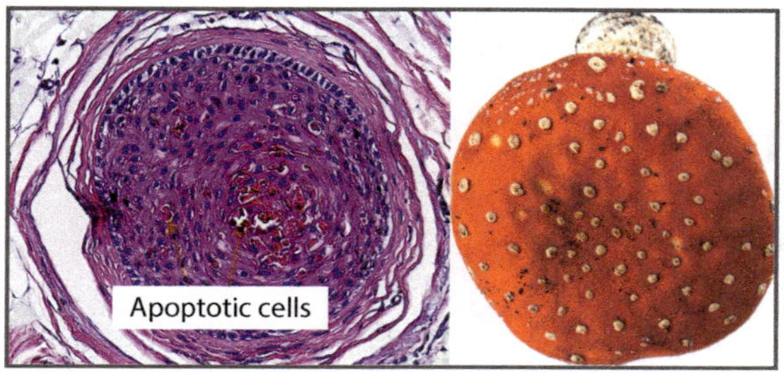

Photomnemonic 1.18 A catagen follicle resembles a fly agaric mushroom because of the apoptotic cells.

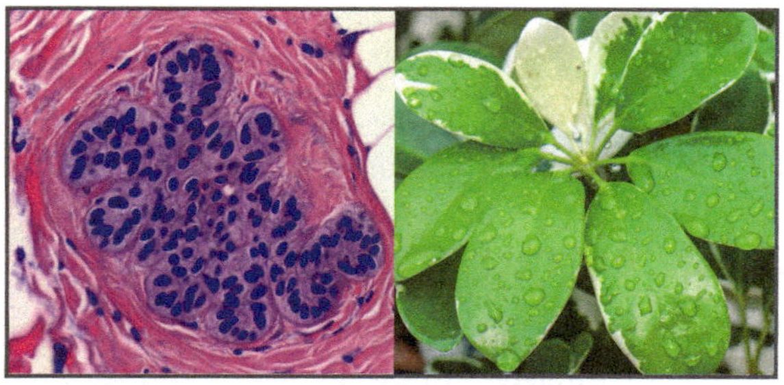

Photomnemonic 1.19 A telogen germinal unit resembles the leaf of the dwarf umbrella tree (*Schefflera arboricola*). It consists of basaloid palisaded epithelial strands after the hair is shed.

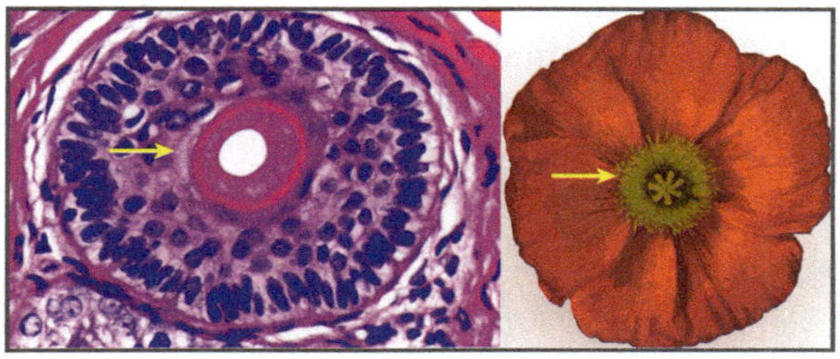

Photomnemonic 1.20 Vellus follicles resemble a poppy flower in cross section. Vellus hairs have a very thin hair shaft (less than 0.03 mm), with a thicker inner root sheath (indicated by the yellow arrow) and a thick outer root sheath.

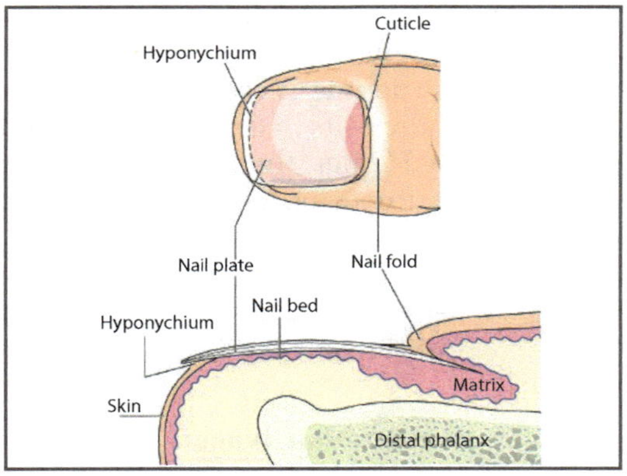

Figure 1.46 Schematic representation of the nail unit.

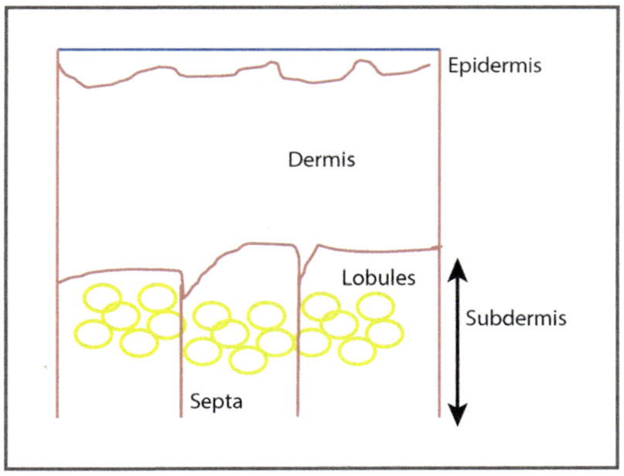

Figure 1.47 Drawing of epidermis, dermis, and subcutaneous fat.

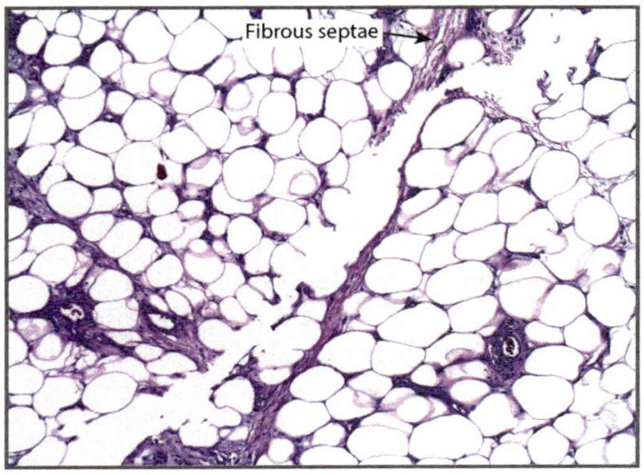

Figure 1.48 Subcutaneous fat: lobules of adipocytes separated by fibrous septae.

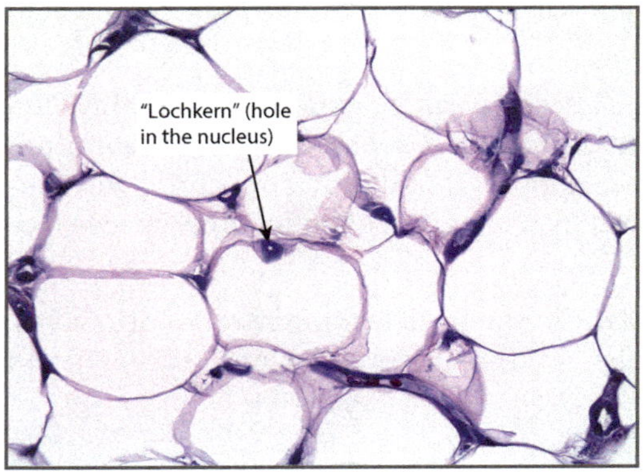

Figure 1.49 High-power view of mature fat shows the eccentric nucleus with the characteristic nuclear "hole."

2 Terminology, special stains, and immunohistochemistry

Mariya Miteva and Jacquelyn Dosal

MOST COMMONLY USED DERMATOPATHOLOGIC TERMS

Orthokeratosis: Thickened basket-weave stratum corneum

Hyperkeratosis: Thickened stratum corneum which appears delicately layered or dense and compact (pink), often with prominent granular layer **(Figure 2.1)**

Parakeratosis: Thickened stratum corneum with retained nuclei of the keratinocytes (incomplete keratinization). Note this is normal on mucous membranes **(Figure 2.2)**

Erosion: Partial loss of epidermis (compare to ulceration, which is complete loss of epidermis/and portion of the dermis)

Acanthosis: Thickening (hyperplasia) of the epidermis

1. *Psoriasiform* – elongated rete ridges of uniform thickness with suprapapillary thinning **(Figure 2.3)**
2. *Pseudoepitheliomatous hyperplasia (PEH)* – extreme hyperplasia of the epidermis and adnexal epithelium, closely simulating squamous cell carcinoma due to pushing bulbously expanded rete ridges, mitoses, and squamous eddies **(Figure 2.4)**
3. *Papillomatosis* – acanthosis with irregular undulated projections above the surface of the skin **(Figure 2.5)**

Atrophy: Decreased thickness of the epidermis (or/and dermis)

Spongiosis: Intercellular edema by stretching the intercellular bridges and separation of the keratinocytes, which appear rhomboid; spongiotic vesicles (blisters) form by coalescing of edematous spaces (see Figure 2.2)

Acantholysis: Complete detachment of keratinocytes which results in intraepidermal clefts, blisters, and bullae; keratinocytes appear round due to loss of intercellular cohesion (desmosomes) (see Figure 2.1)

Dyskeratosis: Abnormal premature/faulty keratinization of individual keratinocytes (or less often group of keratinocytes) which show pycnotic (shrunken) nucleus and pink cytoplasm **(Figure 2.6)**

- *Corps ronds* – "swollen" round cells with normal cytoplasm and perinuclear halo, look like "owl's eye" (in stratum spinosum and stratum granulosum)
- *Corps grains* – "shrunken" oval cells with condensed cytoplasm, look like "plump parakeratosis" (in stratum granulosum and stratum corneum)

Apoptosis: A normal (programmed)/abnormal (premature or faulty) cell death resulting in shrunken keratinocytes with dense and pink (eosinophilic) cytoplasm and condensed nucleus which can be fragmented; they are shed in the dermis as **colloid bodies/Civatte bodies** (eosinophilic deposits in the lower epidermis or upper dermis formed from the intracellular filaments of apoptotic keratinocytes; may entrap immunoglobulin or fibrin)

NB In a 6 mm punch biopsy a normal epidermis has one or two apoptotic cells.

Vacuolar degeneration (vacuolopathy) (Figure 2.7): Damage to the basal layer resulting in small clear spaces (vacuoles) beneath the basal layer. It is often accompanied by apoptotic keratinocytes and **pigment incontinence (Figure 2.8)** (free particles of melanin which drop in the dermis and are engulfed by macrophages (melanophages))

Exocytosis: Benign inflammatory cells or red blood cells in the epidermis, usually accompanied by spongiosis; implies a reactive process **(Figure 2.9)**

Epidermotropism: Malignant cells (lymphocytes, metastatic cells, melanocytes) in the epidermis; implies a malignant process **(Figure 2.10)**

Necrosis: Tissue death involving contiguous cells often with marked inflammatory reaction **(Figure 2.11)**

Ulceration: Complete necrosis of the epidermis and partial/complete necrosis of the dermis **(Figure 2.12, Table 2.1)**. Apoptosis is subtle cellular damage – programmed active form of cell death. There is no inflammatory reaction. Necrosis is a passive form of death involving many contiguous cells (tissue death) with a marked inflammatory reaction

Table 2.1 Types of tissue necrosis

Type	Cause	Effect
Coagulative	Results from interrupted blood supply (ischemia)	General architecture preserved, nuclear changes • Chronic ulcers
Liquefactive	Enzymatic liquefaction of necrotic tissue	Liquefied tissue debris and neutrophils • Abscess
Caseous	Interrupted blood supply and enzymatic liquefaction of necrotic tissue	Amorphous appearance with increased affinity to acidophilic (eosin) dyes • Tuberculoid granulomas
Fibrinoid	Due to deposit of fibrin-like proteinaceous material as part of immune-mediated vasculitis	Smudgy pink appearance in vascular walls • Leukocytoclastic vasculitis

SPECIAL STAINS AND IMMUNOHISTOCHEMISTRY

Understanding colors under the microscope

Synthetic dyes have a coloring part which is either acid (anionic) or basic (cationic). The cationic part has affinity to negatively charged nuclei and ribosomes, and the anionic part has affinity to positively charged cytoplasm, mitochondria, and connective tissue elements.

Hematoxylin and eosin (H&E) is the routine stain in histology. Eosin, which is an acidic stain, colors the cytoplasm of the cells, red blood cells, collagen, and muscle in variations from pink to red (eosinophilic). Hematoxylin acts as a basic stain that colors the "basophilic" structures, such as nuclear heterochromatin and mucins, in blue. The cytoplasm of cells rich in ribonucleoproteins will also stain in blue whereas those with minimal amounts of ribonucleoproteins will be lavender.

SPECIAL STAINS

Definition: Non-H&E stains used to highlight tissue components, microorganisms or foreign materials non-visible/less visible on the H&E sections. The stained component withstands either with its different color (most stains) or peculiar morphology (periodic acid-Schiff stains many elements but highlights the hyphae by their peculiar morphology). Appropriate positive controls are mandatory. Data exists that special stains generally contribute to the diagnosis in only 21.1% of cases: in cases of neoplasm, inflammation, collagen vascular disease, and amyloid, they are helpful in 31.8% but only helpful in 14.7% in cases of infection.

MOST COMMONLY APPLIED SPECIAL STAINS

For infections

PAS (periodic acid-Schiff) – stains in red to purple (magenta) structures containing a high proportion of glycogen (the cells of the outer root sheaths, pagetoid cells in Paget's disease), neutral mucins, basement membranes and blood vessels, as well as fungal walls. Diastase is used to digest the glycogen.

GMS (Gomori methenamine silver) – the most sensitive method for demonstrating hyphae. The fungal walls are outlined in dark brown–black on the green counterstain of the surrounding tissue. GMS highlights degenerated and non-viable fungi that are sometimes refractory with the PAS stain. A disadvantage of the GMS stain is that it masks the color of the fungus, which is important for dematiaceous fungi (in Phaeohyphomycosis, Alternariosis, Chromoblastomycosis).

AFB (acid-fast bacillus or Ziehl–Neelsen) – highlights in bright red the capsule of acid-fast organisms (mycobacteria), which is waxy due to mucolic acids, of high molecular weight, and cannot be penetrated by the routine aqueous dyes. It also stains *Nocardia* spp.

Fite-Faraco – the choice for *Mycobacterium leprae*, which is much less acid- and alcohol-fast than other mycobacteria. The mycobacteria stain in red–purple (magenta).

NB Beware that hair shafts and the eccrine glands may show focal staining with the Fite-Faraco stain!

Brown-Brenn – highlights bacteria: Gram-positive bacteria, *Nocardia*, and *Actinomyces* stain in blue; Gram-negative bacteria stain in red and the background remains yellow.

NB *Nocardia* stains blue with the Brown-Brenn stain, black with the GMS stain, and bright red with the AFB stain.

Warthin-Sterry – a silver stain that highlights the whole organism of *Spirochaetes* spp. in black and the background remains yellow/brownish; it is used in the diagnosis of syphilis, *Bartonella* infections (cat-scratch disease, bacillary angiomatosis, *Borrelia* infections – Lyme disease). Another stain for spirochetes is Steiner's.

Mucicarmine – selectively highlights in red microorganisms that contain polysaccharides in their walls (from muci – mucin, and carmine – dark red) such as the encapsulated yeast-like fungus *Cryptococcus neoformans*.

Giemsa – highlights the *Leishmania* bodies as well as *Histoplasma capsulatum*. The color varies from reddish to blue due to the affinity of the polyanionic part (nucleic acids) to stain blue and the polycationic pink. This stain also labels the cytoplasm of mast cells (purple) and the red blood cells (red).

For the normal components of the skin

Melanin

Fontana-Masson – detects melanin and some neuroendocrine cells. The melanin stains as black granules; the background is pink.

Collagen and muscle

Masson's trichrome – a three-color stain (trichrome): the nuclei stain black, the cytoplasm of the cells and the muscle fibers stain in red, and the collagen stains in blue/green.

PTAH (phosphotungstic acid-hematoxylin) – stains the striated muscle fibers and fibrin in blue–purple

Elastic fibers

The following stains color the elastin:

Orcein – stains elastin dark brown to black

VVG (Verhoeff-van Gieson) – the nuclei and the elastin stain black (by Verhoeff's iron-hematoxyllin stain); the cytoplasm stains in yellow and the collagen in red (by Van Gieson's picro-fuchsin stain).

Mast cells

Toluidine blue – a blue stain that highlights the mast cell granules in red due to the presence of strongly acidic macromolecular carbohydrates. This phenomenon is called metachromasia (change in the color of staining).

Giemsa – see For infections

Leder stain (naphthol AS-D chloracetate) – detects the enzyme chloroacetate esterase which is found in granulocytes (neutrophils) and mast cells. It also highlights degranulated mast cells whereas the other two stains label intact mast cells.

Nerve structures

Bodian's stain – highlights the axons in black.

Lipids (subcutaneous fat)

These stains are used in frozen sections:

Oil-O-red – stains only the most hydrophobic lipids (triglycerides and cholesterol esters)

Sudan black – stains also less hydrophobic lipids such as phospholipids and sphingomyelins

For extraneous deposits in the skin

Amyloid

Congo red – highlights the amyloid deposits from systemic amyloidosis in red, and under polarized light green birefringence is observed

Crystal violet – turns amyloid to purplish-red (metachromasia)

Thioflavin T – causes amyloid and colloid to fluoresce after staining

Calcium

Von Kossa – highlights calcium or calcium salts; works better when large amounts of salts are present, such as in a bone

Alizarin red-S – detects better small calcium particles

Mucin

Alcian blue – identifies mucins and glucosaminoglycans. At pH 2.5 it stains acid mucopolysaccharides (hyaluronic acid) which are deposited in cutaneous mucinoses.

Mucicarmine – see For infections

Colliodal iron – stains the acid mucopolysaccharides in blue–green

Hemosiderin

Perl's potassium ferricyanide and **Prussian blue** – highlight hemosiderin storage complexes in blue

IMMUNOHISTOCHEMICAL MARKERS

Definition: Detecting antigens (proteins) in cells of a tissue section using the principle of applying antibodies which bind specifically to these antigens.

The highlighted component is red or brown depending on the type of chromogen (the reagent that gives the color). It is necessary to know if the stain is nuclear or cytoplasmic to avoid misreading. (A peculiar pattern is the dot-like staining with CK20 of neuroendocrine tumors.) Also compare the results to an H&E-stained section or a negative control of the same block.

MOST COMMONLY APPLIED IMMUNOHISTOCHEMICAL MARKERS

Epithelial markers

Normal epidermis is rich in high molecular cytokeratins (CK) and will not stain with low-molecular cytokeratin markers, such as CAM 5.2, which are positive in Paget's disease.

Pan-cytokeratin (MNF 116) – stains intermediate and low molecular weight cytokeratins.

CAM 5.2 – low molecular cytokeratin, recognizes CK8 and to a lesser extent CK7, is positive in mammary Paget's disease, and useful also in poorly differentiated carcinomas.

CK5/6 – low molecular CK, is positive in spindle cell squamous cell carcinoma (SCC) and in primary versus metastatic adenocarcinoma.

AE1/AE3 – pan-cytokeratin cocktail.

EMA (epithelial membrane antigen) – large cell surface mucoprotein expressed by the glandular and ductal epithelial cells and in most adenocarcinomas. It is positive in SCC, epithelioid sarcoma, Paget's disease, and Merkel cell carcinoma, and negative in basal cell carcinoma (BCC).

CK7 – mammary Paget's disease, metastatic carcinomas (lung, uroepithelial, and colorectal cancer).

CK20 – produces a dotty pattern in Merkel cell carcinoma; positive in colorectal and uroepithelial carcinomas.

BerEP4 – membranous staining; basal cell carcinomas stain positively for BerEP4, in contrast to squamous cell carcinomas, which show no staining. Basosquamous carcinomas show some areas of BerEP4 positivity.

P53 – a nuclear stain which is considered positive if more than 5% of the nuclei are labeled. It distinguishes reactive and metaplastic conditions, which are p53 negative, from malignant neoplasms, which are positive. (Table 2.2)

Table 2.2 Comparison of immunohistochemistry stains for adnexal structures

Stain	Apocrine	Eccrine	Sebaceous
EMA	Positive	Positive	Positive
CEA	Positive	Positive	Negative
S100	Negative	Negative/Positive	Negative
Androgen receptor	Negative	Negative	Positive

Melanocytic markers

MART-1 (MELAN-A) – this is the most sensitive melanocytic marker; however, it is negative in desmoplastic melanoma; it labels the pseudonests in lichenoid actinic keratosis in sun-damaged skin which may be mistaken for melanoma *in situ* (alternative stain: SOX10 with MITF-1).

MITF-1 – a nuclear stain, positive in mast cells, melanocytes, and osteoclasts.

HMB-45 – recognizes melanosomal glycoprotein gp100. Deep melanoma components show at least focal positivity whereas nevi do not show expression in the deeper parts (stratification).

NB Exception – blue nevi stain through with HMB-45.

S100 – acidic protein, present in both the nucleus and the cytoplasm. Less sensitive than MART-1 and HMB-45 for melanocytic lesions, except for desmoplastic melanoma; this is a common marker for neural tissue.

Fibrohistiocytic markers

Histiocytes

Monocytes migrate from the bone marrow to the organs (including skin) where they differentiate into professional histiocytes (macrophages) and antigen-presenting dendritic cells (Langerhans cells in the epidermis and dermal dendritic cells in the dermis). (Table 2.3)

Table 2.3 Useful immunohistochemical markers for the cells of histiocytic lineage

Cells of histiocytic lineage	Immunohistochemistry
Macrophages	CD68, CD163, Factor XIIIa
Epidermal dendritic cells (Langerhans cells)	CD1a, S100, CD207
Dermal (interstitial) dendritic cells	CD163, Factor XIIIa

Fibroblasts

CD34 – defines hematopoetic progenitor cells, dendritic interstitial cells, and endothelial cells; it helps in distinguishing dermatofibroma (negative) from dermatofibrosarcoma (positive). It is positive also in Kaposi's sarcoma and epithelioid sarcoma.

Smooth muscle cells

Desmin – marks myoblasts, myofibroblasts and smooth muscle cells
SMA (smooth muscle actin) – a marker for smooth muscle cells and myofibroblasts; pericytes

Lymphocytic markers

CLA (leukocyte common antigen) – a common marker for hematopoietic cells, stains both T- and B-cells

CD3 – a common T-cell marker

CD4 – a T-helper marker

CD8 – a cytotoxic T-cell marker

CD30 – membranous staining to the lymphocyte activation antigen; positive in Lymphomatoid papulosis, Anaplastic Large Cell Lymphoma, Mycosis Fungoides with transformation and Large B-cell Lymphoma

CD20 – a B-cell marker

CD79a – see Plasma cell markers

Plasma cell markers

CD79a – recognizes B-cell antigen receptor complex associated with protein alpha chain; expressed early in B-cell differentiation (often positive when mature B-cell markers are negative); also expressed in plasma cells

CD138 – B-cell precursors and plasma cells

Plasmocytoid dendritic cells

CD123 – associates with the GM-CSF receptor

Endothelial markers

CD31 – the most sensitive and specific endothelial marker, membranous (not cytoplasmic) stain

> NB It is important not to confuse CD31+ macrophages (granular, membranous expression) with a vascular proliferation.

F.VIII – a common endothelial marker; stains also mast cells and platelets (platelet thrombi)

CD34 – a less sensitive endothelial marker; see Fibroblasts

Podoplanin (D2-40) – the most sensitive marker for lymphatic endothelium; useful in identifying lymphatic invasion by metastases

Neural markers

(Table 2.4)

Table 2.4 Useful immunohistochemical markers for the structural components of the neural tissue

Neural components	Immunohistochemistry
Schwann cells	S100, NSE (neuron-specific enolase), CD57 (Leu-7)
Neurons	NSE, synaptophysin, chromogranin, neurofilaments (NF)
Axons	NSE, NF
Perineural cells	EMA, collagen IV
Neuroendocrine cells	NSE, CD57 (Leu-7), chromogranin, synaptophysin

Cell proliferation markers

Ki67 – a nuclear stain; cytoplasmic expression is not relevant

Panels for most common metastatic tumors of unknown origin

Renal cell carcinoma – CK7, CD10, RCC-Ma

Gastrointestinal malignancy – CD7–, CK20, CDX2

Lung cancer – CK7, TTF1

Breast cancer – CK7, ER, PR
(Table 2.5, Table 2.6, Table 2.7)

Table 2.5 Immunohistochemistry of basal cell carcinoma (BCC) versus squamous cell carcinoma (SCC)

Stain	BCC	SCC
EMA	Negative	Positive
BerEP4	Positive	Negative

Table 2.6 Comparison of immunohistochemistry for melanoma in situ versus Paget's versus pagetoid Bowen's disease

Stain	Melanoma in situ	Paget's	Bowen's
Melanocytic markers (MART-1, S100, HMB-45)	Positive	Negative	Negative
CAM5.2	Negative	Positive	Negative
EMA	Negative	Positive	Positive
CEA	Negative	Positive	Negative

Table 2.7 Primary versus metastatic adenocarcinoma

Stain	Primary	Metastatic
P63	Positive	Negative
CK5/6	Positive	Negative
D2-40	Variable	Negative

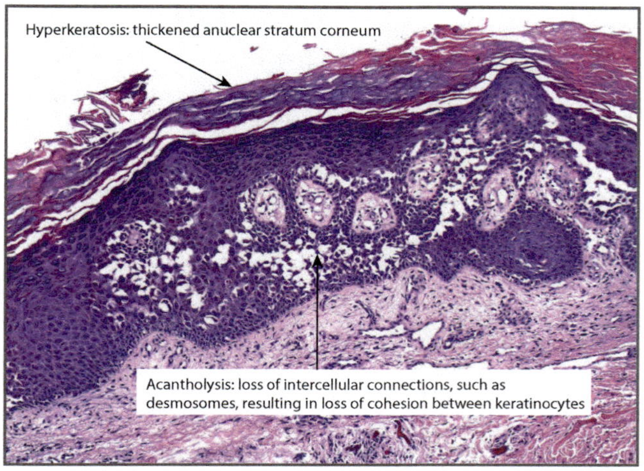

Figure 2.1 A specimen from Hailey-Hailey disease. Note the hyperkeratosis and the acantholysis.

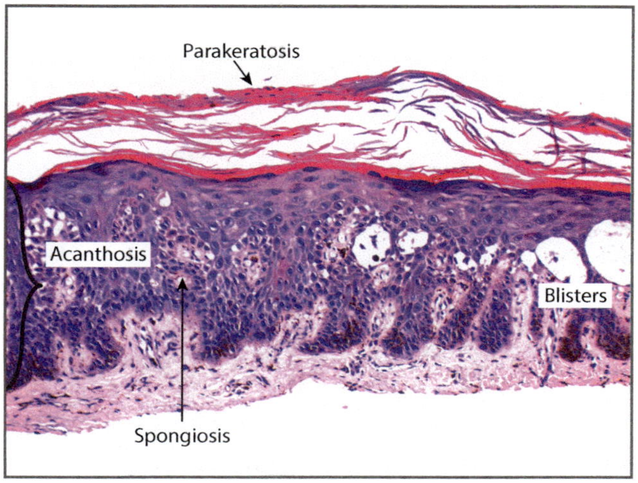

Figure 2.2 The stratum corneum shows parakeratosis (retention of nuclei), acanthosis (thickening of epidermis), and spongiosis (intracellular edema).

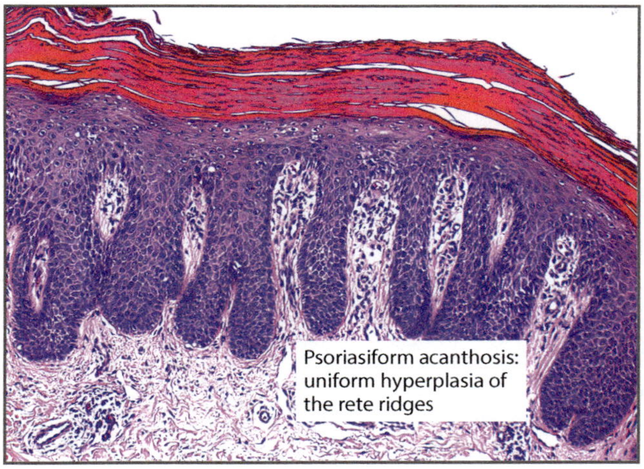

Figure 2.3 Psoriasiform hyperplasia. Note the elongated rete ridges of unified thickness.

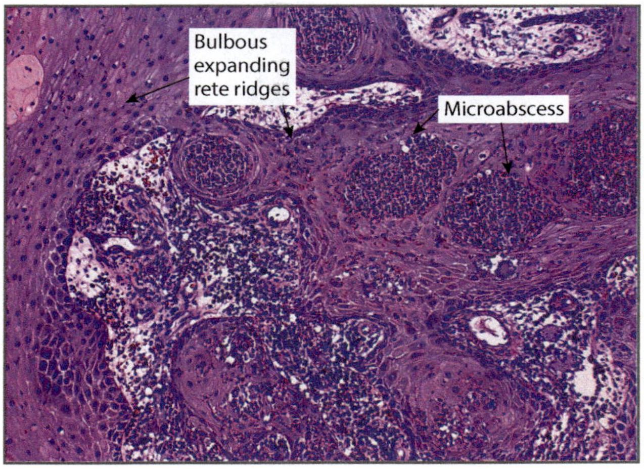

Figure 2.4 Pseudoepitheliomatous hyperplasia in North American blastomycosis. Note the bulbous expanding rete ridges.

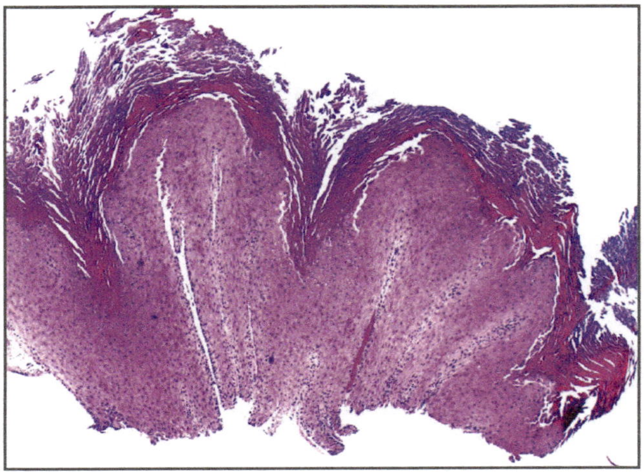

Figure 2.5 Papillomatosis: undulated epidermis.

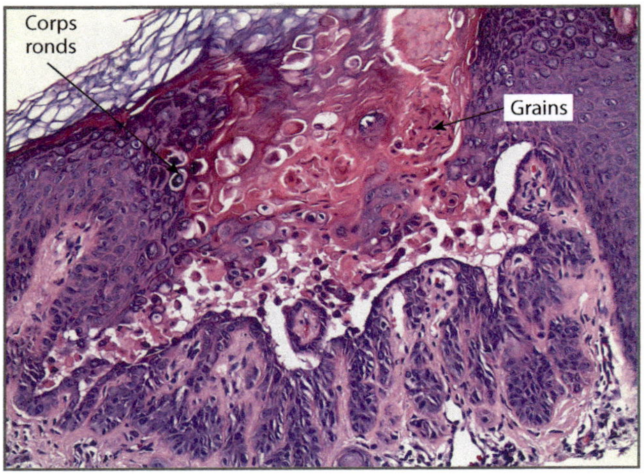

Figure 2.6 Dyskeratosis in Darier disease. Abnormal keratinization occurs prematurely within individual cells or groups of cells below the stratum granulosum.

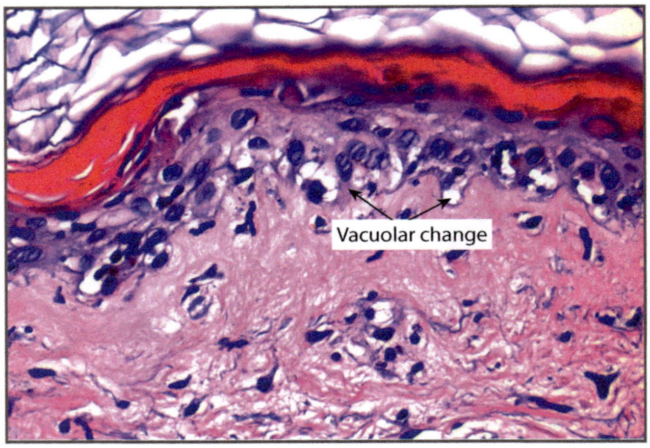

Figure 2.7 Vacuolar degeneration. Note small clear spaces below the basal layer resulting from damage to basal layer keratinocytes.

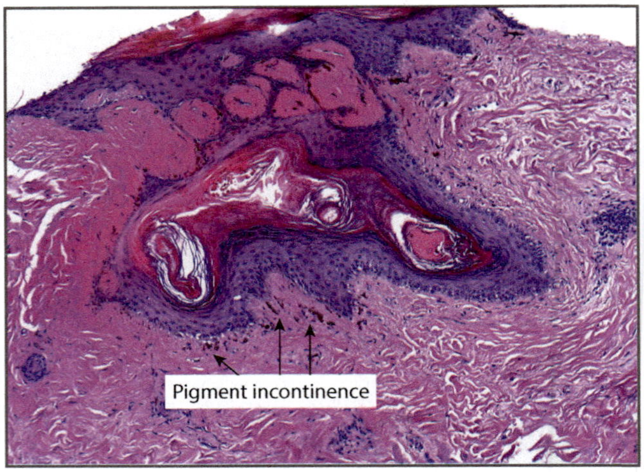

Figure 2.8 Pigment incontinence in discoid lupus erythematosus: melanin engulfed by macrophages.

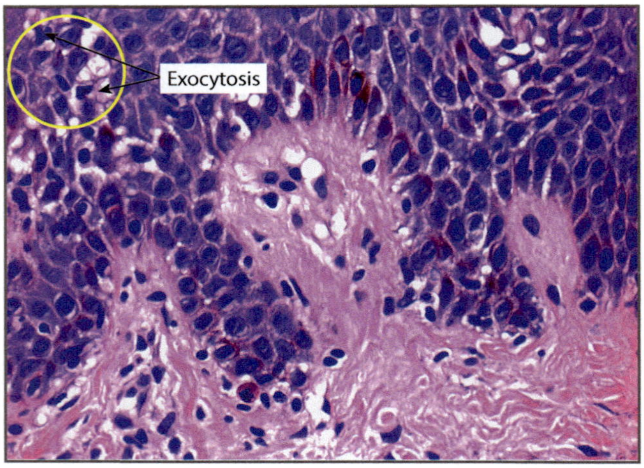

Figure 2.9 Exocytosis: lymphocytes in the epidermis.

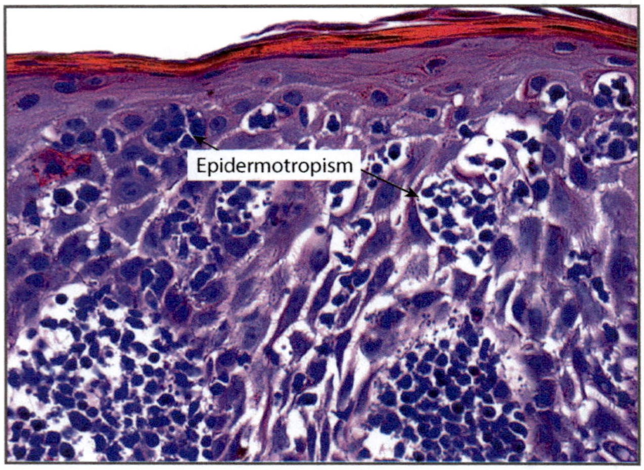

Figure 2.10 Epidermotropism in cutaneous T-cell lymphoma: malignant cells in the epidermis.

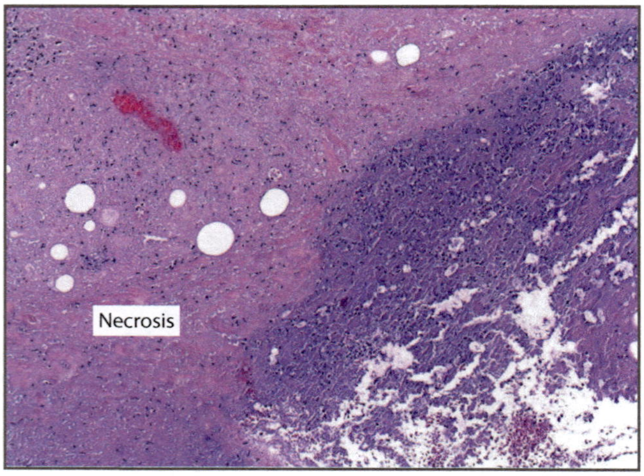

Figure 2.11 Necrosis: pale pink amorphous dead cells with accompanying inflammatory infiltrate.

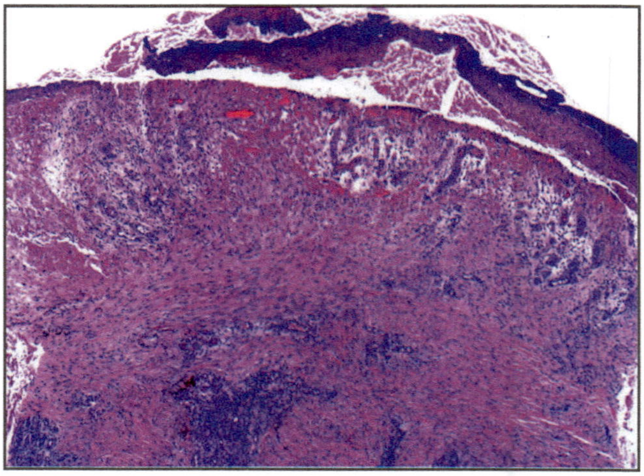

Figure 2.12 Ulceration. Complete loss of the epidermis is accompanied by necrosis.

SECTION II: MOST COMMON DERMATOLOGIC DISORDERS: PATTERN ANALYSIS

3 | Inflammatory dermatoses

SPONGIOTIC PATTERN

Mariya Miteva and Jacquelyn Dosal

Definition: Presence of inter- and intracellular edema (spongiosis) in the epidermis. Intercellular edema results in widening of the spaces between cells, which elongates their intercellular bridges.

(Figure 3.1)

General concepts

NB Spongiosis is a dynamic process – findings depend on the stage of evolution: with time, all spongiotic dermatitides become more psoriasiform and less spongiotic.

(Table 3.1, Figure 3.2)

- In the subacute and chronic stage (when the epidermis has had time to respond to the inflammatory injury), spongiosis often has a parakeratotic cap and a diminished granular layer.
- Inflammatory cells are common at sites of spongiosis (lymphocytes and occasional eosinophils and Langerhans cells) and in perivascular distribution in the superficial dermis (lymphocytes and occasional eosinophils).

Table 3.1 Comparison of acute, subacute, and chronic spongiotic dermatitis

Phase	Histologic features
Acute (*Prototype:* allergic contact dermatitis)	Normal stratum corneum Marked spongiosis (vesicles) No acanthosis
Subacute (*Prototype:* nummular eczema)	Parakeratosis Mild spongiosis Variable hypogranulosis Acanthosis Superficial perivascular infiltrate in the dermis
Chronic (*Prototype:* lichen simplex chronicus)	Compact hyperkeratosis, variable parakeratosis Spongiosis may be subtle Hypergranulosis Psoriasiform acanthosis Superficial perivascular infiltrate Variable papillary dermal fibrosis

NB **Exocytosis** should be distinguished from **epidermotropism**.

- The shape of the spongiotic vesicle has been resembled to a small turned vase with peppered lymphocytes versus a circle with fewer malignant lymphocytes in Pautrier's microabscess.

NB The vase can sometimes be upright.

(Figure 3.3)

- **Ballooning degeneration:** Keratinocytes swell like a balloon and the nucleus is pushed off to the side. Severe ballooning degeneration results in **reticular degeneration**: multilocular balloons explode, leaving behind fragments of cells on background of and intercellular irregular "messy" edema.

NB The differential diagnosis for this pattern is between irritant contact dermatitis and viral exanthem.

(Figure 3.4)

- Pronounced spongiosis may lead to edema in the papillary dermis.

NB Differential diagnosis of papillary dermal edema includes arthropod bite reaction, Sweet's syndrome, allergic contact dermatitis, erythema multiforme, pernio, polymorphic light eruption.

- **Spongiotic mimickers:**
  - Clear cells due to glycogen (outer root sheath of the follicular epithelium, clear cell acanthoma)
  - Pagetoid cells (pagetoid melanoma, Bowen's disease, Paget's disease; metastatic carcinomas)
  - Pallor of the epidermis (in its upper parts) – nutritional and enzymatic deficiencies (necrolytic migratory erythema, acrodermatitis enteropathica, pellagra)
- For the overlap of spongiosis with other inflammatory patterns, see Figure 3.5.

(Figure 3.5)

On low power

(Photomnemonic 3.1)

- Pale and spongy epidermis with various degrees of intercellular edema: mild spongiosis in subacute spongiotic dermatitis; moderate with vesicles in acute spongiotic dermatitis; severe in reticular degeneration in irritant contact dermatitis and viral rash
- Hyperkeratosis or parakeratosis with/without a serum crust (coagulated plasma)
- Variable acanthosis

(Table 3.2)

On high power

Atopic dermatitis

Atopic dermatitis can present as acute, subacute or chronic spongiotic dermatitis.

Table 3.2 Spongiotic disorders classified by the type of predominant cell in the infiltrate

Lymphocytes	Eosinophils	Plasma cells	Neutrophils	Follicular infundibulum	Sweat gland
Allergic contact dermatitis	Pruritic urticarial papules and plaques of pregnancy (PUPPP)	Zoon's balanitis	Pustular psoriasis	Apocrine miliaria (Fox-Fordyce disease)	Miliaria
Nummular dermatitis	Arthropod reaction		IgA pemphigus/ Sneddon-Wilkinson disease	Folliculitis	
Dyshidrotic eczema	Pemphigus vulgaris		Acute generalized exanthematous pustulosis (AGEP)	Follicular mucinosis	
Atopic dermatitis	Bullous pemphigoid, cicatricial pemphigoid		Candidiasis	Seborrheic dermatitis	
Lichen simplex chronicus	Allergic contact/nummular dermatitis				
Seborrheic dermatitis	Herpes gestationis				
Pityriasis rosea	Toxic erythema of the newborn				
Photodermatitis	Incontinentia pigmenti				
Gyrate erythema	Drug eruption				
Stasis dermatitis	Eosinophilic folliculitis (Ofuji's disease)				
Pigmented purpura of Doucas and Kapetanakis type					

Additional features:

- Hyperkeratosis of the acrosyringium: a cap of hyperkeratosis on top of acrosyringium (atopic patients worsen with sweating) **(Figure 3.6)**

Seborrheic dermatitis

- Ortho/hyperkeratotic stratum corneum with shoulder parakeratosis ("S" as seborrheic and shoulder: the parakeratosis is adjacent to and "shoulders" the follicle) **(Figure 3.7A)**
- Acanthosis may be psoriasiform
- Superficial perivascular lymphocytic infiltrate
- Yeast forms of *Pityrosporum* can be found in stratum corneum **(Figure 3.7B)**

> NB In seborrheic dermatitis in HIV note necrotic keratinocytes and plasma cells.

Pityriasis rosea

- Multifocal parakeratosis (in mounts) and angulated parakeratosis ("teapot lid" sign) **(Photomnemonic 3.2)**
- Acanthosis
- Mild spongiosis
- Exocytosis of lymphocytes and red blood cells (red blood cells also in the papillary dermis) **(Figure 3.8)**
- Dyskeratosis in the herald patch

Nummular dermatitis

It is the prototype of subacute spongiotic dermatitis.

Additional features:

- Multifocal spongiosis with exocytosis covered by a scale crust or even ulceration with neutrophils **(Figure 3.9)**
- Irregular acanthosis

Contact dermatitis

It can present as acute, subacute, or chronic spongiotic dermatitis.

Additional features:

1. *Allergic contact dermatitis:*
   - In acute dermatitis: Langerhans cells (S100+ and CD1a+), lymphocytes and eosinophils (eosinophilic spongiosis) in vesicles form "microabscesses" (see Figure 3.3A) **(Figure 3.10)**
   - In chronic dermatitis: eosinophils are in the dermis
2. *Irritant contact dermatitis:*
   - Epidermal necrosis (from individual necrotic keratinocytes to confluent necrosis)
   - Neutrophils predominate over eosinophils (may be absent)
   - Extensive ballooning degeneration and only slight spongiosis (see Figure 3.4)
   - Edema in the papillary dermis

> NB To distinguish between the two:
> Allergic contact dermatitis (hypersensitivity) – eosinophils
> Irritant contact dermatitis (necrosis) – neutrophils

Dyshidrosis (pompholyx)

Acral skin with a confluent spongiosis that forms an intraepidermal macrovesicle/blister **(Figure 3.11)**

> NB Dyshidrosis and tinea pedis can look identical if fungal elements are not noted on H&E. Beware of the dyshidrotic variant of mycosis fungoides.

Lichen simplex chronicus

This is the prototype for chronic spongiotic dermatitis.

Additional features:

- Thick cornified layer (simulating acral skin) in skin bearing hair follicles **(Figure 3.12)**
- Pronounced irregular acanthosis
- Thickened papillary dermis with coarse bundles of collagen arranged in vertical streaks

Prurigo nodularis

The same process as lichen simplex chronicus but shaped as a nodule (inward-pointing lateral rete ridges) **(Figure 3.13)**

- Common central excoriation/ulceration with serum crust and neutrophils
- May be centered around a hair follicle
- Variation: Acanthoma fissuratum

Spongiotic drug eruptions (maculopapular)

All findings are usually mild:

- Mild spongiosis (in the lower half of the epidermis) is the most common pathologic presentation of maculopapular drug eruptions (97% of biopsies)
- Focal parakeratosis
- Mild acanthosis
- Necrotic keratinocytes
- Mild exocytosis (lymphocytes and/or eosinophils)
- Mild perivascular lymphocytic infiltrate (with/without eosinophils)

> NB Drug reaction is usually a constellation of several patterns: spongiotic, lichenoid, psoriasiform associated with necrotic keratinocytes (and eosinophils).

Eccrine miliaria

- **Miliaria cristalina:** Subcorneal vesicle
- **Miliaria rubra:** Spongiotic vesicle in the acrosyringium; spongiosis of the lower portion of the acrosyringium and the dermal duct
  - Variable spongiosis related to the intraepidermal portion of the sweat duct (acrosyringium)

- There may also be edema in the papillary dermis adjacent to eccrine duct
- Neutrophils may be present

NB Distinguish from lichen striatus, which has lichenoid infiltrate with deep dermal infiltrate around eccrine duct.

Stasis dermatitis (venous stasis dermatitis)

It can present as acute, subacute, or chronic spongiotic dermatitis **(Figure 3.14)**.

Additional features:

- Small clusters (lobules) of dilated capillaries (aneurysmatic capillaries) in the papillary dermis with fibrin cuffs (the walls appear thicker and bright pink)
- Fibrosis of dermis
- Red blood cell extravasation and hemosiderin (brown particles of iron from the degraded extravasated red blood cells)

NB Stasis dermatitis may show features for superimposed contact dermatitis with eosinophilic spongiosis.

Arthropod bite reaction

- Eosinophilic spongiosis (focal to extensive macrovesiculation)
- Edema **(Figure 3.15A)**
- Superficial and deep wedge-shaped infiltrate (lymphocytes, eosinophils, neutrophils)
- Flame figures sometimes seen **(Figure 3.15B)**
- Thrombi in spider bites
- Arthropod mouth parts (polarizable due to chitin) sometimes seen

NB Note eosinophils around the sweat glands. About 70% show eosinophils around sweat coils **(Figure 3.15C)**.

Differential diagnosis:

- Allergic contact dermatitis (less likely to have a deep infiltrate)
- Incontinentia pigmenti (dyskeratotic cells)
- Bullous pemphigoid (eosinophils at the basement membrane zone, subepidermal cleft)
- PLEVA (wedge-shaped infiltrate, lymphocyte exocytosis, necrotic keratinocytes, parakeratosis, red blood cell extravasation, interface dermatitis, fewer eosinophils)
- Lymphomatoid papulosis (LyP) (wedge-shaped infiltrate, mostly of lymphocytes although neutrophils and eosinophils may be present, extravasated red blood cells, necrosis)
- Erythema multiforme (may have pronounced edema, a few eosinophils, but has necrotic keratinocytes and intact basket-weave stratum corneum)

Other dermatoses that may show spongiotic pattern

- **Gyrate erythemas** (erythema annulare centrifugum (EAC), erythema repens, erythema marginatum, erythema chronicum migrans): mounds of parakeratosis, tight lymphohistiocytic infiltrate ("sleeve-like") that can be both superficial and deep
- **Viral exanthem:** Focal spongiosis, focal parakeratosis, balloon degeneration
- **Mycosis fungoides** (atypical lymphocytic infiltrate with epidermotropism; slight spongiosis can be found in about 40% of lesions in the patch/plaque stage)
- **Pruritic urticarial papules and plaques of pregnancy (PUPPP):** Mild spongiosis with papillary dermal and superficial perivascular infiltrate containing eosinophils; edema
- **Erythema toxicum neonatorum:** Folliculocentric subcorneal vesicle with eosinophils
- **Incontinentia pigmenti:** (see Chapter 4, Selected genodermatoses)
- **Eosinophilic folliculitis** (eosinophilic pustular folliculitis, Ofuji's disease): Spongiosis in the outer root sheaths with exocytosis of lymphocytes and eosinophils and perifollicular infiltrate

Spongiotic overlaps

"Spongiotic pustular" dermatoses (overlapping spongiotic and psoriasiform patterns)

- **Pustular psoriasis:** Subcorneal spongiotic vesicle with neutrophils (spongiform pustule)
  - Munro microabscess: collection of neutrophils within stratum corneum
  - Spongiform pustule of Kogoj: collection of neutrophils in stratum spinosum
- **Acute generalized exanthematous pustulosis (AGEP):**

NB "Spongiotic psoriasis" with necrotic keratinocytes, and eosinophils: think AGEP!

  - Subcorneal pustules
  - Spongiosis surrounding the pustules
  - Edema in papillary dermis
  - Variable eosinophils in the dermis

NB Differential diagnosis: Candidiasis should be excluded by a PAS stain.

"Spongiotic acantholytic" dermatoses (overlapping spongiotic and acantholytic pattern)

- **IgA pemphigus/Sneddon-Wilkinson disease (subcorneal pustular dermatosis)** (see also Vesicular and bullous disorders); two subtypes:
  - Subcorneal pustular dermatosis (SPD) (the antigen is desmocollin-1)

  - Intraepidermal neutrophilic IgA dermatosis (IEN) (the antigen is desmoglein 1, desmoglein 3)
    - Variable degrees of acantholysis (subcorneal blister with neutrophils in SPD versus suprabasal continuous blister at any level in the epidermis with eosinophils and follicular extension in IEN)
    - Mild spongiosis
    - Mixed perivascular infiltrate (lymphocytes, neutrophils, eosinophils)
- **Grover's disease (spongiotic variant)**: Lentiginous rete ridges, focal acantholysis

Spongiotic dermatitis with plasma cells

- **Zoon's balanitis (balanitis circumscripta plasmacellularis):**
  - Mucosal surface (absent granular layer) with increased amount of small vessels
  - Watery uniform spongiosis with lozenge-/diamond-shaped keratinocytes
  - Dense plasmacytic infiltrate (usually lichenoid)
  - Extravasated red blood cells and hemosiderin

Spongiosis in the follicular infundibulum

- **Fox-Fordyce disease (apocrine miliaria):**
  - Spongiosis and spongiotic vesicles in the follicle at the site of the entrance of the apocrine duct
  - Follicular hyperkeratosis
  - Concomitant findings of subacute to chronic spongiotic dermatitis
- **Folliculitis, eosinophilic:**
  - Mixed infiltrate of lymphocytes, eosinophils, neutrophils, histiocytes within the hair follicle
  - Subtle spongiosis in the follicular epithelium and sometimes the sebaceous lobules
- **Follicular mucinosis:**

NB Note dilated pale follicles that stain blue with special stains for mucin.

  - Mucin and spongiosis within follicular epithelium **(Figure 3.16)**
  - Lymphocytic infiltrate: bland lymphocytes found within the hair follicle (exocytosis) in alopecia mucinosa or atypical (folliculotropism) in follicular mucinosis associated with cutaneous T-cell lymphoma
  - Mucin can be highlighted by Alcian blue or colloidal iron stains

INTERFACE DERMATITIS

Definition: Inflammatory pattern, in which the interface between the basal cell layer and the upper papillary dermis is obscured by leukocytic infiltrate, vacuolar damage, necrosis of keratinocytes, and melanophages in the upper dermis.

1. **Lichenoid interface pattern: ("aggressive pattern"):** Inflammatory cells arranged in a band-like fashion (mostly cytotoxic CD8 lymphocytes) attack the dermoepidermal junction which results in cellular death (apoptotic cells and Civatte bodies) and pigment incontinence.

   NB Associate it with soldiers (the cells) attacking a fortress wall (the epidermis with the junction), leaving dead bodies on the ground (Civatte bodies)

2. **Vacuolar interface pattern ("the washing pattern"):** Focal or contiguous, often discrete vacuoles in the basal cell layer (from intracellular edema) lead to separation at the dermoepidermal junction (artifactual cleft), cellular death (necrotic keratinocytes, Civatte bodies), and pigment incontinence. **(Photomnemonic 3.3)**

NB The inflammatory cell infiltrate is less dense in the vacuolar pattern ("cell-poor") and is usually both perivascular and interstitial with focal involvement of the dermoepidermal junction.

General concepts

NB Cells other than lymphocytes should be rare in most cases of true lichenoid dermatitides.

Lichenoid dermatitis is a dynamic process.

1. **Early lesions:**
   - Focal/discrete vacuolar damage
   - Focal necrotic keratinocytes
   - Preserved basket-weave stratum corneum (fast-developing lesions)
   - Sparse melanin incontinence
2. **Well-developed lesions:**
   - Subepidermal clefting (Max Joseph space) or blister formation due to contiguous vacuolar degeneration
   - Focal or contiguous epidermal necrosis

3. **Late lesions:**
    - Melanophages in the papillary dermis
    - Vascular ectasia with scant inflammation

Satellite cell necrosis: Lymphocytes (CD8+) touching a necrotic keratinocyte on either side, like satellites surrounding a body in space
(Figure 3.17, Photomnemonic 3.4)

NB Acrosyringeal keratinocytic necrosis and eosinophils in the infiltrate: think drug-related erythema multiforme, toxic epidermal necrolysis and drug reaction.

(Table 3.3)

Table 3.3 Distinguishing clues among lichenoid disorders

Clues	Possible disorders
Prominent apoptotic cells not confined to the basal cell layer	Erythema multiforme (EM) Pityriasis lichenoides et varioliformis acuta (PLEVA) Pityriasis lichenoides chronica (PLC)
Subepidermal separation/edema/ vesiculation	Bullous pemphigoid Sweet's syndrome Paraneoplastic pemphigus Bullous lupus erythematous Bullous lichen sclerosis et atrophicus Erythema multiforme Graft-versus-host disease (GVHD)
Presence of deep inflammatory infiltrate	Lichen striatus (around adnexal structures) Drug reaction Secondary syphilis (plasma cells around vessels)
Satellite cell necrosis	Graft-versus-host disease (GVHD) Paraneoplastic pemphigus Erythema multiforme Lichen striatus Regressing flat wart
Atrophic epidermis	Atrophic lichen planus Lichen sclerosis et atrophicus Poikiloderma Graft-versus-host disease (GVHD)
With hemosiderin and extravasated red blood cells in the papillary dermis	Lichen aureus (clinically appears golden because of large amounts of hemosiderin) Lichenoid pigmented purpura of Gougerot and Blum

(continued)

Table 3.3 *(continued)*

Clues	Possible disorders
Predominant inflammatory cells in the band-like infiltrate (other than lymphocytes): • Eosinophils	Urticarial phase bullous pemphigoid
Predominant inflammatory cells in the band-like infiltrate (other than lymphocytes): • Neutrophils	Sweet's syndrome Bullous lupus erythematosus Linear IgA bullous dermatosis Dermatitis herpetiformis Fixed drug eruption (scattered neutrophils only)
Predominant inflammatory cells in the band-like infiltrate (other than lymphocytes): • Plasma cells	Syphilis Zoon's balanitis Lichenoid drug reaction
Predominant inflammatory cells in the band-like infiltrate (other than lymphocytes): • Histiocytes in epithelioid cell infiltrates	Lichenoid and granulomatous dermatitis Lichenoid sarcoidosis Post-herpes zoster reaction

NB For overlap of lichenoid with other inflammatory patterns, see **Figure 3.5**.

On low power

NB **See Definition.**

- Lichen planus is the prototype for lichenoid dermatitis; discoid lupus erythematosus is the prototype for interface dermatitis.
- The classic picture is that of a multicolored sandwich pattern: pink (hyperkeratosis)–purple (hypergranulosis)–pale (squamatized epidermis)–blue (band-like lymphocytes).

On high power

Lichen planus

- Hyperkeratosis **(Figure 3.18)**

NB No parakeratosis.

- Wedge-shaped hypergranulosis
- Irregular saw-tooth acanthosis (pointed rete ridges)
- Necrotic keratinocytes in lower third of the epidermis and Civatte bodies in the papillary dermis
- Basal keratinocytes may be flattened with a "squamatized" appearance
- Usually a dense band of lymphocytes and histiocytes lying parallel in the upper dermis and infiltrating the lower epidermis

Bullous lichen planus

- Subepidermal cleft: separation of the epidermis from the dermis (Max Joseph space) due to extensive vacuolization

NB Lichen planus pemphigoides is a subepidermal blistering disorder caused by autoantibodies against antigens in lamina lucida: BP 180 and a 200kDa antigen): subepidermal blister with eosinophils; no band-like infiltrate.

Hypertrophic lichen planus

- Prominent pseudoepitheliomatous hyperplasia (the epidermis shows thick squamatized bulbous acanthosis) **(Figure 3.19)**
- Prominent hyperkeratosis
- Lichenoid band-like infiltrate

NB Lichen simplex chronicus with a band-like infiltrate: think hypertrophic lichen planus.

Atrophic lichen planus

- Epidermal atrophy instead of saw-tooth acanthosis
- Usually solar elastosis (clue to sun-damaged skin)

Differential diagnosis:

- Lichenoid drug reaction – eosinophils; parakeratosis
- Lichen planus-like keratoses – lentigo or seborrheic keratosis usually present at the border
- Lichen striatus – lymphocytes and histiocytes surrounded by acanthotic epidermis ("ball in a clutch")

Lichen nitidus

- A "ball" of lymphocytes and histiocytes clutched by lateral acanthotic rete ridges (ball in a clutch/ball in a claw) **(Figure 3.20, Photomnemonic 3.5)**
- May have plasma cells and multinucleated giant cells

Lichen striatus

NB Lichenoid inflammation + spongiosis + perieccrine/perifollicular lymphocytic infiltrate restricted to 3–4 dermal papillae: think lichen striatus.

(Figure 3.21)

- Parakeratosis (sometimes)
- Mild spongiosis
- Band-like lymphocytic infiltrate (rarely other scattered cells)
- Necrotic keratinocytes at all layers of the epidermis (sometimes)
- Perieccrine (or rarely perifollicular) lymphocytic infiltrate

Lichenoid drug eruption

- Hyperkeratosis with focal parakeratosis
- Necrotic keratinocytes at all levels of the epidermis
- Band-like lymphocytic infiltrate with variable scattered plasma cells and eosinophils **(Figure 3.22)**

NB Lichenoid drug eruption often presents as a combination of patterns in the same lesion: interface, spongiotic, bullous, superficial and deep perivascular infiltrate pattern with/without vasculitis.

Lichen planus-like keratosis

Similar to lichen planus but showing also **(Figure 3.23)**:

- Focal parakeratosis
- Mid-dermal inflammation
- Necrotic keratinocytes high in the epidermis
- Lentigo or seborrheic keratosis at periphery

NB Distinguish from lichenoid actinic keratosis: keratinocytic atypia and a "flag sign" of alternating pink (parakeratosis)-and-blue (orthokeratosis) stratum corneum (see Chapter 5, Keratinocytic tumors).

Pityriasis lichenoides

Acute: Pyriasis lichenoides et varioliformis acuta (PLEVA)

Note "busy" epidermis **(Figure 3.24)**

- Busy stratum corneum: thick stratum corneum with confluent parakeratosis and neutrophils
- Necrotic keratinocytes in all layers

NB In late lesions the confluent necrotic keratinocytes can form an ulceration.

- Vacuolar damage at the basal layer
- Spongiosis with exocytosis of lymphocytes and red blood cells
- Wedge-shaped infiltrate with lymphocytes and red blood cells

Differential diagnosis:

- Pityriasis lichenoides chronica (similar but "less of everything" and no ulceration)

- Lymphomatoid papulosis (wedge-shaped infiltrate of *atypical* lymphocytes, no red blood cell extravasation)
- Mycosis fungoides (atypia and epidermotropism)
- Arthropod bite reaction (more spongiosis and subepidermal edema; eosinophils around the vessels and along the sweat ducts)

Chronic: Pityriasis lichenoides chronica

Note "less busy" epidermis **(Figure 3.25)**

- Same features but less of everything: parakeratosis, necrotic keratinocytes, spongiosis, extravasated red blood cells
- Predominant superficial perivascular infiltrate
- No ulceration

Erythema multiforme (EM)

- Preserved basket-weave stratum corneum **(Figure 3.26)**
- Necrotic keratinocytes at all levels of the epidermis, including stratum corneum and the acrosyringium (the extent of necrosis depends on the age of the lesion)
- Vacuolar changes in the basal layer with satellite cell necrosis
- Perivascular lymphocytes in the upper dermis (but no band-like infiltrate): early lesions show only tagging of lymphocytes at the dermoepidermal junction, variable eosinophils
- Subepidermal edema (leading to subepidermal blister)

Differential diagnosis:

- Fixed drug eruption (eosinophils, neutrophils, pigment incontinence, deeper infiltrate and melanophages)
- Stevens Johnson–toxic epidermal necrolysis spectrum (confluent necrosis, less inflammation)

Stevens Johnson syndrome–toxic epidermal necrolysis (TEN) spectrum

- Similar to erythema multiforme but shows full thickness necrosis of the epidermis involving the adnexal structures
- Preserved stratum corneum
- Severe vacuolar interface damage with subepidermal cleft/blister (the papillary dermal papillae are preserved and covered by a roof of necrotic epidermis) **(Figure 3.27)**
- Minimal superficial lymphocytic infiltrate with pigment incontinence, sparse eosinophils

> NB The drug-induced dermatoses form a subepidermal blister (compare to the intraepidermal blister in viral infections and pompholyx, and the subcorneal blister in impetigo).

Fixed drug eruption

Similar to erythema multiforme with the following helpful features:

- Hyperkeratosis or parakeratosis (in the course of evolution)
- Prominent Civatte bodies and melanin incontinence with dermal melanophages (except for most acute lesions)
- More dense superficial and deep perivascular infiltrate with eosinophils, but also with neutrophils (EM usually lacks a pronounced band-like infiltrate) **(Figure 3.28)**

Graft-versus-host disease (GVHD)

> NB Each stage of GVHD (acute or chronic) can occur without the other.

Acute GVHD

Think vacuolization!

Four grades:

- Grade 1 – focal or diffuse vacuolization
- Grade 2 – spongiosis, necrotic keratinocytes at all levels (at least 4 per mm of epidermis) and satellite cell necrosis **(Figure 3.29)**
- Grade 3 – partial epidermal clefting
- Grade 4 – complete epidermal separation
- Variable hyperkeratosis and acanthosis or epidermal atrophy (may simulate lichen sclerosis et atrophicus)

> NB Lymphocytic exocytosis and necrotic keratinocytes into the follicular epithelium give an early clue to GVHD.

Chronic GVHD

Think lichenoid!

- **Early:** *Lichenoid* – similar to lichen planus with:
  - columnar epidermal necrosis: small vertical tiers of complete necrosis in the epidermis
- **Late:** *Sclerodermoid* – similar to atrophic lichen planus with:
  - marked dermal sclerosis (the sclerosis starts from papillary dermis and advances downwards compared to scleroderma in which it is the opposite)
  - disappearance of the adnexal structures **(Figure 3.30)**

Discoid lupus erythematosus (DLE)

- Hyperkeratosis (but no parakeratosis)
- Epidermal atrophy, occasionally alternating with irregular acanthosis;
- "Squamatized" epidermis (flat and pale basal cells look like spinous keratinocytes)

- Follicular plugging (hyperkeratosis filling the dilated follicular ostia)
- Vacuolar interface change with necrotic keratinocytes in the basal layer of both epidermis and follicular epithelium **(Figure 3.31)**
- Thickened (wavy) basement membrane
- Civatte bodies and melanophages in the papillary dermis
- Telangiectasia
- Patchy superficial and deep perivascular or nodular lymphocytic infiltrate with plasmocytoid cells, involving also the adnexal structures **(Figure 3.32)**
- Interstitial mucin (positive with colloidal iron and Alcian blue stains)

Hypertrophic lupus erythematosus

Similar to hypertrophic lichen planus. Look for deep dermal perivascular and periadnexal lymphocytic infiltrate.

Tumid lupus erythematosus

- No epidermal involvement; no interface dermatitis
- Superficial and deep patchy perivascular and periadnexal lymphocytic infiltrates **(Figure 3.33)**
- Mucin

NB The diagnosis of tumid lupus excludes systemic lupus erythematosus.

Subacute cutaneous lupus erythematosus (SCLE)

Similar to discoid lupus erythematosus with the following distinguishing features:

- Epidermal atrophy or regular acanthosis (in clinically psoriasiform lesions) **(Figure 3.34)**
- More pronounced vacuolar interface dermatitis with more necrotic keratinocytes (may be found in all levels)
- Edema and mucin in the dermis
- Subtle inflammatory infiltrate

Acute cutaneous lupus erythematosus (systemic lupus erythematosus, SLE)

Early lesions may be non-specific; late lesions are similar to subacute cutaneous lupus erythematosus with the following distinguishing features:

- Focal vacuolar damage with edema and red blood cells in the upper dermis
- Dermal fibrinoid deposits (precipitation of fibrin as blue granular substance among the collagen bundles, similar to leukocytoclastic vasculitis)
- Hyalinization of the fat by pink hyalinized material: fibrin and necrosis in the fat lobules (see Lupus panniculitis)

NB An inflammatory infiltrate is absent.

(Table 3.4)

Table 3.4 Histologic comparison of the types of lupus erythematosus

Feature	SLE/SCLE	DLE
Vacuolar changes	++	+ (including the hair follicles)
Basement membrane thickening	+/–	+
Increased mucin deposition	+	+/–
Periadnexal infiltrate	–	+
Deep dermal infiltrate	–	+
Edema	+	–

Bullous lupus erythematosus

Two patterns:

- **Neutrophilic** (subepidermal blister due to autoantibodies directed against type VII collagen in the anchoring fibrils of lamina densa)

  NB Similar pathology to dermatitis herpetiformis and linear IgA dermatosis.

  - Broad-based subepidermal blister with neutrophils **(Figure 3.35)**
  - Papillary dermal edema
  - Papillary microabscesses with nuclear dust (karyorrhexis: destroyed nuclei of neutrophils)
- **Mononuclear:** Occurs in long-standing systemic lupus erythematosus due to confluent vacuolar damage and separation of the epidermis from the dermis (similar to the pathogenesis of bullous lichen planus)
  - Broad-based subepidermal blister with lymphocytes

Dermatomyositis

NB Dermatomyositis is usually indistinguishable from systemic lupus erythematosus.

(Figure 3.36)

Older lesions (with clinical appearance of poikiloderma):

- Epidermal atrophy
- Marked vacuolar changes in the basal layer
- Band-like lymphocytic infiltrate with melanophages
- Mucin in the dermis

NB The subcutaneous fat may show panniculitis associated with myxoid degeneration of the fat cells and calcification (see Panniculitis).

Lichen sclerosis et atrophicus (LSA)

- Hyperkeratosis with follicular plugging (which leads to disappearance of the adnexal structures) **(Figure 3.37)**
- Atrophy of epidermis with absent rete ridges.
- Stratum corneum is thicker than the epidermis
- Band-like lymphocytic infiltrate of lymphocytes, histiocytes and plasma cells in the superficial dermis (early lesions) which moves down to the mid-dermis (late lesions)
- Subepidermal zone of pallor due to lymphedema and homogenization of the collagen fibers (swollen and pale collagen); in severe lymphedema bullae may form
- Disappearance of the elastic fibers

(Table 3.5)

Table 3.5 Evolution of the histologic findings in lichen sclerosus et atrophicus

Early lesion	Late lesion
Edema Band-like infiltrate in the upper/mid-dermis	Edema or a cleft-like space between epidermis and dermis No band-like infiltrate Homogenized (swollen) collagen

Differential diagnosis: Morphea – square biopsy due to thick collagenous stroma; no edema, no hyperkeratosis; intact elastic fibers on Verhoeff-van Gieson stain (VVG)

Ashy dermatosis (erythema dyschromicum perstans)

- Mild vacuolar interface dermatitis
- Prominent melanin incontinence and melanophages **(Figure 3.38)**

Differential diagnosis: Post-inflammatory hyperpigmentation – melanin incontinence with no interface dermatitis

Poikilodermas

1. Genodermatoses: Bloom's syndrome, Kindler's syndrome, Rothmund-Thomson syndrome, dyskeratosis congenita
2. Dermatomyositis and systemic lupus erythematosus
3. Mycosis fungoides (poikiloderma atrophicans vasculare) and parapsoriasis en plaques

NB The clinical picture of poikiloderma resembles chronic radiodermatitis (erythema, mottled pigmentation, telangiectasia, atrophy)

- Hyperkeratosis
- Epidermal atrophy
- Basal vacuolar change with occasional necrotic keratinocytes and mild band-like lymphocytic infiltrate
- Telangiectasia and edema in the upper dermis
- Melanophages in the upper dermis

Other interface dermatides

- **Secondary syphilis** (see Psoriasiform pattern)

NB Psoriasis with lichenoid infiltrate of histiocytes and plasma cells: think syphilis; look for swollen endothelial cells of blood vessels with/without surrounding plasma cells.

- **Paraneoplastic pemphigus:** Combined interface pattern with acantholytic pattern: heavy band-like infiltrate with necrotic keratinocytes; foci of suprabasal or subepidermal acantholysis

PSORIASIFORM PATTERN

Definition: Inflammatory pattern characterized by regular elongation of the rete ridges and hyperkeratosis.

General concepts

- The clinical counterpart is the papulosquamous lesion.
- Psoriasis is the classic prototype of psoriasiform pattern: regular acanthosis with suprapapillary thinning, hypogranulosis, and hyperkeratosis with retained nuclei of the corneocytes (parakeratosis) **(Figure 3.39)**.

NB **Psoriasiform dermatitides are dynamic** (see below).

1. **Early (evolving or acute) lesions:**
   - Prominent spongiosis
   - Subtle acanthosis
   - Focal parakeratosis
2. **Chronic plaque-type lesions:**
   - Regular acanthosis
   - Confluent hyperkeratosis/parakeratosis
3. **Erythrodermic lesions** often show subtle findings:
   - Less pronounced acanthosis and marked papillary dermal edema

NB Periodic acid–Schiff (PAS) should be considered in any psoriasiform dermatitis to exclude chronic candidiasis and dermatophytosis.

NB Plaque-stage mycosis fungoides shows psoriasiform pattern.

(Table 3.6)

Table 3.6 Distinguishing clues among psoriasiform dermatides

Clues	Possible disorder
Regular acanthosis	Plaque psoriasis Lichen simplex chronicus/Prurigo nodularis Inflammatory linear verrucous epidermal nevus (ILVEN) Granular parakeratosis
Spongiosis	Early psoriasis Lichen simplex chronicus Pityriasis rosea Psoriasiform drug reaction
Neutrophils in the stratum corneum (Munro)	Psoriasis Chronic candidiasis and dermatophytosis Seborrheic dermatitis Clear cell acanthoma ILVEN Psoriasiform keratosis
Follicular plugging	Pityriasis rubra pilaris Seborrheic dermatitis
Alternating ortho- and parakeratosis (patterned parakeratosis)	Pityriasis rubra pilaris Palmoplantar psoriasis ILVEN
Shoulder parakeratosis (hyperkeratosis – and/or parakeratosis alongside the follicular ostia)	With neutrophils: seborrheic dermatitis Without neutrophils: pityriasis rubra pilaris
Collections of neutrophils in the epidermis	Spongiform pustule in stratum spinosum (Kogoj) Pustular psoriasis Acute generalized exanthematous pustulosis (AGEP) Subcorneal pustular dermatosis (SPD)
Pallor of the upper epidermis	Necrolytic migratory erythema Acrodermatitis enteropathica Nutritional deficiency
Plasma cell infiltrate in the dermis	Syphilis
Eosinophils in the dermis	Psoriasiform drug reaction AGEP

NB For the overlap of psoriasiform with other inflammatory patterns, see **Figure 3.5**.

On low power

The regular acanthosis with its elongated and thin rete ridges resembles the Parthenon columns.

(Figure 3.40, Photomnemonic 3.6)

On high power

Guttate psoriasis

- Focal mounds of parakeratosis with neutrophils among orthokeratosis **(Figure 3.41)**
- Much less marked/subtle and irregular acanthosis
- Mild spongiosis in the lower epidermis
- Focal absence of the granular layer
- Superficial perivascular infiltrate around dilated capillaries with extravasated red blood cells but no eosinophils

NB The same features may be seen in treated psoriasis.

Differential diagnosis:
- Pityriasis rosea (more spongiosis, no neutrophils in the parakeratosis)
- Pityriasis lichenoides chronica (heavier dermal lymphocytic infiltrate with epidermotropism and apoptotic keratinocytes, confluent parakeratosis with neutrophils)

Plaque psoriasis

- Regular acanthosis with thin suprapapillary plates
- Diminished granular layer (hypogranulosis or agranulosis)
- Confluent parakeratosis
- "Micropustules": intracorneal neutrophilic collection (Munro microabscess); **(Figure 3.42)**
- Intraepidermal neutrophilic collection (spongiform pustule of Kogoj)
- Mitoses in the basal and suprabasal layers
- Dilated papillary capillaries (tortuous vessels)

Scalp psoriasis

- Irregular acanthosis
- Individual necrotic keratinocytes
- Hypoplastic sebaceous glands
- Increased number of telogen hairs (psoriatic alopecia) **(Figure 3.43)**

Pustular psoriasis

Variations: Rash associated with reactive arthritis; palmo-plantar pustulosis; acute generalized exanthematous pustulosis (AGEP); subcorneal pustular dermatosis (SPD)

- "Macropustules": large collections of neutrophils (Munro or Kogoj) **(Figure 3.44)**

- No prominent acanthosis due to the rapid evolution
- In AGEP (see Spongiotic pattern): spongiosis, eosinophils and neutrophils in the upper edematous dermis
- In SPD (see Spongiotic pattern and Vesicular and bullous disorders): eosinophilic spongiosis, acantholytic cells

Pityriasis rubra pilaris (PRP)

- Alternating ortho- and parakeratosis in horizontal and vertical tiers (sometimes present) **(Figure 3.45)**
- Follicular plugging with shouldering (ortho- and parakeratotic "shouldering" on either side of a follicle)
- Preserved granular layer
- The rete ridges are irregularly elongated and broad among narrow dermal papillae (compare to the thin rete ridges in psoriasis) **(Figure 3.46)**
- Thick suprapapillary plates
- Rare: Acantholysis

> NB Follicular plugging without destruction of the hair follicle: PRP, seborrheic dermatitis, keratosis pilaris; follicular plugging with destruction/involvement of the hair follicle: discoid lupus erythematosus and lichen planopilaris.

Necrolytic migratory erythema (NME)/ Acrodermatitis enteropathica (AE)/Pellagra

> NB A tricolored "French flag-like psoriasis": red (parakeratosis)–white (pale, vacuolated keratinocytes in upper epidermis)–blue (normal lower epidermis).

(Figure 3.47)

- Confluent parakeratosis (later stages)
- Psoriasiform acanthosis (early lesions may show irregular acanthosis)
- Pallor in the upper epidermis (two causes: intracellular edema (NME, AE) or confluent keratinocytic necrosis (pellagra)
- Variable spongiosis (forming bulla or ballooning degeneration in severe acute lesions)
- Scattered necrotic keratinocytes or confluent necrosis

Secondary syphilis

- Concomitant lichenoid and psoriasiform patterns (occasionally also granulomatous)
- Parakeratosis with a scale crust with neutrophils
- Broad band-like infiltrate of mononuclear cells (plasma cells, histiocytes, lymphocytes)
- Superficial and deep perivascular infiltrate of lymphocytes and plasma cells **(Figure 3.48)**
- Swollen endothelial cells with small or missing lumina (plump cells obscure the lumina)

> NB Any "psoriasis" with plasma cells in a lichenoid pattern should exclude syphilis **(Figure 3.49)**.

Inflammatory linear verrucous epidermal nevus (ILVEN)

- Sharply demarcated two alternating components in the horizontal direction:
  - *Depressed orthokeratosis* with preserved granular layer
  - *Elevated parakeratosis* with absent granular layer, overlying mild spongiosis and exocytosis of lymphocytes

  (Figure 3.50, Photomnemonic 3.7)
- Acanthosis; thin epidermal hyperplasia or thickened "tabled" rete ridges (papillomatosis)
- Frequent neutrophils in the stratum corneum

Clear cell acanthoma

> NB Sharply demarcated pale psoriasis: think clear cell acanthoma (compare to palor only in the upper epidermis in necrolytic migratory erythema, acrodermatitis enteropathica and pellagra).

- Psoriasiform acanthosis
- Slightly enlarged, pale cells (due to glycogen vacuoles) **(Figure 3.51)**
- Confluent parakeratosis with serum crust and neutrophils (neutrophils may form microabscesses)

Other psoriasiform dermatides

- **Pityriasis rosea** (see Spongiotic pattern)
- **Chronic candidiasis and dermatophytosis** (see Chapter 4, Infections): PAS-positive fungal organisms
- **Lichen simplex chronicus (LSC)/prurigo nodularis (PN)** (see Spongiotic pattern): LSC is a broad plaque; PN is a papule or nodule, but they are otherwise similar: think of acral stratum corneum on hair-bearing skin
- **Seborrheic dermatitis** (see Spongiotic pattern): Often facial skin with many follicles and sebaceous glands and pityrosporum; shoulder parakeratosis
- **Granular parakeratosis:** Confluent layered parakeratosis with retained keratohyaline granules
- **Psoriasiform keratosis:** Solitary lesion, indistinguishable from plaque psoriasis
- **Mycosis fungoides** (see Chapter 5, Cutaneous lymphoid neoplasms): Atypical lymphocytes and band-like infiltrate of atypical lymphocytes in the upper dermis

SUPERFICIAL AND DEEP PERIVASCULAR DERMATITIS

Definition: Group of disorders with various clinical presentations (usually there is no scale clinically) and a common histologic pattern of superficial or superficial and deep perivascular infiltrate.

General concepts

- Most disorders with superficial and/or superficial and deep perivascular infiltrate present with concomitant features of epidermal involvement, vasculitis or lichenoid infiltrate and are therefore discussed in the corresponding chapters.

- NB If the infiltrate is distributed only around the upper vascular plexus, it appears "flat-bottomed" **(Figure 3.52A)**; if it is distributed also around the lower vascular plexus, it appears wedge-shaped **(Figure 3.52B)**.

- NB Perivascular and periadnexal infiltrate with lymphocytes is a clue to lupus erythematosus (look for interface change and mucin); perniosis (edema); arthropod bite reaction (eosinophils around the sweat glands).

(Table 3.7)

Table 3.7 Most common dermatoses with superficial and deep perivascular infiltrate

Without epidermal change	With epidermal change
Urticaria	Gyrate erythemas:
Urticaria pigmentosa	• erythema annulare centrifugum
Dermal hypersensitivity reaction	Pityriasis lichenoides
Perniosis	Pityriasis lichenoides and varioliformis acuta
	Arthropod bite reaction
	Wells' syndrome
	Connective tissue disorders:
	• subacute lupus erythematosus
	• systemic lupus erythematosus
	• dermatomyositis
	Polymorphous light eruption (PMLE)
	Viral exanthem

On low power

- Invisible dermatosis (urticaria)
- Blue patches in a perivascular distribution (polymorphous light eruption (PMLE), arthropod bite reaction)
- Tight blue sleeves or cuffs in a perivascular distribution (deep gyrate erythemas)
- With edema only: urticaria
- With edema and blue patches: perniosis, PMLE
- Edema with a dense infiltrate of eosinophils: eosinophilic cellulitis (Wells' syndrome) **(Photomnemonic 3.8)**

On high power

Urticaria

The pathologic features may be subtle or even invisible.

- Normal epidermis

NB If the epidermis is even slightly involved, consider dermal hypersensitivity reaction which has otherwise similar histologic features.

- Mild dermal edema
- Slightly dilated capillaries
- Sparse perivascular and interstitial infiltrate of lymphocytes, eosinophils, mast cells, and neutrophils (early lesions may contain mostly neutrophils: distinguish neutrophilic urticaria from neutrophilic urticarial syndrome: see Neutrophilic dermatoses *per se*) **(Figure 3.53)**
- Vasculitis is not a feature (see Urticaria vasculitis)

Gyrate erythemas: erythema annulare centrifugum

Superficial type ("scaly")

- Mild spongiosis with mounds of parakeratosis
- Superficial coat sleeve-like infiltrate of lymphocytes **(Figure 3.54)**

Deep type ("classic")

- No epidermal involvement
- Superficial and deep perivascular cuffed-like infiltrate of lymphocytes

Wells' syndrome

- Intraepidermal or subepidermal blisters
- Possible edema
- Main feature: dense infiltrate of eosinophils from the top to the bottom (see Photomnemonic 3.8)
- Flame figures (collagen impregnated with eosinophilic (red) granules **(Figure 3.55)**

GRANULOMATOUS DERMATITIS

Definition: Granulomatous dermatitis encompasses a large group of inflammatory and non-inflammatory dermatoses showing two patterns of inflammation on pathology: 1) nodular – discrete or compact aggregates of cells separated by relatively normal dermis; and 2) diffuse – dispersed cells among collagen bundles usually filling the entire specimen.

(Table 3.8)

Table 3.8 Nodular and diffuse granulomatous dermatitis categorized by the type of predominant cells

Clues	Possible disorders
Nodular	
With predominant lymphocytes	Pseudolymphoma Lymphoma Tumid lupus erythematosus Jessner's lymphocytic infiltration
With predominant neutrophils	Ruptured cyst Dissecting cellulitis Hidradenitis suppurativa Leukocytoclastic vasculitis Granuloma faciale Erythema elevatum diutinum Churg–Strauss syndrome Sweet's syndrome Pyoderma gangrenosum
With eosinophils	Lymphoma
With predominant histiocytes (sarcoidal granulomas)	With interface dermatitis: • lichen nitidus • sarcoidosis In the dermis: • sarcoidosis • Crohn's disease • Melkersson–Rosenthal syndrome • tuberculoid leprosy • foreign body • granulomatous rosacea

(continued)

Table 3.8 *(continued)*

Clues	Possible disorders
With predominant histiocytes (tuberculoid granulomas)	Foreign body Tattoo Tuberculosis cutis Atypical mycobacterial infection Leishmaniasis Late secondary syphilis Granulomatous rosacea Perioral dermatitis Lupus miliaris disseminatus faciei
With predominant histiocytes (palisaded granulomas)	Granuloma annulare Actinic granuloma Necrobiosis lipoidica Necrobiotic xanthogranuloma Rheumatoid nodule Gout Cat scratch disease Churg–Strauss syndrome Wegener's granulomatosis Epithelioid sarcoma Palisaded neutrophilic granulomatous dermatitis
With predominant histiocytes (interstitial granulomas)	Interstitial granuloma annulare Interstitial granulomatous dermatitis
With predominant histiocytes and neutrophils in the center (suppurative granulomas)	Ruptured cyst Foreign body Bacterial infections (botryomycosis; blastomycosis-like pyoderma; cat-scratch disease; lymphogranuloma venereum) Tuberculosis cutis (scrofuloderma) Atypical mycobacterial infection Actinomycosis Nocardiosis Deep fungal infections Majocchi's granuloma Kerion Crohn's disease

(continued)

Table 3.8 *(continued)*

Clues	Possible disorders
Diffuse	
With predominant lymphocytes	Pseudolymphoma B-cell lymphoma Mycosis fungoides
With predominant neutrophils	Ruptured cyst Acne/acne keloidalis Dissecting cellulitis Hidradenitis suppurativa Leukocytoclastic vasculitis Churg–Strauss syndrome Granuloma faciale Erythema elevatum diutinum
With predominant eosinophils	Eosinophilic cellulitis Arthropod bite reaction
With eosinophils and plasma cells	Pseudolymphoma
With plasma cells	Infections Granuloma inguinale Lymphogranuloma venereum
With mast cells	Urticaria pigmentosa
With abnormal leukocytes	Leukemia cutis Lymphoma
With predominant Langerhans cells	Langerhans cell histiocytosis
With predominant histiocytes	Interstitial granuloma annulare
With predominant histiocytes and neutrophils	Foreign body Ruptured cyst Pyoderma gangrenosum Bacterial infections (botryomycosis; blastomycosis-like pyoderma; cat-scratch disease; lymphogranuloma venereum) Tuberculosis cutis Atypical mycobacterial infections Deep fungal infections Majocchi's granuloma
With predominant histiocytes and foamy histiocytes	Benign cephalic histiocytosis Generalized eruptive histiocytoma Silicone/paraffin granuloma Xanthelasma Xanthoma

General concepts

The dermal infiltrates are characterized by predominant monocytes (macrophages).

NB Epithelioid cells are monocytes which collect and form granulomas because they have little phagocytic activity. They can fuse to form giant cells.

- **Sarcoidal ("naked") granulomas:** Collections of macrophages with few/no surrounding lymphocytes **(Figure 3.56)**
- **Tuberculoid ("dressed") granulomas:** Like naked granulomas but rimmed by lymphocytes
- **Palisading granulomas:** Collections of macrophages around a central area of necrobiosis (degenerated and pale blue–gray collagen) or necrosis with secondary accumulation of mucin or fibrin **(Figure 3.57, Photomnemonic 3.9)**
- **Caseating granulomas:** Palisading granulomas with more pronounced central necrosis (caseation: homogenous infarct-like necrosis due to macrophage death)
- **Suppurative granulomas:** Palisading granulomas with collections of neutrophils in the center **(Figure 3.58)**
- **Foreign body granulomas:** Collections of macrophages and giant cells with mixed-cell infiltrate (neutrophils, plasma cells) around foreign material (follicle, foreign objects, injectable fillers, suture, gout) **(Figure 3.59)**

NB Granulomas with other inflammatory cells (neutrophils, plasma cells) and caseating granulomas should be stained for infections; foreign body granulomas should be polarized.

- Additional cells in the granulomas can help in narrowing the differential diagnosis (see Table 3.8)

On low power

NB Pale collections in the dermis (histiocytes have ample cytoplasm) are a clue to a granulomatous disorder. They resemble clouds in the sky **(Photomnemonic 3.10)**.

On high power

Granuloma annulare (GA)

- **Palisading GA:** Pale histiocytes surround a zone of necrobiosis and mucin **(Figure 3.60A)**

- **Interstitial GA** (busy dermis):
  - Histiocytes splayed in the interstitial space between collagen bundles **(Figure 3.60B)**
  - Lymphocytes around vessels and mucin **(Figure 3.60C)**

Differential diagnosis: Drug reaction (epidermal involvement; no mucin); morphea (sclerosis); metastatic disease (Indian filing)

- **Sarcoidal GA:** Naked granulomas with mucin

NB Colloidal iron and Alcian blue highlight the mucin.

Differential diagnosis: *Necrobiosis lipoidica* (sclerosis, layered granulomas, plasma cell collections, no mucin); *Epithelioid sarcoma* (geographic necrosis in the dermis, cytologic atypia)

Actinic granuloma (actinic granuloma of O'Brien, annular elastolytic granuloma)

NB Palisading granuloma on sun-damaged skin: think actinic granuloma.

- Palisading granuloma-like in GA but without mucin and necrobiosis **(Figure 3.61A)**
- Solar elastosis
- Giant cells phagocytizing elastic fibers (elastolysis: highlighted by the VVG stain) **(Figure 3.61B)**

Necrobiosis lipoidica

NB Busy slide: rectangular shape of the biopsy (due to sclerosis) with full thickness involvement of the dermis and subcutis (from top to bottom and from side to side) but "most action" is in the lower two-thirds of the biopsy.

- The granulomatous inflammation is in horizontal tiers and can be:
  - Palisading **(Figure 3.62A, Photomnemonic 3.11)**
  - Interstitially scattered macrophages, giant cells and/or foamy histiocytes
- Degeneration of collagen (necrobiosis) but no mucin (compare to GA)
- Sclerosis (rectangular biopsy, compare to GA: inward retraction of the biopsy)

Additional helpful features:
- Cholesterol clefts
- Lymphoid follicle-like aggregates of lymphocytes or plasma cells **(Figure 3.62B)**
- Thickening of blood vessel walls with/without occlusion

Rheumatoid nodule

NB Pink palisading granuloma in the deep dermis and subdermis.

- Large zone of pink fibrinoid necrosis in the center (no mucin: compare to GA) **(Figure 3.63)**
- Rim of palisading elongated histiocytes and foreign body giant cells
- Proliferation of blood vessels and fibrosis in surrounding stroma

NB Lymphocytes, neutrophils, and nuclear dust are common.

Differential diagnosis:
- GA (mucin, fewer giant cells and no fibrosis)
- Necrobiosis lipoidica diabeticorum (NLD) (busy slide, necrobiosis of collagen with tiered granulomas, plasma cells)
- Epithelioid sarcoma (geographic necrosis: looks like coalescing rheumatoid nodules, and atypical cells)
- *Cryptococcus* infection (deep palisading granulomas with necrotic debris and organisms)

Lupus miliaris disseminatus faciei (acne agminata)

- Large focus of pale homogenous pink necrosis in the center surrounded by macrophages (caseating granuloma) **(Figure 3.64)**
- May be perifollicular

Granulomatous rosacea

Two types of granulomas on background of classic rosacea features: 1) sebaceous hyperplasia, 2) telangiectasia, and 3) edema:

- Non-caseating tuberculoid granulomas (more than 90% of cases) **(Figure 3.65)**
- Sarcoidal granulomas

NB Giant cells may be present around ruptured follicles.

Cutaneous Crohn's disease

1. **Adjacent lesions (perianal/peristomal/perioral):** Pseudoepitheliomatous hyperplasia with suppurative granulomas
2. **Metastatic (at sites discontinuous to the gastrointestinal tract):** Non-caseating sarcoidal granulomas close to the epidermis in lichenoid arrangement

Additional features:
- Dense infiltrate of lymphocytes and plasma cells **(Figure 3.66)**

- May extend from papillary dermis to subcutaneous fat
- Granulomatous vasculitis

Granulomatous cheilitis (Melkersson–Rosenthal syndrome)

- Small and scattered sarcoidal granulomas **(Figure 3.67)**
- Nodular infiltrate of lymphocytes and plasma cells
- Telangiectasia and edema

NB Absent granular layer and cornified layer are clues to mucosal surface.

Palisaded neutrophilic granulomatous dermatitis (PNGD)

Three stages:

1. **Early:** Resembles LCV with broad cuffs of fibrin in the vessel walls
2. **Developed:** Resembles palisading GA but with a bluish hue due to neutrophils, nuclear dust, and fibrin mixed with mucin **(Figure 3.68)**
3. **Late:** Resembles NLD with splayed neutrophils and nuclear dust; fibrosis

Sarcoidosis

"Naked" granulomas with no/minimal lymphocytes surrounding the granuloma

NB 40% of cases may have mild lymphocytic infiltrate **(Figure 3.69A)**.

- No necrosis
- Possible fibrin
- In later lesions fibrosis forms from the periphery of the granulomas
- In the subcutaneous type of sarcoidosis (Darier-Roussy sarcoidosis) the granulomas involve the subcutaneous fat **(Figure 3.69B)**

NB *Lichenoid arrangement* of sarcoidal granulomas is a clue to sarcoidosis; *perineural arrangement* is a clue to tuberculoid leprosy.

Asteroid bodies (star-like "asteroid" collagen entrapped in giant cell)

Schaumann bodies (oval, calcified body within the cytoplasm of a giant cell) **(Figure 3.69C)**

Neither type of body is specific to sarcoidosis.

FOREIGN BODY (FB) GRANULOMAS

GENERAL CONCEPTS

- **Endogenous materials:** Ruptured follicles and cysts (keratin granuloma, pilonidal cyst)
- **Exogenous materials:** Pigments (tattoo), silica (dirt, soil or glass), talc, suture material, zirconium (deodorants), beryllium (fluorescent light manufacturing), intralesional steroid, injectable substances (implants/fillers)
  - *Polarizable:* Talc (needle-shaped blue–green or yellow–brown), nylon suture, starch (Maltese cross), silica (variable-shaped), wood, some fillers (bovine collagen, polymethylmetacrylate)
  - *Sarcoidal granulomas:* Beryllium, zirconium, silica

NB Nodular collections of epithelioid histiocytes and giant cells, and knife marks (linear diagonal artifacts through the granuloma in the dermis) are clues to FB reactions.

Ruptured follicle (keratin granuloma), pilonidal cyst

NB This is the most common FB granuloma.

- Follicular-associated FB granuloma (mixed inflammation of macrophages, giant cells, neutrophils, plasma cells) **(Figure 3.70)**
- Keratin debris/polygonal keratin fragments (in ruptured cysts) or naked hair shafts (in pilonidal cyst, acne keloidalis nuchae) free in the dermis or within giant cells
- Fibrosis and sclerosis in older lesions (acne keloidalis nuchae)

Tattoo

Intra- or extracellular, irregularly shaped clumps of compact black material (melanin is never that compact and black) **(Figure 3.71A)**

- **Granulomatous reaction** (two types):
  - FB granulomas
  - Sarcoidal granulomas
- **Non-granulomatous reaction:**
  - Allergic contact dermatitis (most common cause is mercury red) and photodermatitis (cadmium yellow)
  - Lichenoid: hypertrophic lichen planus **(Figure 3.71B)**
  - Perivascular inflammation with pigment-containing macrophages
  - Pseudolymphoma and lymphoma
  - Keratoacanthoma **(Figure 3.71C)**
  - Infections

Monsel's solution for hemostasis

- Jagged clumps of coarse brown pigment in giant cells (positive with iron stains (Perl's))

- NB Look for scar tissue.

Injectable fillers

Silicone and paraffin

- Many ovoid/round cavities of varying size, which remain after silicone has been lost during processing (Swiss cheese) **(Figure 3.72A, Photomnemonic 3.12)**
- Histiocytes (usually foamy) and giant cells among the cavities
- Bundles of sclerotic collagen, fibrosis
- Usually involves the subdermis (lobular panniculitis)

NB The FB reaction to the solid silicone elastomers presents with diffuse granulomatous inflammation and fibrosis; the FB reaction to liquid silicone oil/gel presents with sparse inflammation (siliconoma) and no well-developed granulomas **(Figure 3.72B)**.

Hyaluronic acid

- Blue "splashed" patchy substance in the dermis (colloidal iron and Alcian blue positive) **(Figure 3.73)**
- FB granulomas

Low-power diagnosis of injectable fillers based on their shape and color

- Bluish material in the dermis – hyaluronic acid, polyacrylamide gel, polyalkylamide gel
- Alcian blue/colloidal iron positive – hyaluronic acid and polyacrylamide gel
- Suppurative granulomas – polyalkylamide and polyacrylamide
- Polarizable fillers – bovine collagen and Sculptra® (poly-L-lactic acid)
- "Suture material-like" – Sculptra® (poly-L-lactic acid)
- "Swiss cheese-like" – paraffin and silicone
- "Popcorn-like" – Bioplastique® (polyvinylpyrrolidone silicone suspension)
- "Balloon-like"– Artecoll®, Arteplast® (polymethyl methacrylate)
- "Broken glass-like"– Dermalive® (hydroxyethylmetacrylate, hyaluronic acid in acrylic hydrogel)
- Swiss cheese with sparse inflammation – silicone oil or gel
- Swiss cheese with granulomatous inflammation and fibrosis – solid silicone elastomers

Other foreign materials

- **Aluminium (vaccines):** Granular violaceous to gray particles in macrophages: "purple macrophages"
- **Triamcinolone depot:** Palisading granuloma around acellular pale granular material with clear spaces **(Figure 3.74)**
- **Gel foam** (a hemostatic device applied to bleeding surfaces): Angulated bluish purple material filling a skin defect **(Figure 3.75)**

VESICULAR AND BULLOUS DISORDERS

Definition: Wide variety of blistering dermatoses which can be categorized on pathology by the level of the blisters (in the epidermis or beneath) and the absence or presence of a predominant type of inflammatory cell.

General concepts

Blister: A cavity in or beneath the epidermis containing fluid, plasma, inflammatory cells

- *Vesicle* – a blister less than 0.5 cm
- *Bulla* – a blister more than 0.5 cm

Pustule: A vesicle with prominent neutrophils or eosinophils with fluid/plasma

Microabscess: A small aggregate of lymphocyte and/or eosinophils

Cleft: A slit-like space in the epidermis, or between the epidermis and dermis

Epitope: Part of an antigen that is recognized by antibodies, B- and T-cells; **epitope spreading:** immune responses to endogenous epitopes arise secondary to the release of self antigens during a chronic autoimmune or inflammatory response; this causes hybrid (with overlapping features) bullous dermatoses

Bullous dermatoses are dynamic:

- If biopsied in "pre-bullous" (urticarial) stage, bullous pemphigoid may be confused with other eosinophilic dermatoses such as arthropod bite reaction.

NB Direct immunofluorescence (DIF) is helpful early as antibody-target interaction precedes the bullous reaction.

- A blister several days old may be present at a higher level due to epidermal growth (re-epithelialization).

(Table 3.9)

Table 3.9 Classification of bullous dermatoses by the level of the blister and the inflammatory infiltrate

Characteristics of the blister	Possible disorders
Subcorneal	Pemphigus foliaceus (PF) Staphylococcal scalded skin syndrome Bullous impetigo Subcorneal pustular dermatosis (SPD)/ Sneddon-Wilkinson disease SPD-like IgA pemphigus Transient neonatal pustular dermatosis Erythema toxicum neonatorum Pustular psoriasis Acute generalized exanthematous pustulosis Miliaria Dermatophytosis
In the spinous layer	Spongiotic dermatides Pemphigus vulgaris (early lesions) Pemphigus foliaceus Pityriasis rosea Incontinentia pigmenti Herpes virus infection Hailey-Hailey disease Grover's disease
Suprabasal	Hailey-Hailey disease (dilapidated brick wall) Darier's disease Pemphigus vulgaris (broad) Grover's disease (focal) Friction blister
Subepidermal without cells (cell poor)	Porphyria cutanea tarda (PCT) Pseudoporphyria Toxic epidermal necrolysis
Subepidermal with eosinophils	Bullous pemphigoid Pemphigoid gestationis Arthropod bite reaction
Subepidermal with neutrophils	Epidermolysis bullosa acquisita (eosinophils predominate in neonates) Anti p-105 and p-200 pemphigoid (neutrophils) Dermatitis herpetiformis (papillary dermal microabscesses) Linear IgA bullous dermatosis Bullous Sweet's syndrome Bullous pyoderma gangrenosum Bullous lupus erythematosus
Subepidermal with lymphocytes	Paraneoplastic pemphigus (lichenoid) Stevens–Johnson syndrome/Toxic epidermal necrolysis Bullous fixed drug eruption (lymphocytes and eosinophils) Lichen planus pemphigoides (lymphocytes and necrotic keratinocytes) GVHD (lymphocytes and necrotic keratinocytes; satellite cell necrosis) Polymorphous drug eruption
Eosinophilic spongiosis	Incontinentia pigmenti Bullous pemphigoid Pemphigus (early) Arthropod bite reaction Allergic contact dermatitis

On low power

- Empty space/s at subepidermal, intraepidermal or subcorneal level (cell-poor blisters)
- "Busy space(s)" at subepidermal, intraepidermal, or subcorneal level (cell-rich blisters)

NB In subtle cases always study the margins of the biopsy to find the cleft.

On high power

PEMPHIGUS GROUP

Pemphigus vulgaris (PV)

Target for antibodies: The extracellular epitopes of the desmogleins (DSG1 (upper epidermis), DSG3 (lower epidermis and the outer root sheath of hair follicles) and DSG3 (mucosal epithelium)) and the desmocollins **(Figure 3.76)**

Direct immunofluorescence (DIF): Intraepidermal IgG in a "Swiss-cheese"/"chicken-wire" pattern; IgA in IgA pemphigus

- Suprabasal bulla with intact roof and a floor of prominent dermal papillae protruding as villi lined by detached basal cells **(Figure 3.77, Photomnemonic 3.13)**
- Acantholytic cells

NB The acantholysis involves the hair follicles; DIF can be done on plucked hairs.

NB Early lesions may show only eosinophilic spongiosis or neutrophilic spongiosis.

Pemphigus vegetans

- Pseudoepitheliomatous hyperplasia **(Figure 3.78)**
- Eosinophilic spongiosis and intraepidermal eosinophilic microabscesses
- Subtle suprabasal cleft with acantholytic cells and eosinophils

Pemphigus foliaceus (PF)

- Flaccid flat cleft between stratum corneum and stratum granulosum (the blister "sits on top of the epidermis") **(Figure 3.79)**

  NB The roof of the blister may be missing.

  - With dyskeratotic granular keratinocytes
  - With acantholytic keratinocytes

Additional helpful features:
- Hypergranulosis at the edge of the specimen
- Neutrophils in varying degrees
- The acantholysis goes down the hair follicles

Differential diagnosis:
- Pemphigus vulgaris: suprabasal blister; no dyskeratotic cells
- Staphylococcal scalded skin syndrome: may look identical, DIF is negative
- Bullous impetigo: bacteria, DIF is negative

  NB Impetiginized PF may show identical histologic features to bullous impetigo.

- Superficial pustular dermatosis (SPD): dome-shaped pustule (compare to the flaccid flat pustule in PF)

Pemphigus erythematosus

The same features as pemphigus foliaceus combined with interface dermatitis (as in lupus erythematosus)

DIF: Intercellular IgG with granular deposition of IgG and IgM at the dermoepidermal junction

IgA pemphigus

- **Subcorneal pustular dermatosis (SPD)-like IgA pemphigus:** The antigen is desmocollin 1
  - Subcorneal vesiculopustule with minimal acantholysis
- **Intraepidermal neutrophilic dermatosis (IEN):** The antigen is desmoglein 1 (DSG1) or desmoglein 3 (DSG3)
  - Large, spread dome-shaped subcorneal or intraepidermal pustule with neutrophils and eosinophils **(Figure 3.80)**
  - Acantholysis
  - In the dermis: variable neutrophilic microabscesses and perivascular infiltrate of lymphocytes, eosinophils and neutrophils

NB SPD: smaller, subcorneal blister with no acantholysis; IEN: spread blister with acantholysis, low in the epidermis.

DIF: Intercellular IgA deposition differentiates SPD-like IgA pemphigus from SPD (Sneddon–Wilkinson disease)

Paraneoplastic pemphigus

NB Overlapping features of pemphigus (pemphigus vulgaris/pemphigus foliaceus) with an interface pattern (lichen planus, erythema multiforme).

DIF on rat bladder epithelium: IgG (variable IgM, IgA too) and C3 in intercellular and linear/granular junctional deposition

- Suprabasal acantholysis
- Vacuolar interface dermatitis, necrotic keratinocytes, lichenoid infiltrate of lymphocytes and variable melanophages in the upper dermis

OTHER BULLOUS DISORDERS

Hailey-Hailey disease

- Epidermal hyperplasia due to downward elongation of the rete ridges **(Figure 3.81)**
- Spread and full-thickness acantholysis (along the entire length of the epidermis and at least in half of its thickness) can be compared to a "dilapidated brick wall" **(Photomnemonic 3.14)**
- Early lesion: suprabasal cleft with protruding villi (dermal papillae covered by one or several layers of keratinocytes)

Differential diagnosis:
- From pemphigus: no hair follicle involvement, no eosinophils
- From Darier's disease: minimal dyskeratosis, some acantholytic cells are dyskeratotic but have preserved nucleus and cytoplasm

Darier's disease (keratosis follicularis)

NB Darier's disease is the classic example for *acantholytic dyskeratosis*: the keratinocytes lose the intercellular bridges (acantholysis) followed by premature keratinization (corps ronds – round dyskeratotic cells and corps grains – flattened dyskeratotic cells) (see Chapter 1).

- Suprabasal acantholysis (lacunae) with protruding villi **(Figure 3.82)**
- Dyskeratosis (corps ronds in spinous and granular layer and corps grains in the parakeratotic cornified layer)

Additional features:
- Papillomatosis
- Hypergranulosis
- Multiple foci in one specimen
- Involves the hair follicles: keratotic plugs with dyskeratotic cells (remember it from the name: keratosis follicularis)

NB Warty dyskeratoma shows identical features, but it is a solitary lesion (see Chapter 5, Keratinocytic tumors).

Grover's disease

- Small foci of intraepithelial acantholysis with dyskeratosis (usually limited to a few rete ridges)
- Acanthosis "pointing" to the central focus of dyskeratosis and acantholysis

Six main types:
- Hailey-Hailey type
- Darier's type **(Figure 3.83A)**
- Pemphigus type (suprabasal in PV type and in the upper epidermis in PF type) **(Figure 3.83B)**
- Lichenoid type (with lichenoid, lymphocytic inflammation)
- Spongiotic type (acantholytic cells in spongiotic vesicles)
- Lentiginous type (elongation of rete ridges with hyperpigmentation)

DIF: Negative

NB Possible clues for Grover's disease: more than one pattern in the same specimen; focal involvement of the epidermis; lentiginous rete ridges and eosinophils in the dermis.

(Table 3.10)

Table 3.10 Comparing the acantholysis and dyskeratosis pattern in pemphigus, Hailey-Hailey disease, Grover's disease, and Darier's disease

Disease	Acantholysis	Dyskeratosis
Hailey-Hailey	Broad and thick: "dilapidated brick wall" No hair follicle involvement	No/minimal: pink cytoplasm, preserved nucleus
Darier's	Suprabasal (lacunae) with protruding villi Involves hair follicles	Corps ronds/ corps grains
Grover's	Focal (2–3 rete ridges)	+/–
Pemphigus	Suprabasal Involves hair follicles	No

Bullous pemphigoid (BP)

1. Early lesions (urticarial, pre-bullous phase)
   - Eosinophilic spongiosis
   - Edema
   - Perivascular and interstitial eosinophils with lymphocytes and neutrophils
2. a) Blisters on erythematous skin are cell-rich
   - Eosinophils aligned along the dermoepidermal junction **(Figure 3.84A, Photomnemonic 3.15)**
   - Subepidermal bulla with eosinophils
   - Eosinophils in the papillary dermis (eosinophilic abscesses)
   - Preserved dermal papillae (festooning)

   b) Blisters on normal skin are cell-poor

NB Older blisters show an intraepidermal split (due to epidermal regeneration) **(Figure 3.84B)**.

DIF: Linear C3 > IgG deposition at the dermoepidermal junction

Salt split skin: C3 and IgG on the roof of the blister (80%) and on both roof (lower basal keratinocytes) and floor (superior aspect of the dermis) (20%)

Pemphigoid gestationis (herpes gestationis)

NB Same features as bullous pemphigoid with additional features:
- variable necrotic keratinocytes in the basal layer
- marked papillary dermal edema with "teardrop-like" papillae.

DIF: Linear C3 (and less often IgG) at the dermoepidermal junction

Mucous membrane (cicatricial) pemphigoid (MMP)

- Subepidermal blister with fibrin and inflammatory cells
- Edema and variable often lichenoid inflammation in the dermis: lymphocytes, eosinophils, histiocytes, plasma cells

NB Plasma cells prevail in oral lesions.

- Lamellar dermal fibrosis (scar) in older lesions

NB Subepidermal blister overlying inflammation (with plasma cells and eosinophils) in a scar: think MMP **(Figure 3.85)**.

DIF: Identical to BP

Epidermolysis bullosa acquisita

Cell-free variant

Trauma-induced blisters on dorsal hands, feet, knees, and elbows which heal with scars and milia) – identical to PCT (see below):

- Subepidermal blister
- Preserved dermal papillae (festooning)
- Scar and milia (miniature infundibular cyst with stratified epithelial wall) **(Figure 3.86)**

Inflammatory variant

- Bullous pemphigoid-like: identical to BP
- Dermatitis herpetiformis-like: identical to DH (see below)

DIF: Linear C3 and IgG along the dermoepidermal junction

Salt split skin: Deposit of complement and IgG on the floor of the blister (compare to BP)

Dermatitis herpetiformis (DH)

- Multiloculated subepidermal collections of neutrophils and eosinophils in the dermal papillae (papillary microabscesses) **(Figure 3.87)**

> NB Variable necrotic keratinocytes overlying microabscess.

- The rete ridges are usually spared among the abscesses (compare to linear IgA)
- Fibrin and edema in the papillae (they are bluish and smudged)
- Nuclear dust (karyorrhexis)
- As lesions age, eosinophils increase

DIF: Granular IgA in dermal papillae on immunofluorescence ("snow hills')

IIF: IgA antiendomysial antibodies

Linear IgA bullous dermatosis (LAD)

- Broad-based subepidermal blister with neutrophils (and eosinophils) and fibrin along the entire dermoepidermal junction

> • NB Note lost rete ridges in the cavity (compare to DH) **(Figure 3.88)**.

- Less often microabscesses in the papillary dermis

> • NB Neutrophils lining the dermoepidermal junction are a clue to LAD.

DIF: Linear IgA deposition along the dermoepidermal junction

PCT

- Cell-poor subepidermal blister
- Very well-preserved dermal papillae projecting into the blister (festooning "decorated with garland" papillae)
- The papillae appear "solid" due to thickened papillary vessels with hyalinization (compare to the "soft" teardrop-like papillae in BP and pemphigoid gestationis) **(Figure 3.89)**
- Caterpillar bodies: pink basement membrane material which resembles dyskeratotic cells along the roof of the blister (stains positive with collagen IV, which is a stain for basement membrane)
- Dermal sclerosis

DIF: C3 in thickened blood vessels and focally at the dermoepidermal junction

> NB Other forms of porphyria (and pseudoporphyria) have identical features.

VASCULAR DISEASE

> **Definition:** A large group of disorders characterized by vascular injury and/or inflammation of the vessel walls.

General concepts

Vascular injury:

1. *Primary* – the pathologic process occurs in the vessels
2. *Secondary* – the vessels are "victims" involved secondarily by the adjacent inflammation and ulceration

This results in:

- Endothelial swelling
- Endothelial necrosis
- Red blood cells extravasation
- Leukocytes extravasation
- Luminal thrombosis
- Fibrin deposition in the walls (rim of pink hyaline material)
- Frank fibrinoid necrosis

Vasculitis: Combination of clear vascular injury with inflammation of the vessel walls (inflammatory cells: neutrophils, lymphocytes or macrophages)

- *Neutrophilic vasculitis:* neutrophils in the infiltrate
- *Lymphocytic vasculitis:* limited vascular injury with absent fibrinoid necrosis and presence of lymphocytes in the infiltrate

> NB Most cutaneous vasculitides involve small blood vessels and are neutrophilic or known also as necrotizing or leukocytoclastic (from cytoclasia: nuclear dust, karyorrhexis of the neutrophils' nuclei).

Vasculopathy: Vascular injury with intraluminal fibrin and/or thrombi but without inflammation

Pesudovasculitis and pseudovasculopathy: Closely mimic vasculitis and vasculopathy; arise due to dense inflammation, trauma and/or ulceration of the surrounding tissue

NB Usually only the vessels in a focal area are involved (compare to the normal vessels outside the affected area) and the fibrinoid deposition is perivascular rather than intravascular.

Purpura: Leakage of red blood cells in the dermis; the purpura becomes palpable if inflammation is present too

The vascular disease is dynamic: vascular injury → purpura + inflammatory infiltrate → palpable purpura + vascular occlusion → necrosis and/or ulceration

NB Any vessel visible on 2× magnification is a large vessel.

NB The diagnosis of small-vessel vasculitis requires the presence of fibrin in the vessel walls; in medium- and large-vessel vasculitis fibrin may be absent.

(Table 3.11)

Table 3.11 The most common vasculitides classified by the size of the vessel

Type	Possible disorders
Small-vessel vasculitis	Leukocytoclastic (neutrophilic, necrotizing) vasculitis (LCV) • Henoch-Schönlein purpura (HSP) (IgA-dominant immune deposits) • acute hemorrhagic edema of infancy Urticarial vasculitis Microscopic polyangiitis (few or no immune deposits) Essential cryoglobulinemic vasculitis (cryoglobuin deposits) Wegener's granulomatosis Churg–Strauss syndrome
Medium-vessel vasculitis	Polyarteritis nodosa (necrotizing vasculitis of medium-size arteries)
Large-vessel vasculitis	Giant cell arteritis (granulomatous inflammation of the temporal artery) Takayasu arteritis

On low power

- **Neutrophilic vasculitis:** Pink and smudged (indistinct) vessels due to fibrin in the walls, "blurry dermis, like covered by a veil": red dots, lakes of red dots (red blood cells extravasation) and blue dots (nuclear dust)
- **Lymphocytic vasculitis:** "Blue cuffs or sleeves" around vessels (lymphocytes), red dots, lakes of red dots in the dermis (red blood cells extravasations)
- **Vasculopathy:** Clogged vessels in the dermis

How to approach vascular disease

1. Vasculitis versus vasculopathy (vascular injury with inflammation versus vascular injury only)
2. Primary vascular injury (all vessels are affected) versus secondary (only focally affected vessels and adjacent tissue ulceration, inflammation)
3. Size and type of vessels (small/postcapillary venules in the upper dermis, medium or large in the lower dermis)
4. Type of predominant infiltrates (neutrophils, lymphocytes, eosinophils, macrophages)

NB Late stage leukocytoclastic vasculitis shows only lymphocytes.

5. Rule out infection (special stains)

On high power

SMALL-VESSEL VASCULITIS

Leukocytoclastic vasculitis (LCV)

- The small vessels in the upper dermis have thick walls due to edema, fibrin, and neutrophils **(Figure 3.90A)**
- Occlusion of the lumen by swollen endothelial cells and/or thrombi (made of fibrin, red blood cells, platelets, and neutrophils)
- Bluish fibrin exudates in the adjacent dermis
- Nuclear dust and red blood cells in the dermis **(Figure 3.90B)**
- If edema is present, subepidermal blister may form
- If neutrophils are densely packed, subepidermal pustules may form (pustular vasculitis)

NB Resolving lesions show mild perivascular lymphocytes and eosinophils and busy dermis: interstitial fibroblasts and histiocytes.

DIF: IgM, IgG, C3 in vessel walls

Henoch–Schönlein purpura

- Identical features to LCV
- DIF shows granular IgA deposition within the small vessels

Urticarial vasculitis (UV)

NB Subtle findings: there is minimal vasculitis with increased vascular permeability.

- Mild vascular damage: swollen endothelial cells and sparse infiltrate of neutrophils, lymphocytes, and eosinophils **(Figure 3.91A)**
- Edema of the upper dermis **(Figure 3.91B)**
- Florid LCV findings are rare (more common in hypocomplemententemic UV)

Cryoglobulinemia and cryoglobulinemic vasculitis

- **Type I** – monoclonal immunoglobulins (IgM) (underlying hematologic disorder: multiple myeloma, leukemia, lymphoma)
- **Type II** – mixed monoclonal (IgM) and polyclonal immunoglobulins (IgG) (autoimmune disorders as connective tissue disease, Sjögren's syndrome, or infections: hepatitis C and B)
- **Type III** – polyclonal immunoglobulins IgM and IgG (same conditions as in type II)

NB Type I is an occlusive vasculopathy; Types II and III are cryoglobulinemic vasculitis.

Type I

- Hyaline occlusions in small and medium-sized vessels (PAS-positive cryoglobulin precipitates) **(Figure 3.92)**
- Red blood cell extravasations
- No vasculitis

Types II and III

- LCV of both small and medium-sized vessels with occlusive thrombi in the lumina

Connective tissue disease-associated vasculitis

NB LCV of both small and medium-sized vessels.

- Interface dermatitis in lupus erythematosus
- LCV or lymphocytic vasculitis in Sjögren's syndrome

ANCA-associated vasculitides

ANCA (antineutrophil cytoplasmic antibodies) against antigens in the cytoplasm of neutrophils: c-ANCA (cytoplasmic) and p-ANCA (perinuclear)

NB Granulomatous infiltrate of the vessel walls (granulomatous vasculitis) is uncommon in skin lesions; in skin lesions the granulomas are extravascular.

Wegener's granulomatosis (granulomatosis with polyangiitis (GPA))

c-ANCA (levels reflect disease activity)

- Half of the biopsies show non-specific features
- LCV of small and medium-sized vessels
- Blue granulomas with suppurative necrosis: extravascular palisading histiocytes around necrobiotic collagen impregnated with fibrin and nuclear dust **(Figure 3.93)**

Churg–Strauss syndrome

p-ANCA (levels correlate with disease activity)

- LCV of small and medium-sized vessels
- Red granulomas: palisading histiocytes, variable giant cells around necrobiotic collagen impregnated with degranulated eosinophils
- The infiltrate can be rich in eosinophils

Localized fibrosing small-vessel vasculitides

Granuloma faciale (GF)

- Grenz zone
- LCV in the upper dermis (the process involves the upper two-thirds of the dermis) **(Figure 3.94A)**
- Perivascular and interstitial dense polymorphous infiltrate: eosinophils, lymphocytes, neutrophils, and histiocytes **(Figure 3.94B)**
- The infiltrate spares the adventitial dermis (this is the papillary dermis with the periadnexal dermis)
- Mild nuclear dust and fibrin can be found

Erythema elevatum diutinum

NB Similar features to granuloma faciale but does not have a Grenz zone, and neutrophils prevail over eosinophils.

Early lesions:

- LCV of small vessels with prominent fibrin in the vessel walls (toxic hyaline)
- "Busy" cellular dermis: neutrophils with nuclear dust and fibrin, mixed inflammation

Later lesions:

- Laminated concentric fibrosis around small blood vessels ("onion-like") **(Figure 3.95)**
- Fibrosis in the dermis in a storiform pattern
- Extracellular lipids (xanthomatization of the dermis)

NB Older lesions may look like dermatofibroma or Kaposi's sarcoma with small foci of neutrophilic vasculitis.

MEDIUM-VESSEL VASCULITIS

Polyarteritis nodosa (PAN)

NB PAN is a vasculitis of the medium-sized arteries but in the skin it may also involve small vessels.

Early lesions:
- LCV of arteries in the deep dermis and subcutaneous fat: usually one vessel shows florid full-thickness inflammation of the wall (neutrophils with leukocytoclasia, eosinophils) and fibrinoid necrosis **(Figure 3.96)**

Older lesions:
- Intimal proliferation
- Thrombosis
- Fibrosis

NB VVG stains the elastic lamina to confirm that the involved vessel is an artery; the internal and external elastic lamina can be destroyed.

LARGE-VESSEL VASCULITIS

Giant cell (temporal) arteritis
- Lymphohistiocytic inflammation of the entire vessel wall of the affected artery
- Fragmentation of the elastic lamina and elastophagocytosis by giant cells

Takayasu's arteritis

NB Indistinguishable from PAN.

- Small and medium arteries of the subcutaneous fat
- Fibrinoid necrosis of the entire vessel wall with inflammation of neutrophils and lymphocytes

VASCULOPATHIES

Vasculopathies are a group of vascular diseases characterized by vascular injury in the absence of vasculitis.
- **Early lesions** may show only red blood cell extravasations (purpura).
- **Developed or older lesions** show intravascular thrombi; in severe cases hemorrhagic infarcts with epidermal and derma necrosis occur (ulcers) **(Figure 3.97)**.

Cryoglobulinemia
See Leukocytoclastic vasculitis (LCV) above

Atrophie blanche
- The superficial vessels are increased in number and have thick pink walls due to fibrin deposition **(Figure 3.98)**
- Minimal inflammation (lymphocytes)
- Red blood cell extravasation
- In late stages:
  - Dermal sclerosis
  - Occlusion of the vessels by intimal proliferation and/or fibrin thrombi which stain PAS positive

Degos disease
- Epidermal atrophy with hyperkeratosis
- Wedge-shaped cone of necrosis in the dermis with a vessel showing vascular damage with fibrin thombi at its base
- Mucin (early – in the cone of necrosis; late – in the margins of normal dermis)

Calciphylaxis
- Calcium deposition in the small blood vessels in the subcutaneous fat (calcifying panniculitis is possible)
- The calcium is deposited in the media
- Proliferation of the intima with luminal occlusion by thrombi **(Figure 3.99)**

Differential diagnosis: Pancreatic panniculitis (look for ghost cells)

NB Thrombi may be present in non-involved vessels too.

Lymphocytic vasculitis
- Limited (mild) vascular injury: endothelial swelling, minimal fibrinoid necrosis **(Figure 3.100)**
- Lymphocytes surround vessels and invade vessel walls ("blue handcuffs")
- Red blood cell extravasations

Most common dermatoses showing lymphocytic vasculitis:
- Perniosis
- Pigmented purpuras
- Arthropod bite reactions
- Drug reactions
- Connective tissue disorders
- Infections (viral)
- Infestations (scabies)
- Pityriasis lichenoides (PLEVA and PLC)
- Lymphomatoid papulosis and other lymphomas
- Polymorphous light eruption
- Behçet's disease

Pigmented purpura
- A lymphocytic perivascular infiltrate limited to the papillary dermis **(Figure 3.101)**
- Mild vascular injury: only endothelial swelling with/without lymphocytic infiltrate

NB The adjacent affected vessels are connected by a cuff of lymphocytes.

- Dermal hemorrhage with hemosiderin

Additional features, depending on the type:
- Lichenoid or band-like infiltrate (lichen aureus: with scattered hemosiderin laden macrophages; Gougerot and Blum: more dense infiltrate)
- Spongiosis and parakeratosis (Doucas and Kapetanakis)
- Prominent telangiectasia (Majocchi's disease)

Perniosis

The clue for perniosis is acral skin (thick stratum corneum).

In the epidermis:

- Acanthosis with spongiosis
- Vacuolar degeneration at the dermoepidermal junction
- Scattered necrotic keratinocytes to confluent necrosis

In the dermis:

- Edema in the upper dermis
- Lymphocytic vasculitis of the superficial and deep vessels
- Deep perieccrine lymphocytic infiltrate

NB The combination of spongiosis, edema, and deep perieccrine lymphocytic infiltrate favors perniosis over lupus erythematosus and erythema multiforme.

PANNICULITIS

Definition: Heterogeneous group of disorders which present clinically as subcutaneous erythematous nodules and histologically as inflammation and necrosis of the subcutaneous fat.

General concepts

- Panniculitides are dynamic: although they are classified as predominantly septal or lobular, over time they become mixed; lower magnification is the best approach to assess for septal and lobular distribution.
- Inflammation in early lesions consists mostly of neutrophils; in older lesions it consists mostly of lymphocytes, histiocytes, and foamy macrophages.
- Septal involvement results in widening of the septa due to edema, hemorrhage, inflammation, and fibrosis.
- Lobular involvement results in fat necrosis, inflammation, and later fibrosis within the lobules.
- **Fat necrosis** presents in different forms:
  1. *Lipophagic:* Most common but least specific (foamy macrophages are laden with lipid products from the dead adipocytes)
  2. *Hyaline* (the hyaline material among adipocytes makes them appear "mummified"): Lupus panniculitis
  3. *Membranous* (late-stage fat necrosis, which appears as "frost on the window") **(Figure 3.102, Photomnemonic 3.16)**
  4. *Ischemic* (anucleated small adipocytes in the center of the lobule due to small vessel vasculitis)

NB Fat necrosis with saponification is specific for pancreatic panniculitis (free fatty acids from enzyme-induced lipolysis bind with calcium and form blue (basophilic) soapy deposits.

- There are no vascular connections between the adjacent fat lobules and therefore large-vessel vasculitis in the septa does not cause inflammation in the lobules whereas vasculitis of the small capillaries in the lobules leads to ischemic necrosis and inflammation in the lobule.
- When large vessels are involved, distinguishing between an artery and a vein is crucial: arteries have compact muscular layers and their thick internal elastic lamina stains with VVG.

- NB Always check for foreign bodies, organisms, calcium, and crystals.

- NB Erythema nodosum and erythema induratum of Bazin comprise 90% of all panniculitides.

(Table 3.12)

Table 3.12 Classification of the panniculitides

Type		Possible disorders
Septal panniculitis	With vasculitis	1. **Of the small vessels:** LCV 2. **Of the large vessels:** • *arteries:* polyarteritis nodosa (PAN) • *veins:* superficial thrombophlebitis
	Without vasculitis	1. **With lymphocytes mostly:** Erythema nodosum 2. **With histiocytes mostly (granulomatous infiltrate):** Infection (tuberculosis or syphilis) • *with radial granulomas:* erythema nodosum • *with naked granulomas:* sarcoidosis (Darier-Roussy) • *with mucin:* subcutaneous granuloma annulare 3. **With degenerated collagen, foamy histiocytes, and cholesterol clefts:** Necrobiotic xanthogranuloma

(continued)

Table 3.12 *(continued)*

Type		Possible disorders
		4. **With sclerotic collagen:** Scleroderma/morphea Eosinophilic fasciitis
Lobular panniculitis	With vasculitis	1. **Of the small vessels:** Erythema nodosum leprosum 2. **Of the large vessels:** Erythema induratum of Bazin
	Without vasculitis	1. **Without inflammation:** • *with needle-shaped crystals:* sclerema neonatorum, subcutaneous fat necrosis of the newborn • *with vascular calcification:* calciphylaxis 2. **With lymphocytes mostly:** • *with lymphoid follicles, plasma cells and nuclear dust:* lupus profundus • *with plasma cells*: dermato-myositis • *with atypical lymphocytes:* lymphoma, leukemia 3. **With neutrophils mostly:** Infections (bacteria, fungi or protozoa) • *with extensive fat necrosis and saponification:* pancreatic panniculitis • *with neutrophils splayed among collagen of the dermis:* alpha-1 antitrypsin deficiency • *with foreign bodies:* factitial panniculitis 3. **With macrophages:** Lipodermatosclerosis Sarcoidosis 4. **With sclerosis:** Lipodermatosclerosis Eosinophilic fasciitis (late stage)

On low power

- **Lobular panniculitis** shows inflammation and necrosis within the lobules resembling honeycomb with bees **(Photomnemonic 3.17)**.
- **Septal panniculitis** shows edema, inflammation, and hemorrhage in the thickened septa resembling a log with fungi **(Photomnemonic 3.18)**.
  - *Lupus panniculitis:* collections of lymphocytes and lymphoid follicles in the lobules resembling moss on a river stone **(Photomnemonic 3.19)**
  - *Lipomembranous panniculitis:* frost on the window (see Photomnemonic 3.16)
  - *Sclerema neonatorum and subcutaneous fat necrosis of the newborn:* stack of needles **(Photomnemonic 3.20)**
  - *Pancreatic panniculitis:* blue soap foam **(Photomnemonic 3.21)**

On high power

Some of the most common panniculitides are discussed below.

SEPTAL PANNICULITIDES

Erythema nodosum (EN)

Early lesions:

- Septal edema with polymorphous cell infiltrate: neutrophils (even clusters if neutrophils) and eosinophils may predominate; the infiltrate may extend into the adjacent lobules **(Figure 3.103A)**

- NB Miescher's radial granulomas are considered specific for EN: well-defined nodular aggregation of histiocytes around a central jagged (stellate or banana-shaped cleft); they can be found at any stage of EN **(Figure 3.103B)**.

- Rarely paraseptal and septal blood vessels show edema and inflammation of the vessel walls with separation of the muscular layers (venulitis)

Late lesions:

- Fibrosis, sparse lymphocytes, histiocytes and giant cells in the septa
- Paraseptal granulation tissue and foamy histiocytes

Superficial migratory thrombophlebitis

- A large vein with a thrombosed lumen within a septum of the upper subdermis **(Figure 3.104)**
- Inflammatory infiltrate in the vessel wall (early: neutrophils; later: lymphocytes)

NB PAN is the differential diagnosis:

- The inflammation and fibrinoid necrosis of the wall are more prominent than the thrombosis.
- The involved vessel is a septal artery (VVG stains the elastic lamina) (see Vascular disease).

LOBULAR PANNICULITIS

Erythema induratum of Bazin (EIB) (nodular vasculitis)

The evolution of the lesions goes through several phases:

1. Small- and medium-vessel vasculitis with thrombosis in the lobules →
2. Ischemic (caseous) fat necrosis →

3. Granulomatous inflammation forms to clear the tissue damage →
4. Fibrosis
   - Fibrinoid necrosis and lymphohistiocytic inflammation in the vessel walls (vasculitis) **(Figure 3.105)**
   - Caseous fat necrosis which may extend to the dermis and result in ulceration
   - Lymphocytes, epithelioid histiocytes and giant cells forming granulomas between the fat cells
   - Later stage: septal and lobular fibrosis

NB Mycobacterial stains are negative.

Lupus panniculitis/Lupus profundus (LP)

NB Lobular panniculitis with DLE features (interface dermatitis, periadnexal infiltrate and mucin deposition in the dermis): think lupus panniculitis.

- Lymphocytes and plasma cells rim the fat cells in the lobules (but can also be found in the septa and in the dermis) (see Photomnemonic 3.19)
- Lymphoid follicles in more than 50% of the cases **(Figure 3.106A)**

NB Hyalinization with fibrin and lymphoid follicles in the lobules: think lupus panniculitis.

The hyalinization involves several components:

- Sclerotic collagen in the septa (glassy and pink septa)
- Blood vessels and adnexal structures
- Fat necrosis

(Figure 3.106B)

Differential diagnosis:

1. *Cutaneous lymphoma:* Careful search for cytologic atypia, a panel of immunostains, and gene rearrangement may help to distinguish from other disorders:
   - Subcutaneous T-cell lymphoma of alpha/beta phenotype
   - Subcutaneous T-cell lymphoma of gamma/delta phenotype
   - NK T-cell lymphoma
2. *Panniculitis in dermatomyositis:*
   - More common LCV of the small vessels in the lobules with lymphocytic vasculitis of the arterioles in the septa
   - Lipophagic necrosis with foamy histiocytes
   - Calcifications of the deep tissue

Lipodermatosclerosis/Sclerosing panniculitis (LDS)

Venous insufficiency → stagnation in the lobular capillaries → ischemia and necrosis in the center of the lobules

NB Stasis dermatitis is a constant finding in both early and late-stage LDS.

- Clusters of aneurysmatic (dilated) capillaries with/without fibrin (pink) cuffs in upper dermis
- Fibrosis
- Hemosiderin deposition

Early stage:

- Sparse inflammatory infiltrate of lymphocytes in the septa
- Ischemic necrosis: pale and small anucleated adipocytes
- Red blood cell extravasation and hemosiderin in the necrotic area

Late stage:

- Thick and fibrotic septa
- Lipophagic fat necrosis (foamy macrophages) and lipomembranous necrosis (fatty microcysts lined by feathery remnants of lipid material in arabesque pattern/frost on the window) **(Figure 3.107)** (see also Figure 3.102 and Photomnemonic 3.16)
- Patchy chronic inflammation

NB Lipomembranous necrosis is a key feature of chronic LDS but is not specific; it can be seen in other panniculitides too:
- Erythema nodosum
- Morphea
- Necrobiosis lipoidica
- Traumatic panniculitis

Factitial and traumatic panniculitis

Etiology:

1. Blunt trauma (traumatic panniculitis mostly in women on the calves or thighs)
2. Injections of fillers/foreign materials (factitial panniculitis)
3. Cold temperature (physical panniculitis)
   - Mostly lobular panniculitis with mild infiltrate of lymphocytes and histiocytes in the lobules

Additional features:

- Foamy macrophages and giant cells are common (factitial): look for angulated or round vacuoles in their cytoplasm as a clue to injectable foreign material "Swiss-cheese pattern" (silicone, paraffin or other materials) **(Figure 3.108)**
- Different size of microcysts in the fat with/without lipomembranous changes (traumatic)
- Dermal changes of edema, lymphocytic vasculitis extending in the fat similar to pernio (cold)

Pancreatic panniculitis

NB A lobular panniculitis with intense necrosis with ghost remnants only: think pancreatic panniculitis.

- Acellular remnants of adipocytes which look angulated and bigger than the normal adipocytes, and have granular blue cytoplasm due to saponification (ghost cells) **(Figure 3.109)** (see Photomnemonic 3.21)
- Ghost cells are grouped in clusters in the center of the lobule
- Dystrophic calcification
- Granulomatous infiltrate (foamy macrophages and giant cells) in late lesions

Subcutaneous fat necrosis of the newborn/ Sclerema neonatorum

Common feature: Lobular panniculitis in neonatal age characterized by needle-shaped clefts arranged radially in the adipocytes (see Photomnemonic 3.20) **(Table 3.13)**

Table 3.13 Comparison between subcutaneous fat necrosis of the newborn and sclerema neonatorum

Subcutaneous fat necrosis of the newborn	Sclerema neonatorum
Full-term babies	Low-weight premature newborns
Begins in first month of life in healthy babies	Begins in first days of life in severely ill babies
Good prognosis	Poor prognosis
On pathology: • lobular panniculitis on low power • dense mixed inflammation and necrosis • needle-shaped crystals in adipocytes • calcification is common	On pathology: • little abnormality of the fat on low power • no/minimal inflammation and necrosis • needle-shaped crystals in adipocytes • no calcification

Neutrophilic lobular panniculitis

NB Alpha-1 antitrypsin deficiency panniculitis and infective panniculitis are similar; special stains are needed for the diagnosis.

NB Most common infectious organisms cause lobular panniculitis due to secondary (hematogenous) spread in immunocompromised individuals. (Primary infections involve the dermis.)

- **Bacteria:** *Streptococcus pyogenes, Staphylococcus aureus, Pseudomonas, Klebsiella*, and *Nocardia*
- **Mycobacteria:** *M. tuberculosis* and atypical mycobacteria (Buruli ulcer)
- **Fungal organisms:** *Candida, Fusarium, Histoplasma, Cryptococcus neoformans, Actinomyces israelii, Sporothrix schenkii, Aspergillus* and dematiaceous fungi (*Fonsecaea pedrosoi, Phialophora verrucosa, Cladosporium carrionii*, or *Fonsecaea compacta*)

(Table 3.14)

Table 3.14 Comparison between alpha-1–antitrypsin associated panniculitis and infective panniculitides

Alpha-1 antitrypsin deficiency associated panniculitis	Infective panniculitis
Splaying of neutrophils among collagen in the dermis (early); no granulomas Blood vessels may be thrombosed Special stains are negative	Suppurative granulomas Severe necrosis of the fat lobules possible Deep dermal necrosis (later) and severe necrosis of the fat lobules Clue: focality (necrotic lobule adjacent to a normal one) Blood vessels are thrombosed with/without organisms Special stains are positive for the culprit organism

Lipoatrophy

Localized diffuse generalized loss of fat leading to depressed and thinner (shrunken) appearing skin (classic example is the iatrogenic-induced lipoatrophy due to intralesional steroid infiltration)

- Early lesions may have inflammatory pattern with foamy macrophages and necrosis
- In developed lesions everything is "shrunken" **(Figure 3.110)**
- Smaller (shrunken) adipocytes
- Smaller (shrunken) lobules
- Increased number of small vessels in the subdermis

NEUTROPHILIC DERMATOSES *PER SE*

Definition: Group of dermatoses characterized by dermal neutrophilic infiltrates and variable vascular damage with leukocytoclasia.

General concepts

- Perivascular and interstitial neutrophilic infiltrate in the dermis and subdermis
- Usually the vascular injury is secondary to the surrounding inflammation/necrosis and there is no clear leukocytoclastic vasculitis (LCV) (only focal areas of vessels are involved, no fibrinoid necrosis; fibrin can be present but only perivascular not intravascular

- NB Exceptions: Behcet's disease, erythema elevatum diutinum and granuloma faciale.

- Negative special stains and cultures for infectious organisms
- Clinical improvement on systemic immunosuppressive treatment

(Table 3.15)

Table 3.15 The most common dermatoses characterized by neutrophilic infiltrates

Clues	Possible disorders
With LCV	Granuloma faciale Erythema elevatum diutinum Behçet's disease
With band-like infiltrate	Sweet's syndrome
With follicular involvement	Pyoderma gangrenosum Folliculitis
With sparse neutrophils throughout dermis	Neutrophilic urticarial dermatosis
With atypical myeloid cells/ neutrophils	Leukemia cutis
With vesicles and bullae	Dermatitis herpetiformis Linear IgA dermatosis

On low power

Sea of red–blue dots (neutrophils, leukocytoclasia) in the dermis; when the infiltrate is dense, it is often arranged in an abscess-like pattern

On high power

Sweet's syndrome

Dermal edema with band-like infiltrate of neutrophils: think Sweet's **(Figure 3.111)**

NB The differential diagnosis of edema includes also pernio, contact dermatitis, erythema multiforme, PMLE, and arthropod bite reaction.

- Edema in the upper dermis; if the edema is severe, it forms subepidermal blisters
- The epidermis shows no change (20%) or variable degrees of spongiosis, exocytosis of neutrophils and keratinocyte necrosis (80%)
- Band-like and diffuse dermal infiltrate of neutrophils

NB Immature neutrophils (so-called bands with a curved instead of a lobed nucleus) are common **(Figure 3.112)**.

- Vascular injury but no true LCV (more common in long-standing lesions)
- Neutrophils in the subdermis: more common in associated malignancy

NB Look for atypical cells to exclude leukemia cutis.

Histiocytoid Sweet's syndrome

A variant of Sweet's syndrome

- Upper dermal edema with uniform infiltrate of histiocyte-like cells **(Figure 3.113A)**
- Similar to leukemia cutis with the presence of atypical monocytes with reniform nuclei (blast-like cells) **(Figure 3.113B)**
- A panel of myeloid stains must be applied (MPO, CD43, CD68, CD15, and CD34)
- Leukemic cells are absent in peripheral blood tests and in the bone marrow, and the lesions resolve dramatically with systemic corticosteroid use

NB Leukemia cutis should be excluded in all cases of histiocytoid Sweet's syndrome.

Pyoderma gangrenosum (PG)

- It is a diagnosis of exclusion: non-specific pathologic features
- Early lesions: neutrophilic infiltrate involving follicular structures

- Developed lesions: extensive, dense diffuse mixed-cell infiltrate with predominant neutrophils ("abscess-like") throughout the dermis

NB If PG involves the subcutaneous fat, the infiltrate changes to granulomatous.

- Secondary vascular injury
- Epidermal and dermal necrosis (in ulcerative PG)

Behçet's disease

Most common clinical findings are: oral and genital ulcers, uveitis, superficial thrombophlebitis, cutaneous pustules (induced by minor trauma: pathergy)

Early lesions:
- Leukocytoclastic vasculitis (possible pustular vasculitis, see LCV)
- Dense diffuse infiltrate of neutrophils with lymphocytes; histiocytes in the dermis

Late lesions: Lymphocytic vasculitis

Neutrophilic urticarial dermatoses

A spectrum of autoimmune connective disorders (adult-onset Still's disease, systemic lupus erythematosus and Schnitzler syndrome) characterized clinically by urticarial rash and histologically by neutrophilic infiltrates
- The epidermis is intact or with variable vacuolar alteration along the dermoepidermal junction
- Edema
- Interstitial and perivascular neutrophilic infiltrate with leukocytoclasia but no vasculitis **(Figure 3.114)**

NB The infiltrate extends from the top to the bottom of the specimen, including the subcutaneous fat (compare to the sparse neutrophils in the upper dermis in the neutrophilic subtype of urticaria (see Urticaria)).

SPONGIOTIC PATTERN

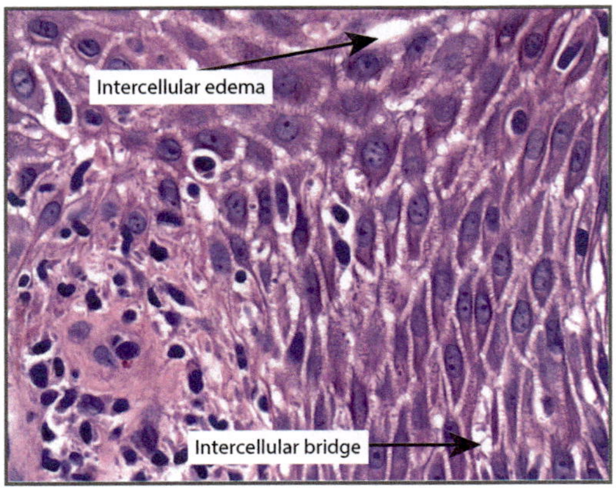

Figure 3.1 Keratinocytes are stretched apart by intercellular edema, highlighting the intercellular bridges.

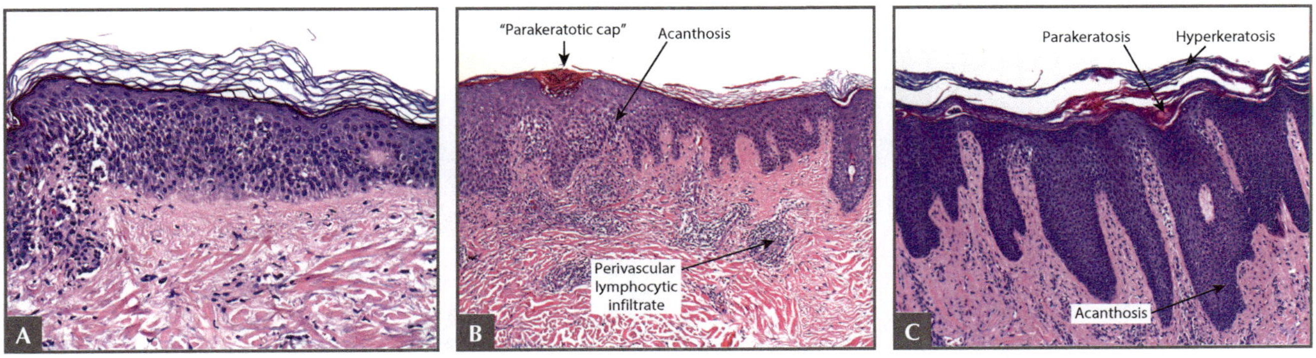

Figure 3.2 Spongiotic dermatitis. **A** Acute spongiotic dermatitis: note the marked spongiosis without parakeratosis and acanthosis. **B** Subacute spongiotic dermatitis: note the development of parakeratosis, acanthosis, and perviascular infiltrate in comparison to acute spongiotic dermatitis. **C** Chronic spongiotic dermatitis: note the thick hyperkeratosis with focal parakeratosis, pronounced acanthosis but only scarce spongiosis.

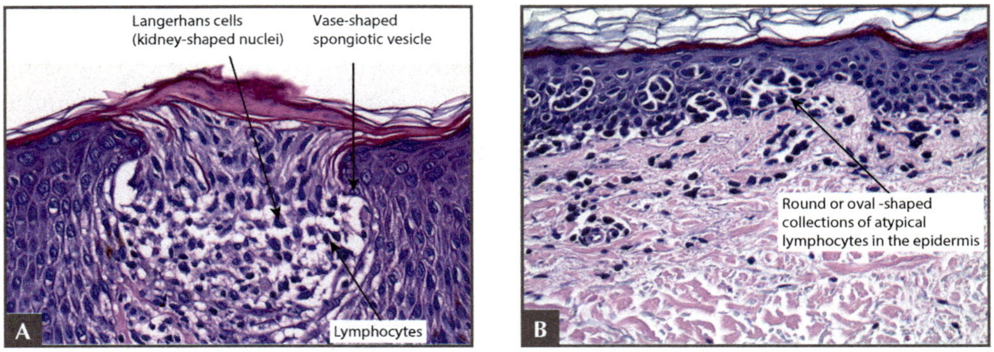

Figure 3.3 A A spongiotic vesicle has the shape of an upright vase. Note the presence of lymphocytes (exocytosis) and Langerhans cells. **B** Mycosis fungoides: note the round or oval shape of the Pautrier's microabscesses.

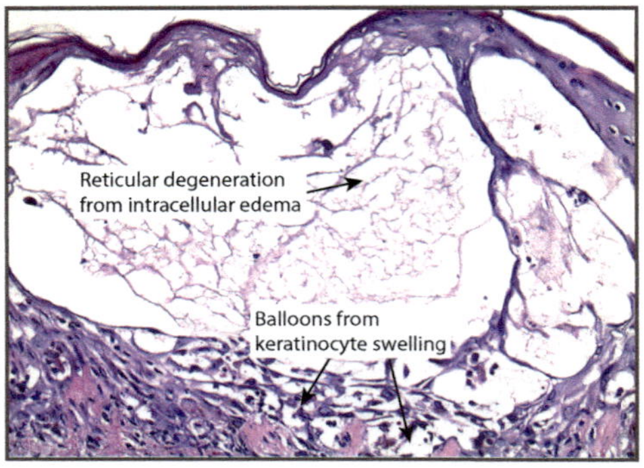

Figure 3.4 Ballooning degeneration evolving into reticular degeneration in viral exanthem.

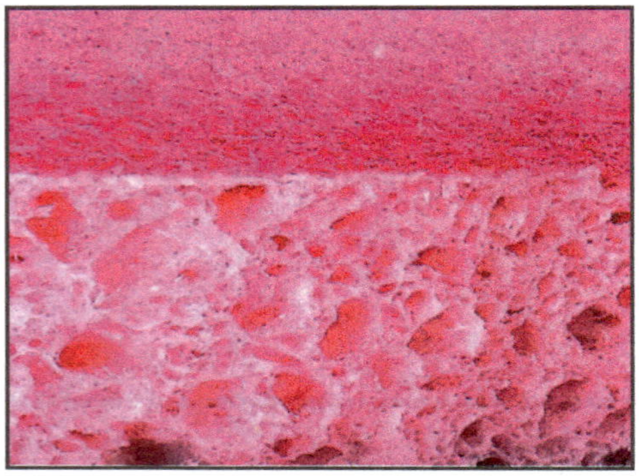

Photomnemonic 3.1 The pores in the sponge resemble the spaces in the epidermis formed by the intercellular edema.

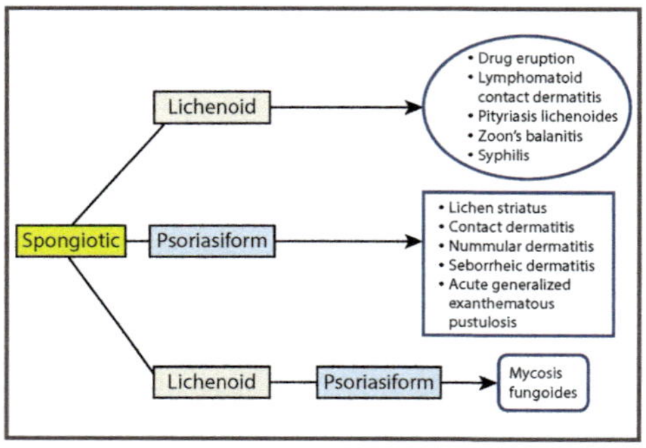

Figure 3.5 Spongiosis: overlap with other inflammatory patterns.

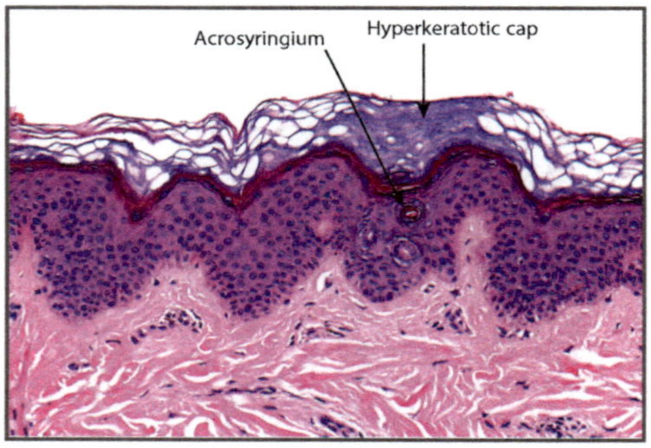

Figure 3.6 A hyperkeratotic cap covers the acrosyringium in atopic dermatitis.

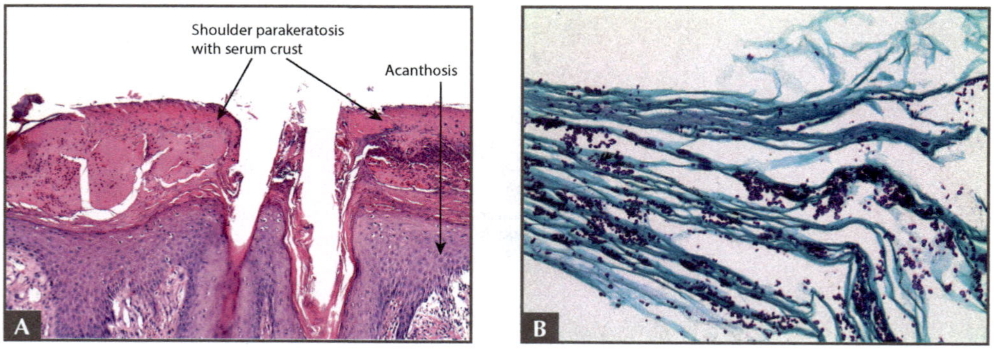

Figure 3.7 Seborrheic dermatitis. **A** Seborrheic dermatitis on the scalp: note the psoriasiform acanthosis, shoulder parakeratosis, and normal sebaceous glands; there is also a serum crust. **B** Yeast and spores of *Pityrosoporum* in the parakeratotic layer in seborrheic dermatitis (PAS stain).

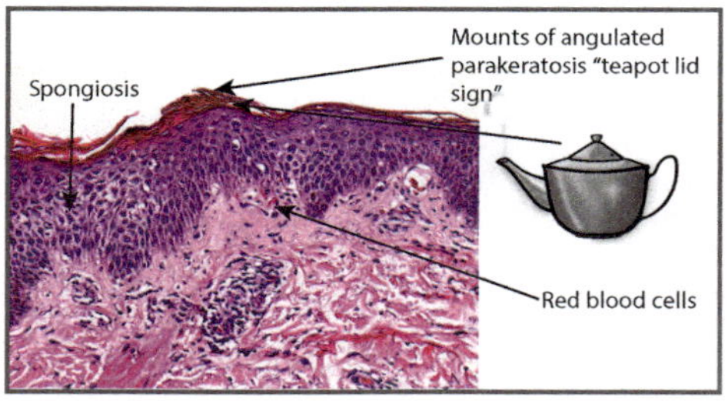

Photomnemonic 3.2 Pityriasis rosea, with mounds of angulated parakeratosis resembling the lid of a teapot ("teapot lid sign").

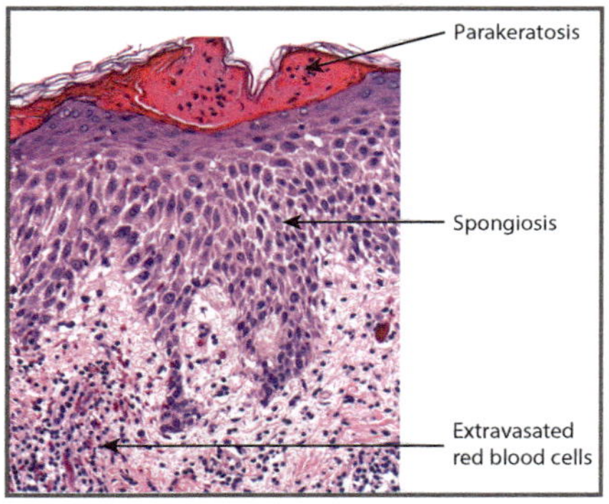

Figure 3.8 The vertical triad of angulated parakeratosis on top of spongiosis and red blood cell extravasation in the dermis suggests pityriasis rosea. Note also the acanthosis.

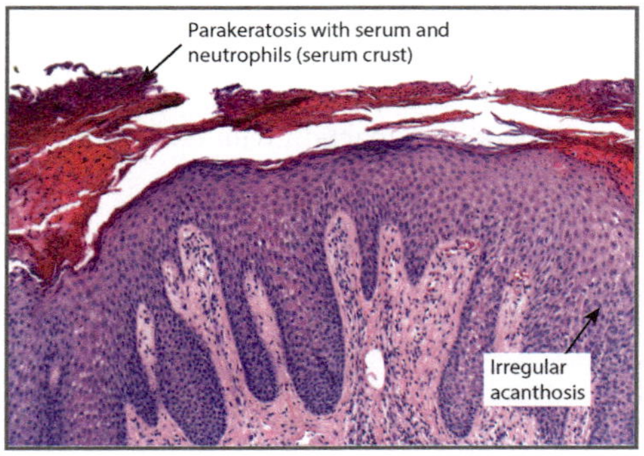

Figure 3.9 Nummular dermatitis showing parakeratosis with serum and neutrophils (serum crust) plus irregular acanthosis.

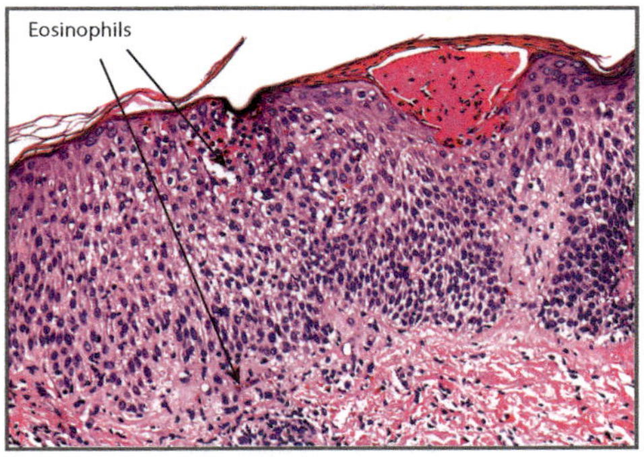

Figure 3.10 Eosinophilic spongiosis in allergic contact dermatitis.

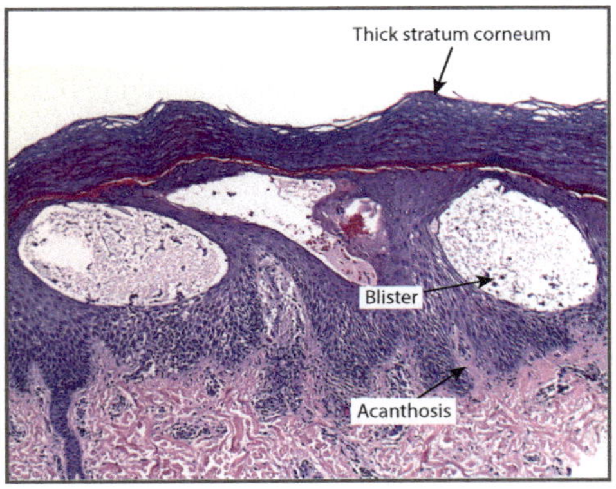

Figure 3.11 Pompholyx (dyshidrotic eczema). Note the pronounced spongiosis with blister formation.

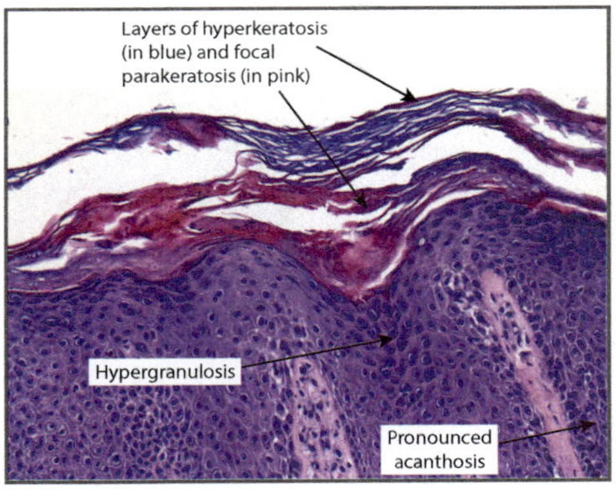

Figure 3.12 Lichen simplex chronicus: note the "acral look" of this lesion due to the thick stratum corneum.

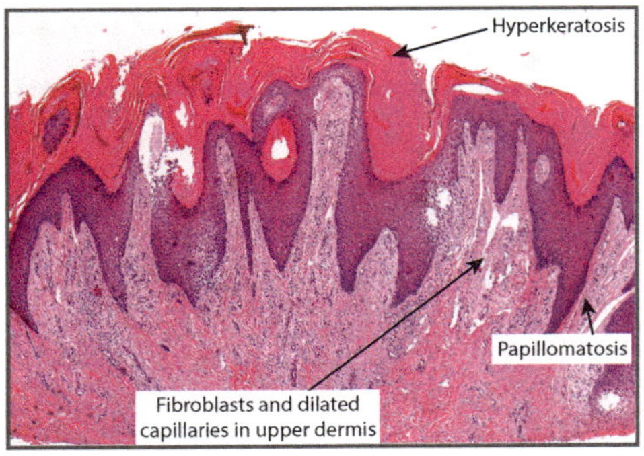

Figure 3.13 Prurigo nodularis: note the inward-pointing rete ridges and the presence of dilated capillaries and fibroblasts in the upper dermis.

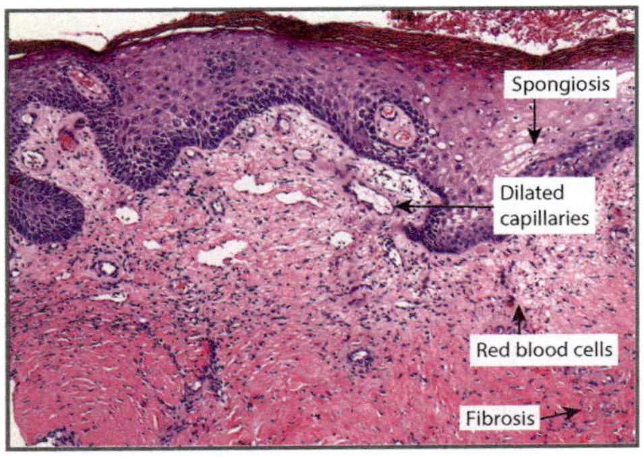

Figure 3.14 Stasis (venous) dermatitis: subacute spongiotic dermatitis. Clusters of dilated capillaries in the upper dermis with red blood cell extravasation, and fibrosis in the lower dermis, are clues to venous disease.

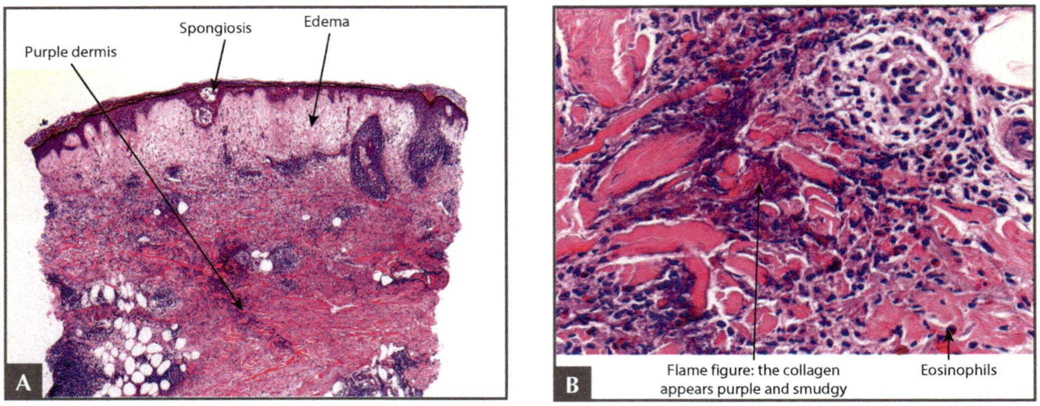

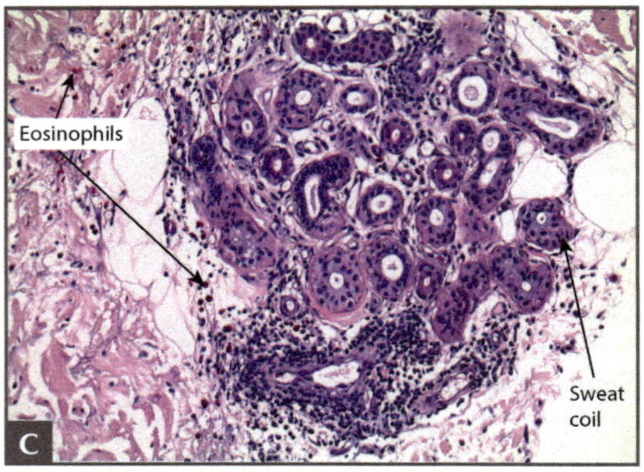

Figure 3.15 Arthropod bite reaction.
A Arthropod bite reaction with edema. **B** Flame figure in an arthropod bite reaction.
C Eosinophils around the sweat coils and ducts are a clue to an arthropod bite reaction.

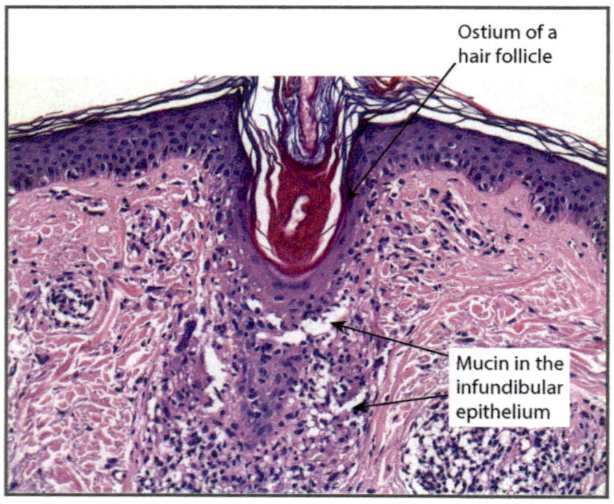

Figure 3.16 Follicular mucinosis. Note that the clear spaces within the follicular infundibulum are collections of mucin: compared to spongiosis there is no preservation of the keratinocyte bridges (compare to Figure 3.1).

INTERFACE DERMATITIS

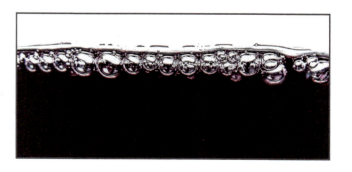

Photomnemonic 3.3 Vacuolar interface pattern resembles bubbles on a wine surface.

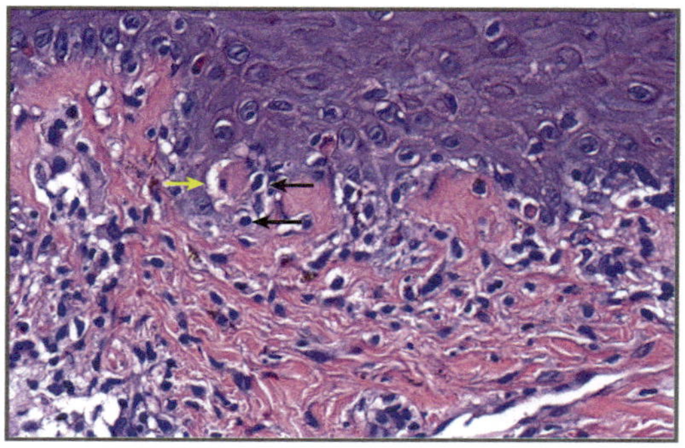

Figure 3.17 Satellite cell necrosis in GVHD. A necrotic keratinocyte (yellow arrow) is surrounded by two lymphocytes (black arrows) at the dermoepidermal junction.

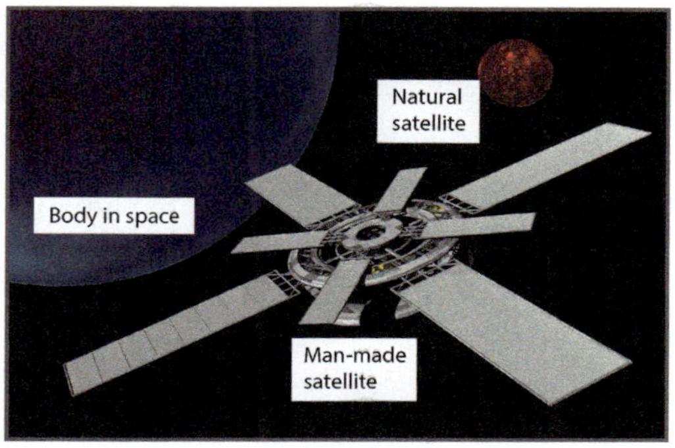

Photomnemonic 3.4 A satellite.

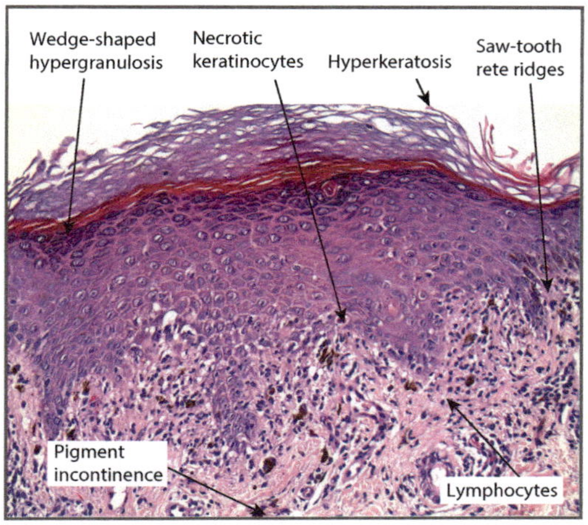

Figure 3.18 Lichen planus.

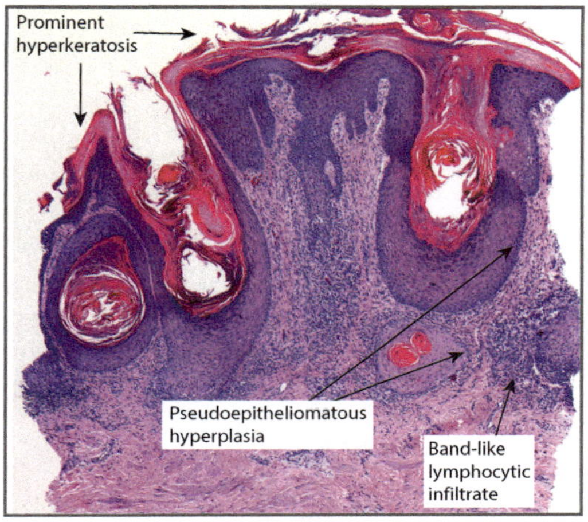

Figure 3.19 Hypertrophic lichen planus: note the thick bulbous expansion of the epidermis (pseudoepitheliomatous hyperplasia) covered by thick hyperkeratosis. There is also lymphocytic band-like infiltrate.

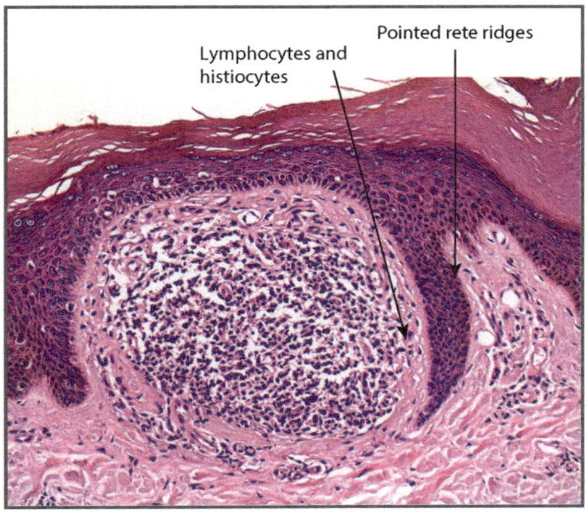

Figure 3.20 Lichen nitidus: A round aggregate of lymphocytes and histiocytes is locked by two adjacent rete ridges at the dermoepidermal junction. The thick stratum corneum is a clue to acral skin.

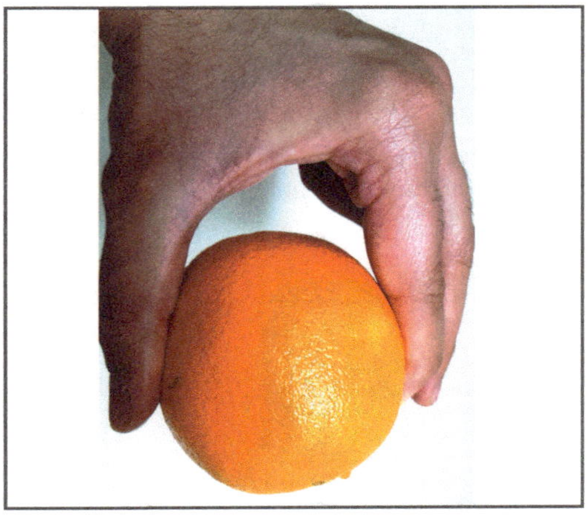

Photomnemonic 3.5 Lichen nitidus: "ball in a clutch."

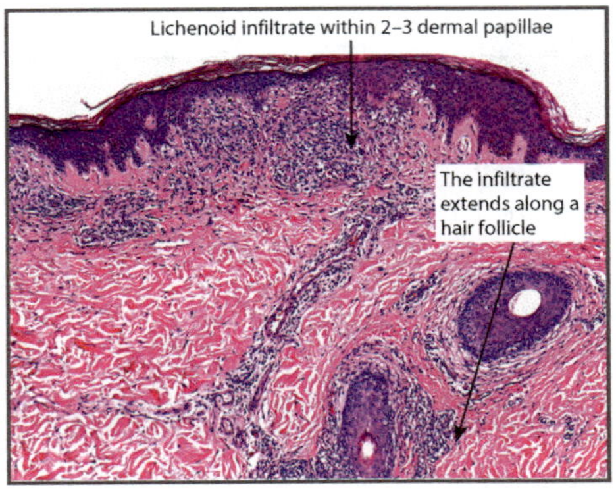

Figure 3.21 Lichen striatus. Note that the lichenoid infiltrate is present only at a portion of the dermoepidermal junction and it stretches down around the blood vessels and a hair follicle.

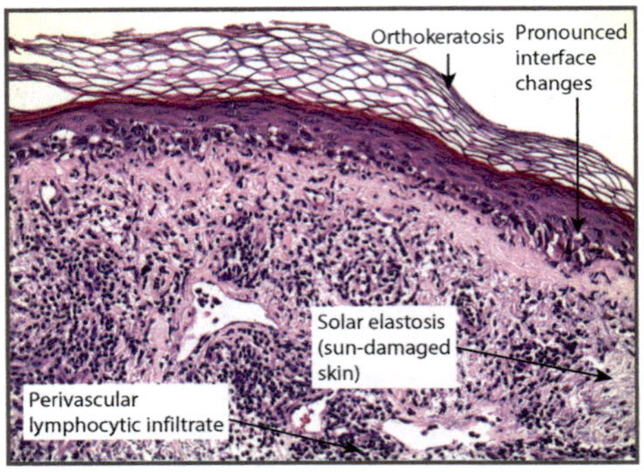

Figure 3.22 Lichenoid drug reaction: there is a combination of pronounced interface pattern and a superficial and deep perivascular pattern.

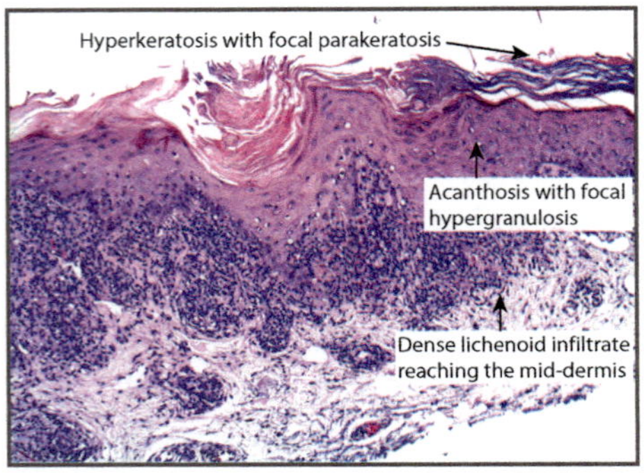

Figure 3.23 Lichenoid keratosis (lichen planus-like keratosis) can be indistinguishable from lichen planus on pathology.

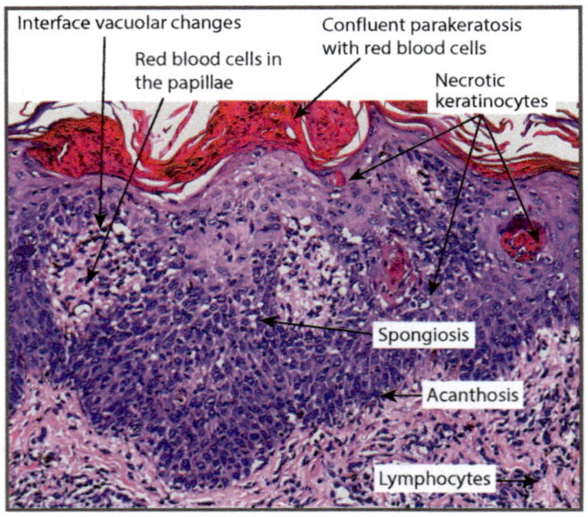

Figure 3.24 PLEVA: a busy epidermis and a busy stratum corneum.

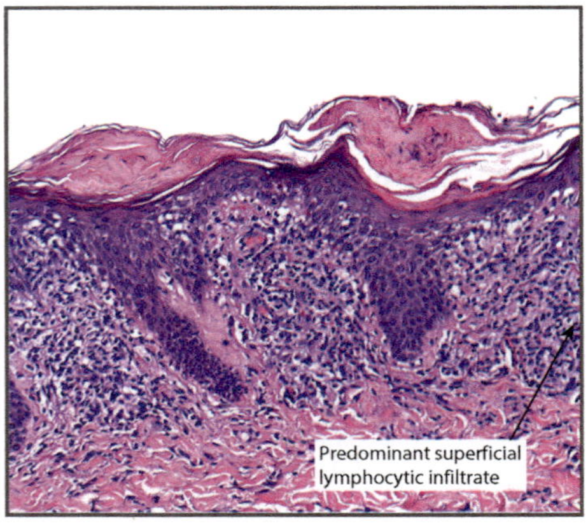

Figure 3.25 Pityriasis lichenoides chronica (PLC): there is a "busy" stratum corneum. Note the less pronounced acanthosis, spongiosis, and interface pattern compared to PLEVA.

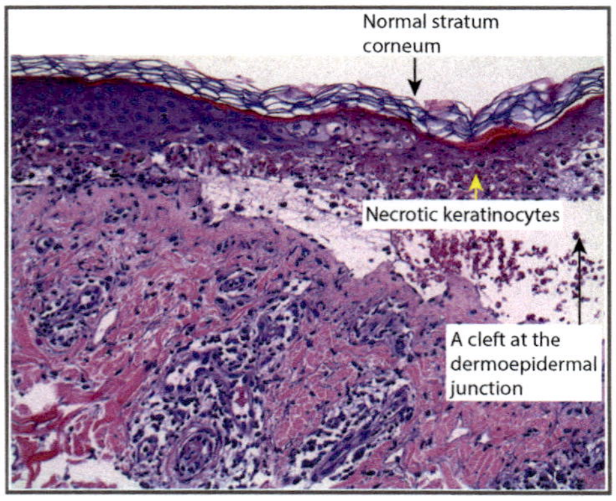

Figure 3.26 Erythema multiforme (EM): note the preserved basket-weave stratum corneum, the necrotic keratinocytes at all levels of the epidermis leading to a cleft at the dermoepidermal junction. There is no band-like infiltrate.

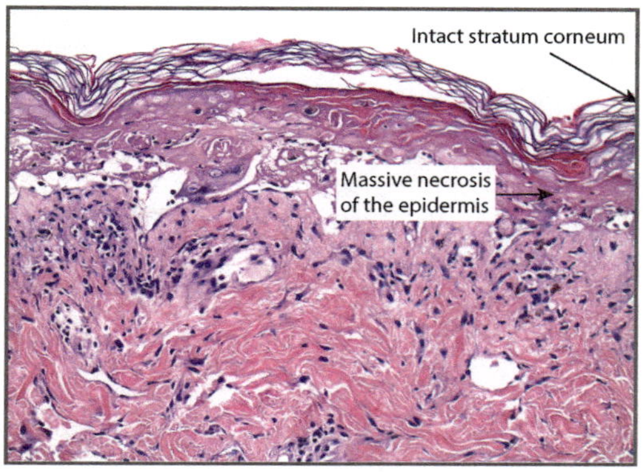

Figure 3.27 Toxic epidermal necrolysis: the epidermis shows a confluent mass of necrotic keratinocytes.

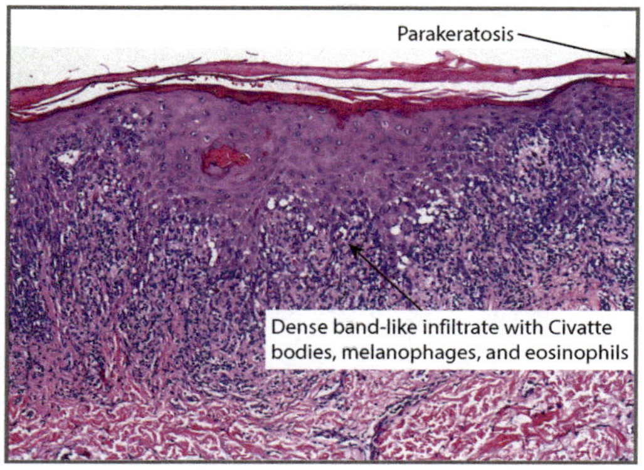

Figure 3.28 Fixed drug eruption: note the presence of parakeratosis and dense band-like infiltrate with numerous Civatte bodies, melanophages, and eosinophils compared to EM.

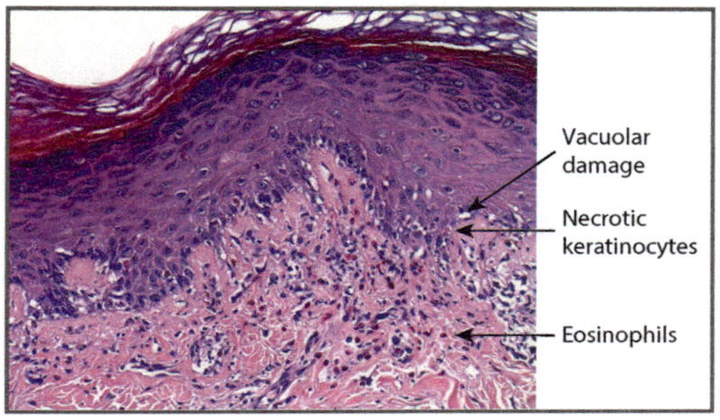

Figure 3.29 Acute graft-versus-host disease (GVHD): vacuolization at the dermoepidermal junction with necrotic keratinocytes at all levels of the epidermis, satellite cell necrosis, and eosinophils in the dermis.

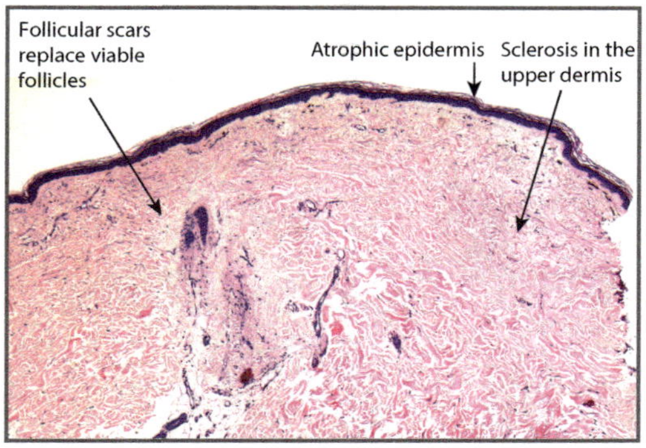

Figure 3.30 Sclerodermoid (lichen sclerosus and atrophicus-like) GVHD: upper dermal sclerosis and disappearance of the adnexal structures.

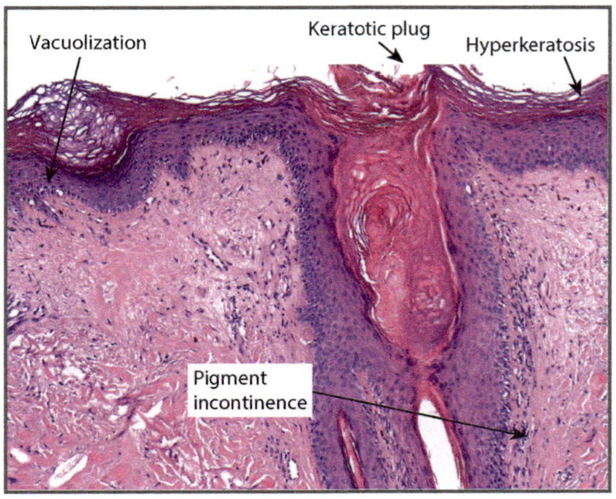

Figure 3.31 Discoid lupus erythematosus. Note the dilated infundibulum with the keratotic plug, the thickened basement membrane, and the interface changes involving also the follicular epithelium.

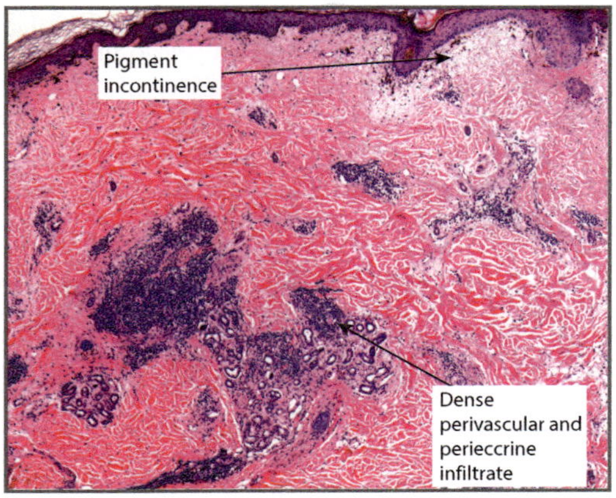

Figure 3.32 Discoid lupus erythematosus: there is dense periadnexal infiltrate.

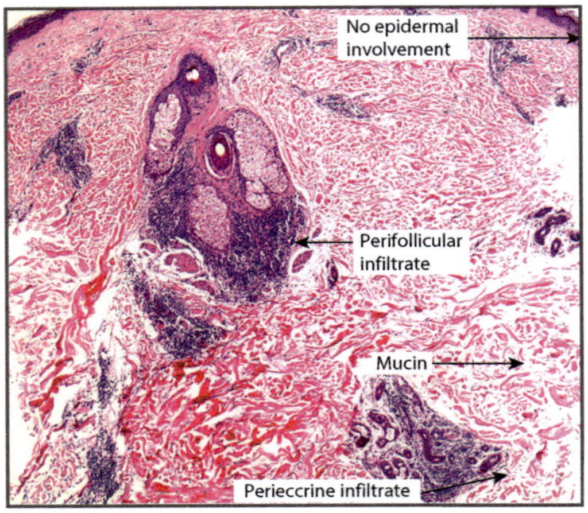

Figure 3.33 Tumid lupus erythematosus: there is no junctional involvement, the dermis looks pale due to deposition of mucin, and the infiltrate may extend deep around the adnexal structures.

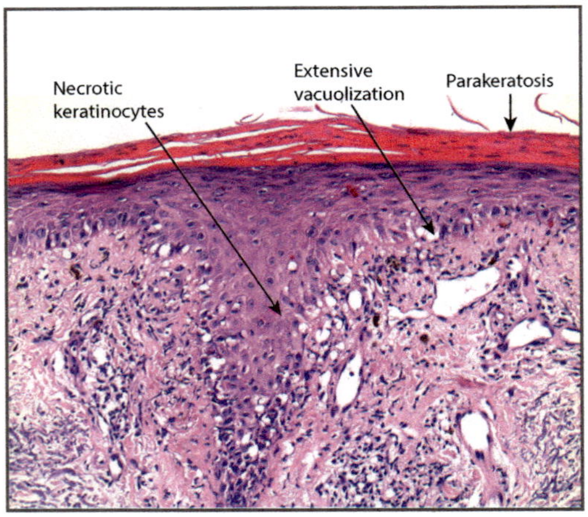

Figure 3.34 Subacute cutaneous lupus erythematosus. In this specimen from a psoriasiform lesion, note the parakeratosis and the pronounced interface change.

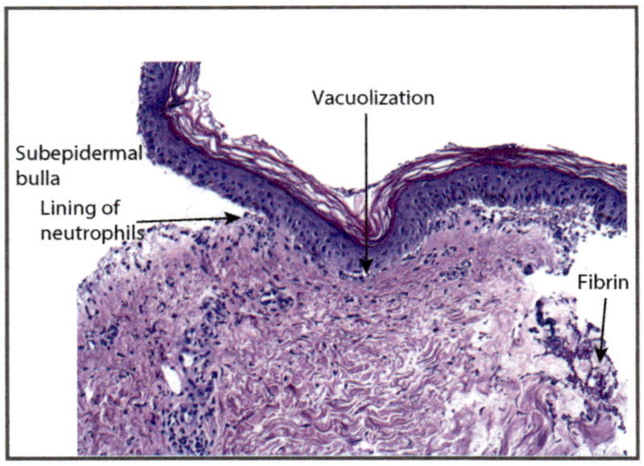

Figure 3.35 Bullous lupus erythematosus: there is a pronounced subepidermal blister with neutrophils lining its floor; there is also fibrin in the dermis.

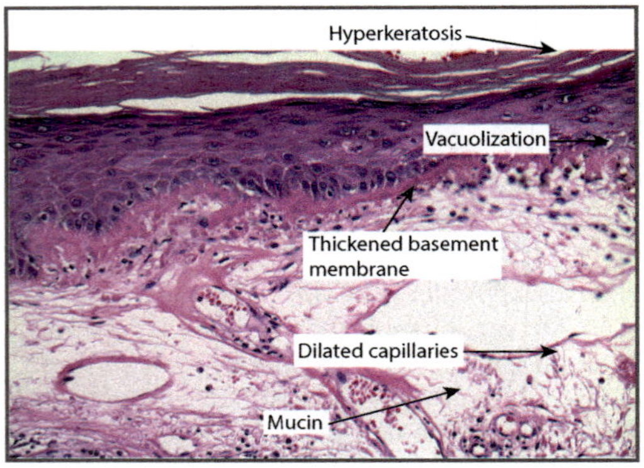

Figure 3.36 Dermatomyositis. This image is indistinguishable from lupus erythematosus. Note the vacuolization, the thickened basement membrane, the increased mucin in the dermis, and the dilated capillaries.

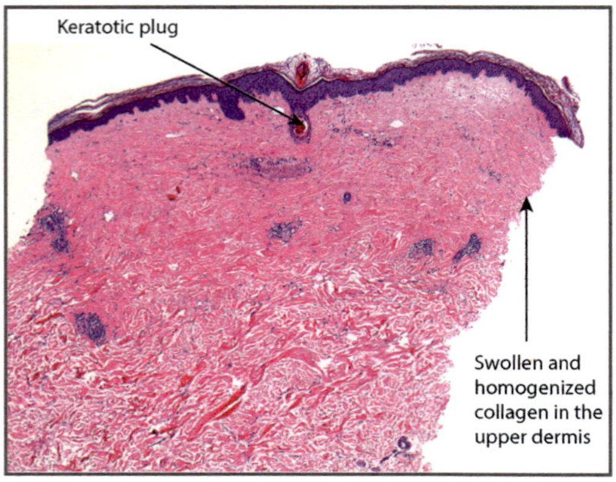

Figure 3.37 Lichen sclerosis et atrophicus (LSA): The stratum corneum is as thick as the thinned epidermis, and there are homogenized pale collagen bundles in the upper dermis.

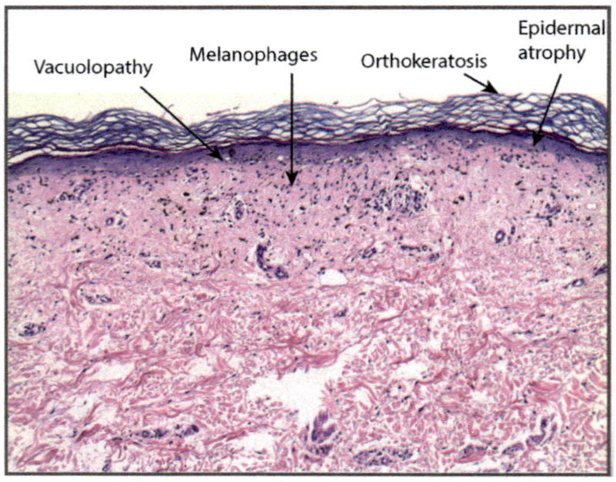

Figure 3.38 Ashy dermatosis: the epidermis is atrophic, and there is mild vacuolar change at the dermoepidermal junction with numerous melanophages in the papillary dermis.

PSORIASIFORM PATTERN

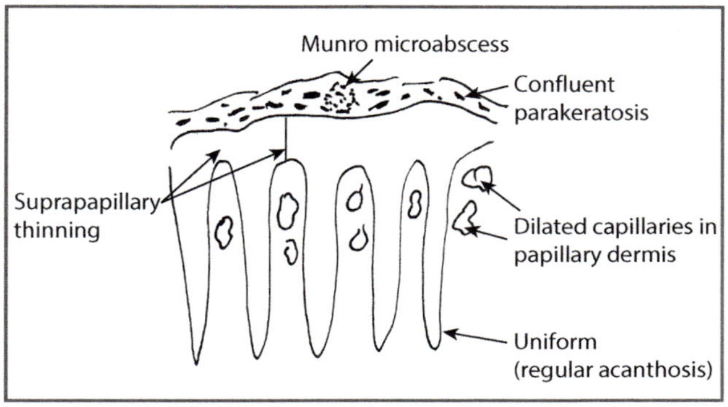

Figure 3.39 Psoriasis is the classic prototype of the psoriasiform pattern.

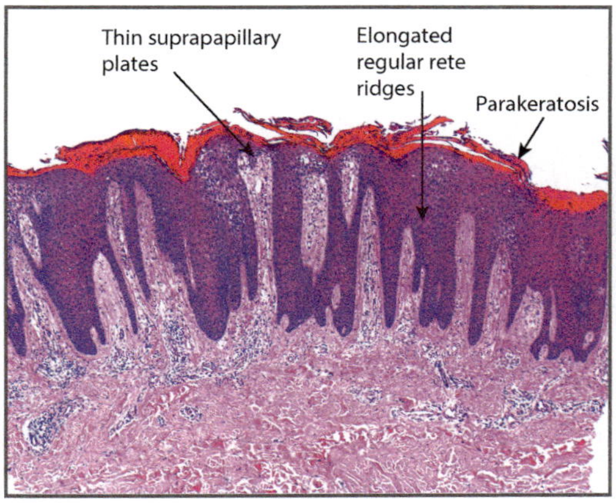

Figure 3.40 Psoriasis is characterized by regular acanthosis of the rete ridges with suprapapillary thinning, hypogranulosis, and parakeratosis.

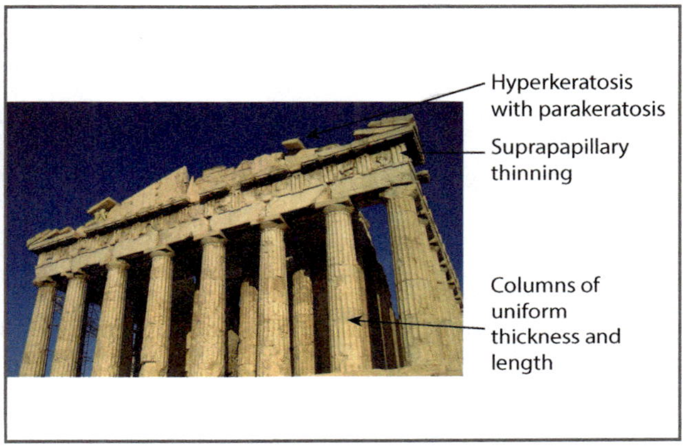

Photomnemonic 3.6 The regularly elongated and thin rete ridges in psoriasis resemble columns in the Parthenon.

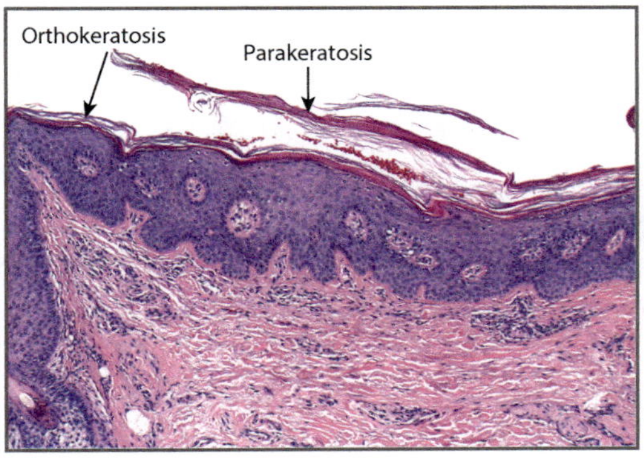

Figure 3.41 Guttate psoriasis: note the much less pronounced acanthosis as well as the mounds of parakeratosis with orthokeratosis.

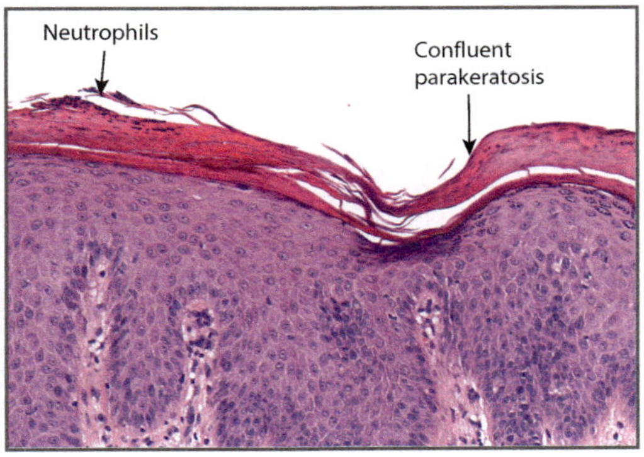

Figure 3.42 Plaque psoriasis: note the absence of granular layer and the confluent parakeratosis with neutrophils (Munro microabscess).

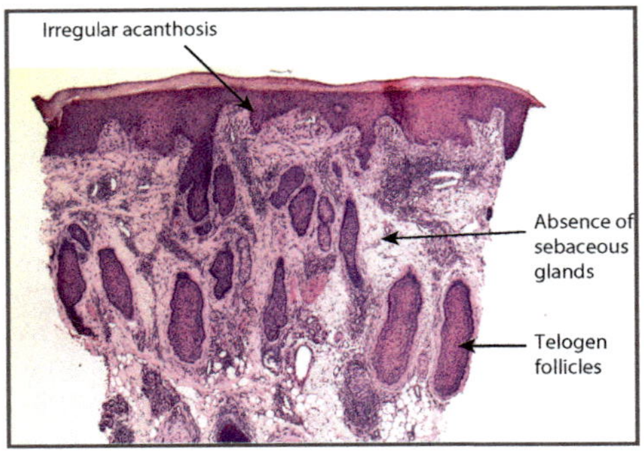

Figure 3.43 In scalp psoriasis there is irregular acanthosis, increased telogen count, and the sebaceous glands are atrophic or absent.

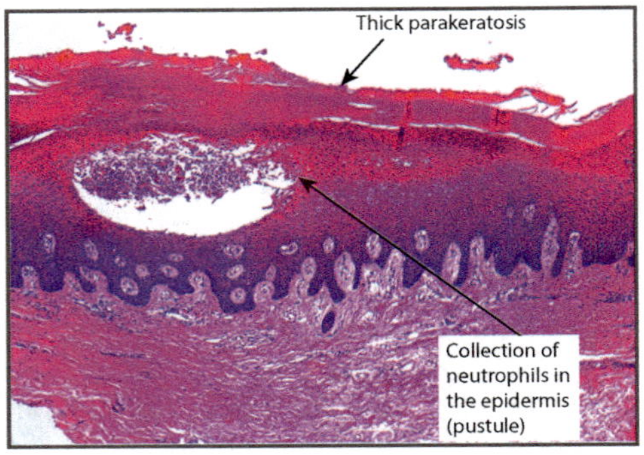

Figure 3.44 Palmo-plantar pustular psoriasis: there is a large pustule of Kogoj in the spinous layer.

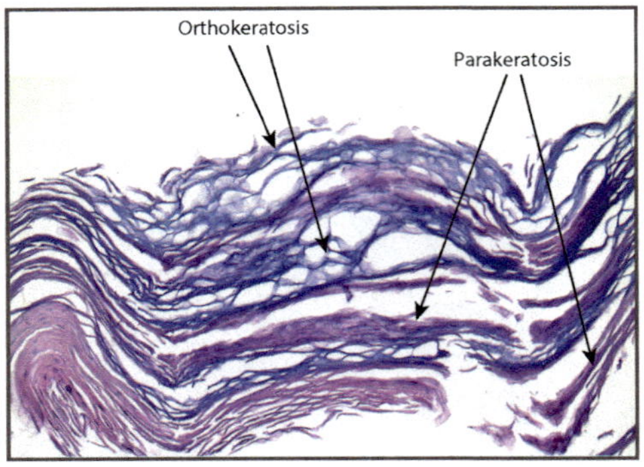

Figure 3.45 Pityriasis rubra pilaris: the scale shows the checkerboard pattern of alternating orthokeratosis and parakeratosis in horizontal and vertical tiers.

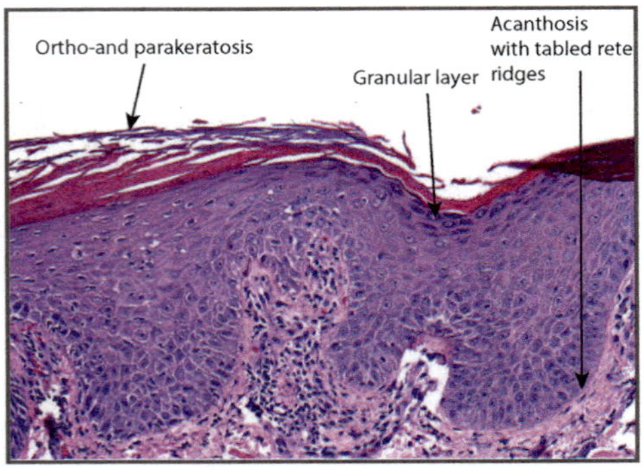

Figure 3.46 Pityriasis rubra pilaris: note the thick tabled rete ridges and alternating ortho- and parakeratosis.

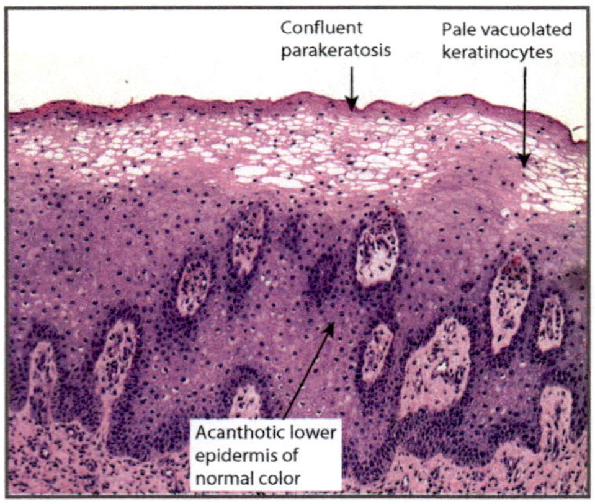

Figure 3.47 Nutritional dermatosis (zinc deficiency): note the tricolored layers of the epidermis, which is also acanthotic.

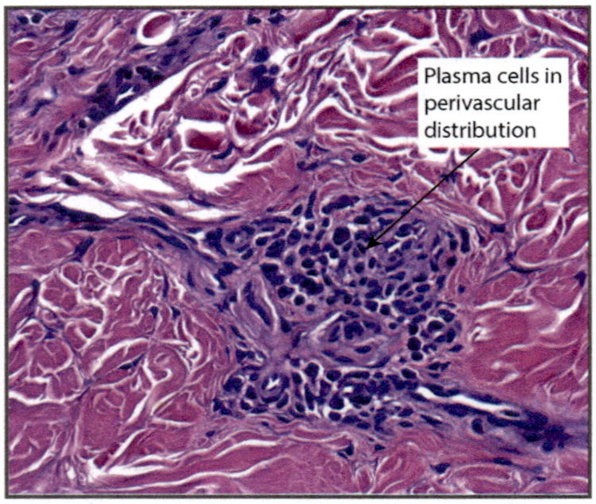

Figure 3.48 Syphilis: there is perivascular infiltrate of plasma cells in the dermis.

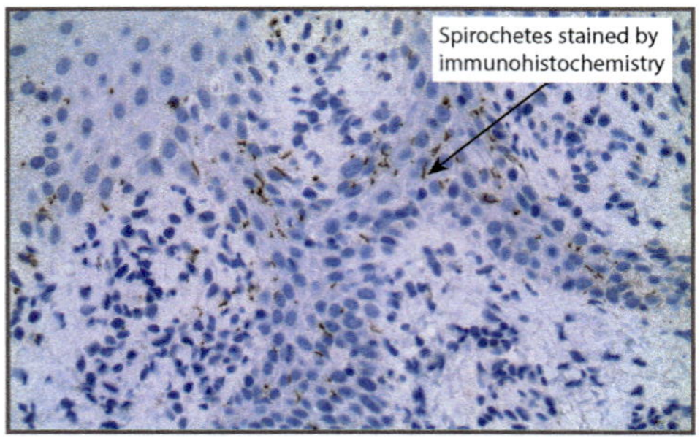

Figure 3.49 Anti-*Treponema pallidum* antibody stains the spirochetes in the acanthotic epidermis in syphilis.

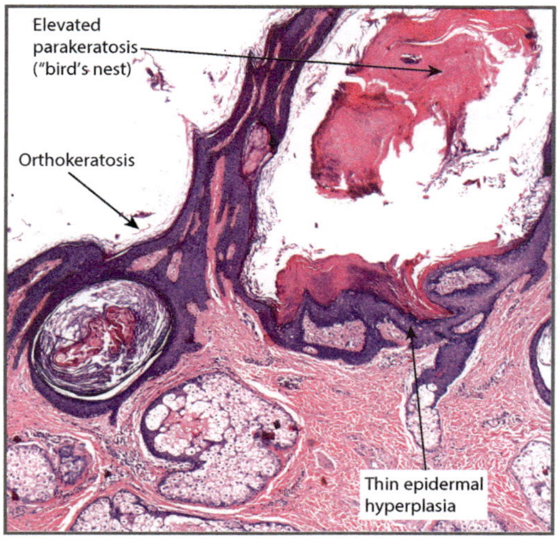

Figure 3.50 Inflammatory linear verrucous epidermal nevus (ILVEN): there is acanthosis with alternating depressed orthokeratosis and elevated parakeratosis.

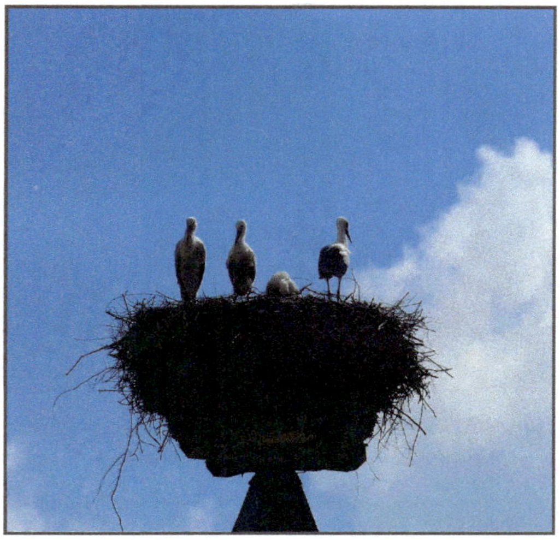

Photomnemonic 3.7 Elevated parakeratosis in ILVEN resembles a bird's nest.

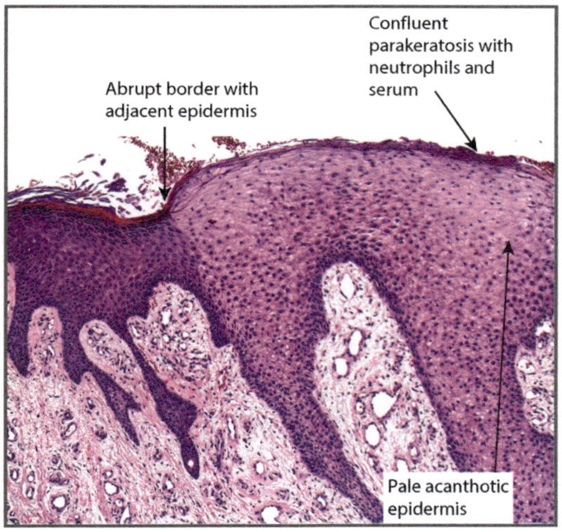

Figure 3.51 Clear cell acanthoma: there is pale acanthosis covered by confluent parakeratosis with neutrophils.

SUPERFICIAL AND DEEP PERIVASCULAR DERMATITIS

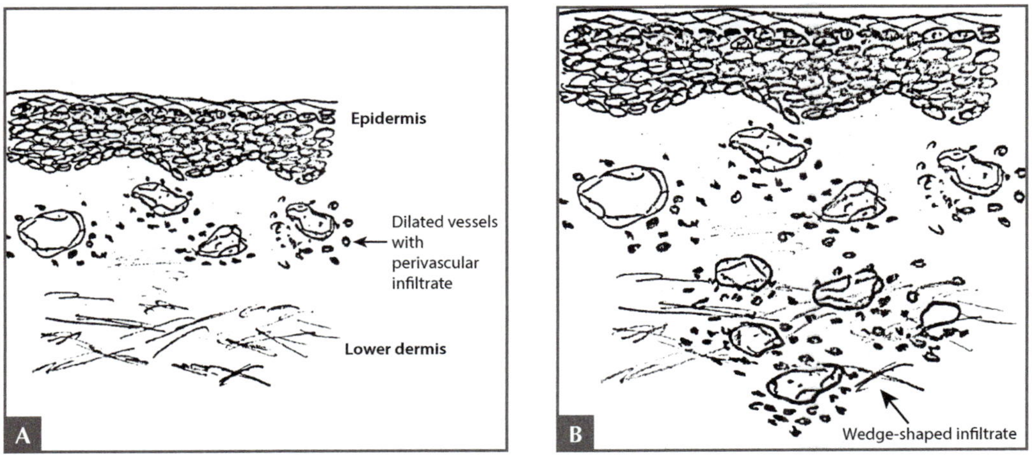

Figure 3.52 Superficial and deep perivascular dermatitis. **A** The superficial perivascular infiltrate is flat-bottomed. **B** The superficial and deep perivascular infiltrate is wedge-shaped.

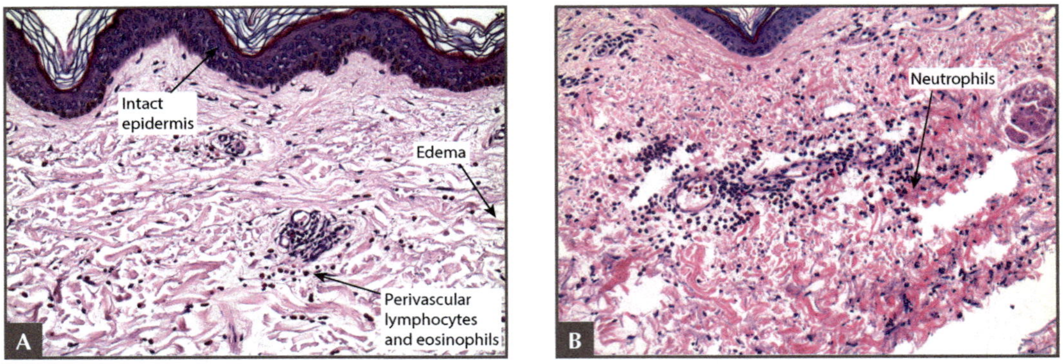

Figure 3.53 Urticaria. **A** In urticaria there is a subtle perivascular infiltrate of lymphocytes and eosinophils. **B** In neutrophilic urticaria the neutrophils are sparse and mainly in the upper dermis.

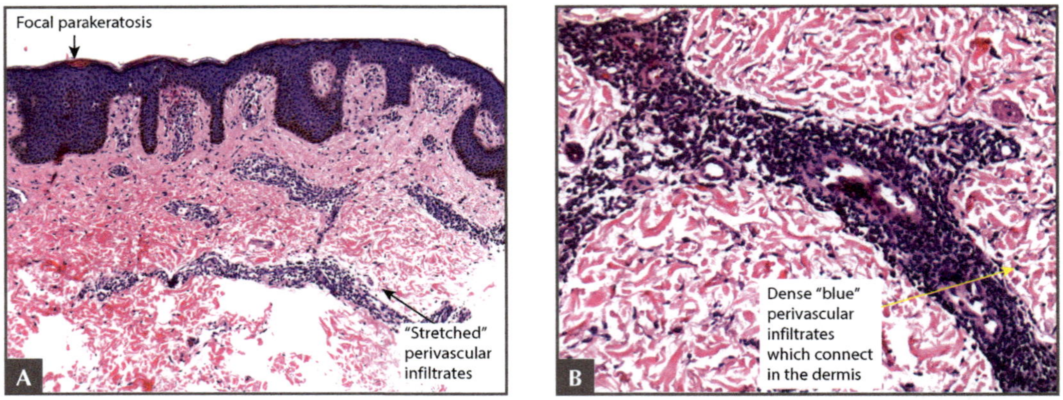

Figure 3.54 Erythema annulare centrifugum. **A** Superficial type: note the epidermal involvement. **B** Deep type: there are deep, tight perivascular infiltrates resembling a blue coat sleeve.

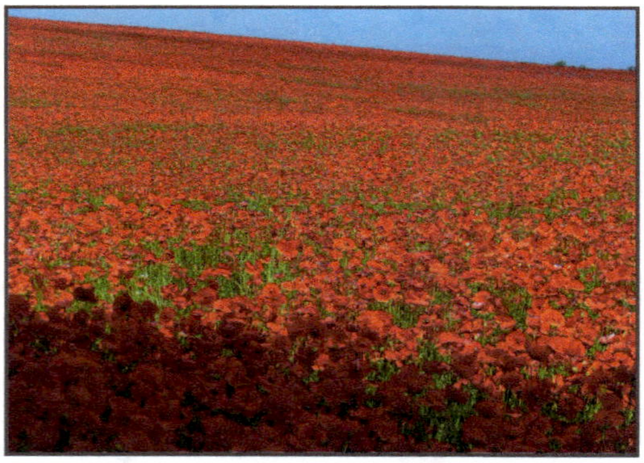

Photomnemonic 3.8 A dense infiltrate of eosinophils in Well's syndrome resembles a red poppy field.

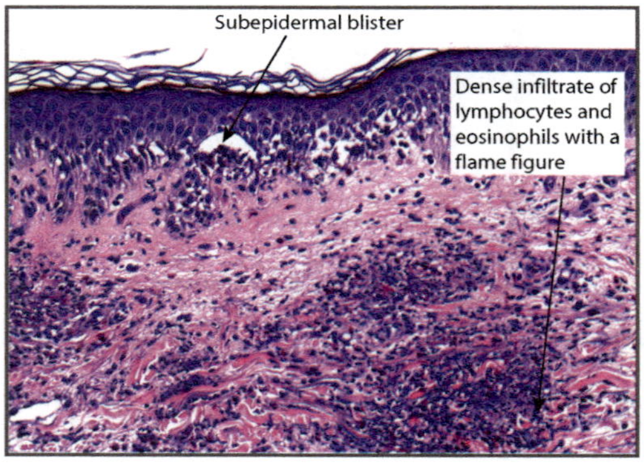

Figure 3.55 Wells' syndrome (eosinophilic cellulitis): note the flame figure in the dermis.

GRANULOMATOUS DERMATITIS

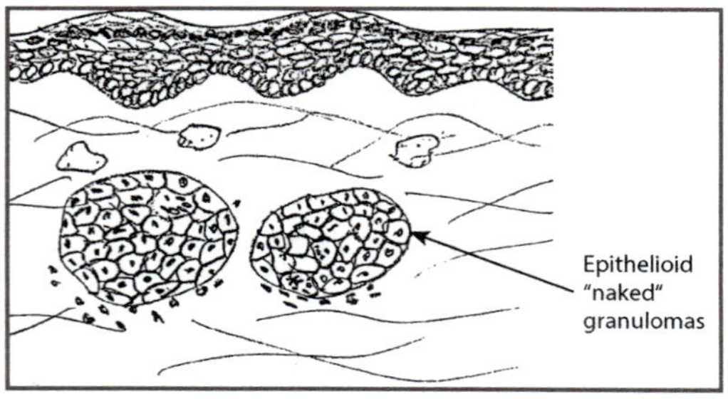

Figure 3.56 Sarcoidal granulomas are aggregates of epithelioid cells without or with a sparse mantle of lymphocytes.

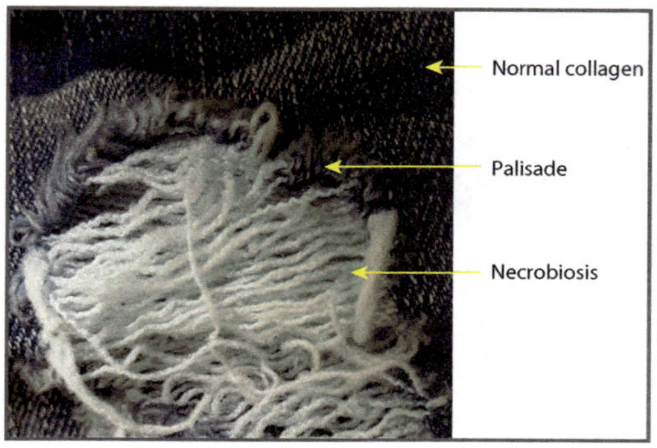

Photomnemonic 3.9 A palisading granuloma resembles a ripped patch on jeans.

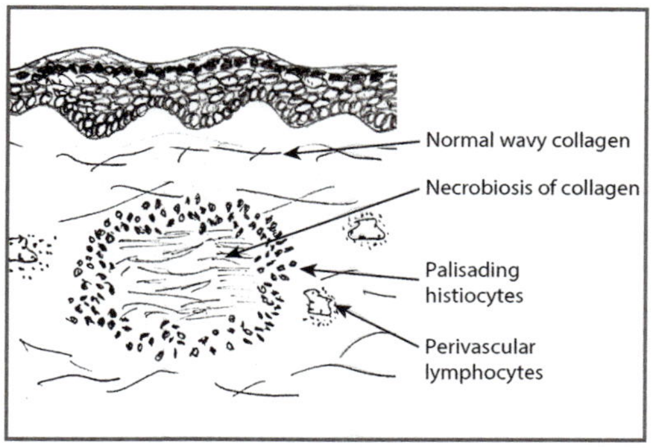

Figure 3.57 Palisading granulomas usually show central necrobiosis and a palisade of histiocytes.

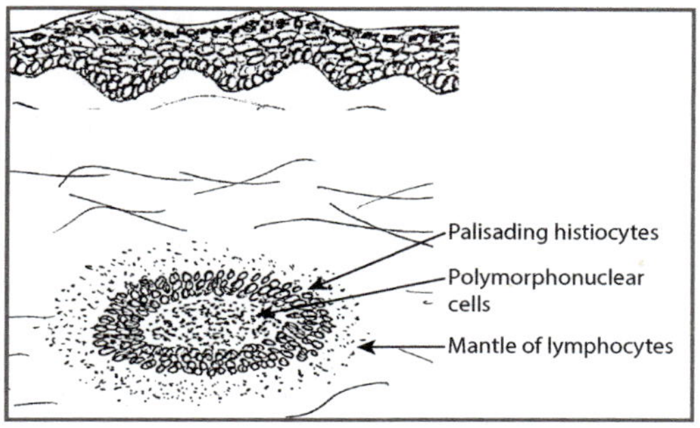

Figure 3.58 Suppurative granulomas are organized in layers: neutrophils form the core, surrounded by a palisade of histiocytes and an outer mantle of lymphocytes.

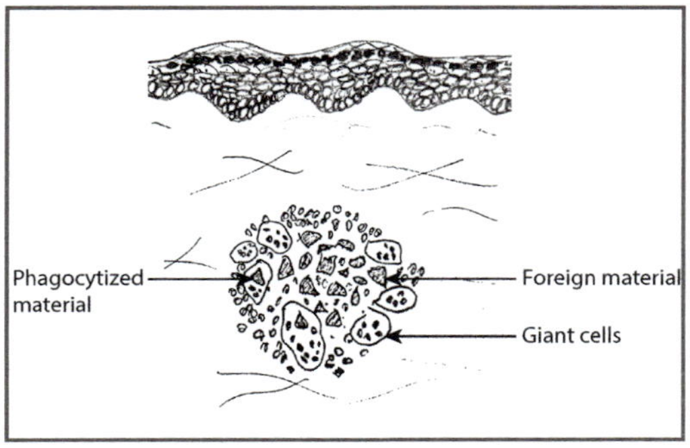

Figure 3.59 Foreign body granulomas are aggregates of histiocytes and giant cells among and around foreign material.

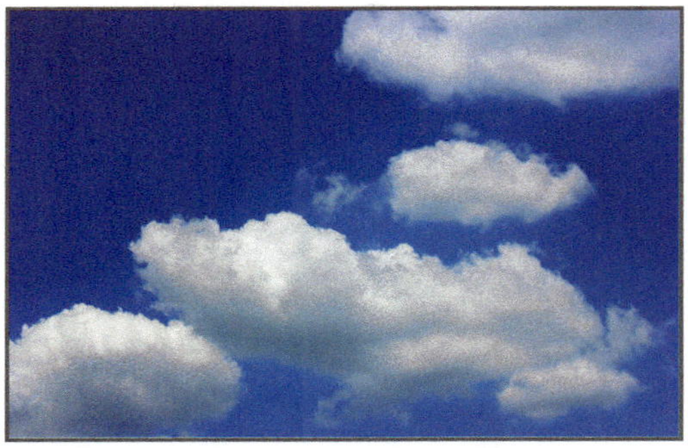

Photomnemonic 3.10 Granulomas are pale aggregates because they are composed of histiocytes which have a pale cytoplasm.

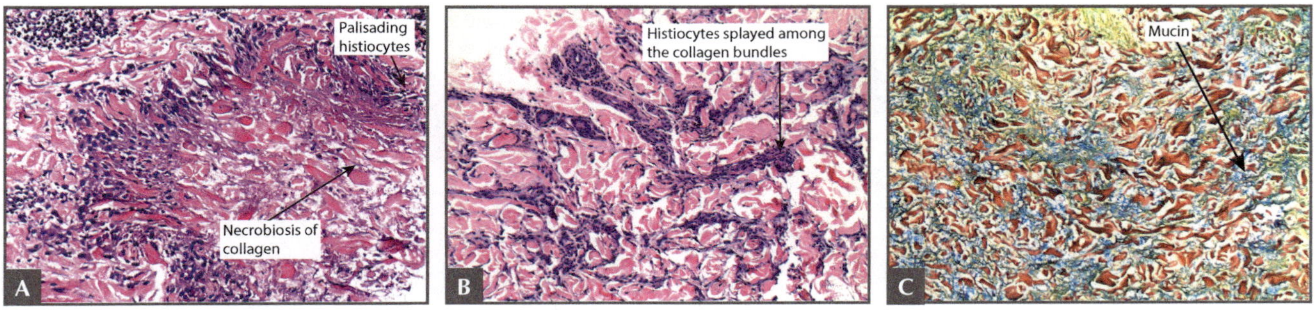

Figure 3.60 Granuloma annulare (GA). **A** Palisading GA: the collagen is degenerated and shows a pale hue due to presence of mucin. **B** Interstitial GA: there are histiocytes splayed among the collagen bundles. **C** Colloidal iron highlights the interstitial deposition of mucin in a case of interstitial GA.

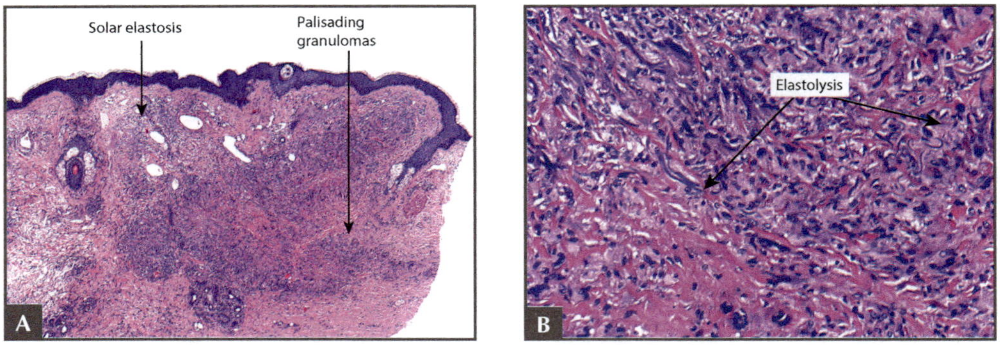

Figure 3.61 Actinic granuloma. **A** Actinic granuloma showing a palisading granuloma on a background of solar elastosis. Note the absence of necrobiosis. **B** Elastolytic granuloma showing elastolysis: the elastic tissue is fragmented and phagocytized.

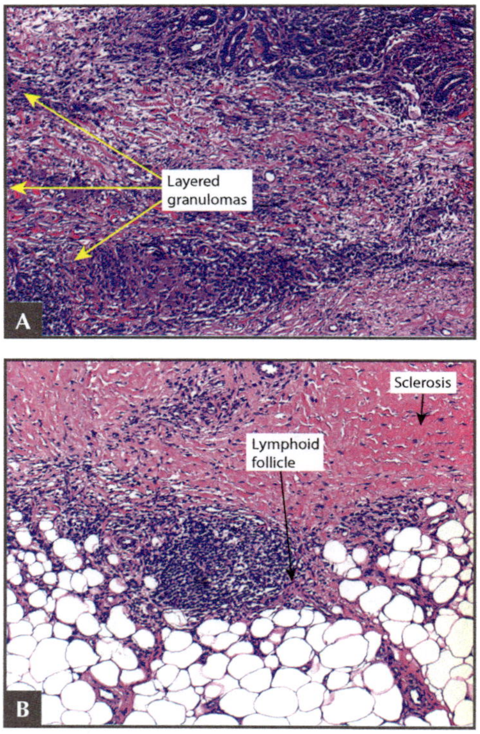

Figure 3.62 Necrobiosis lipoidica (NLD). **A** Layered histiocytic infiltrate (tiered granulomas) in the sclerotic dermis. **B** Note the lymphoid follicles in the deep dermis.

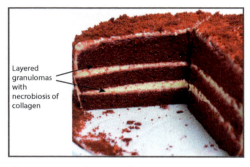

Photomnemonic 3.11 The tiered arrangement of the granulomatous infiltrate in NLD resembles a layered cake.

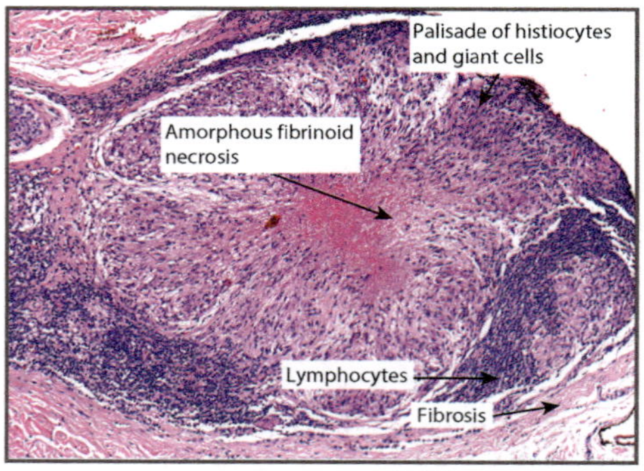

Figure 3.63 Rheumatoid nodule. The granuloma is in the deep reticular dermis and shows pronounced fibrinoid necrosis in the center.

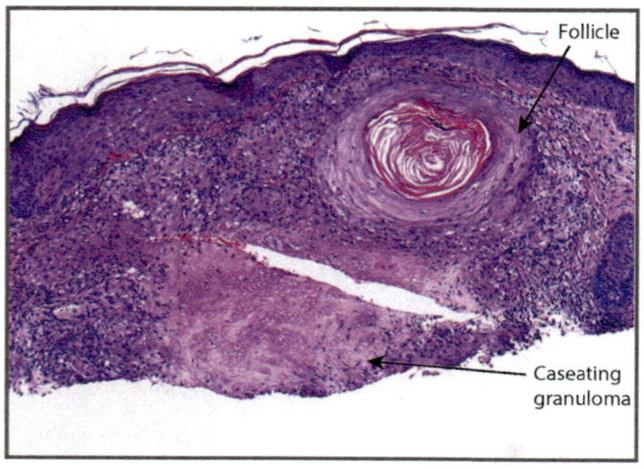

Figure 3.64 Lupus miliaris disseminatus faciei: there is a perifollicular caseating granuloma.

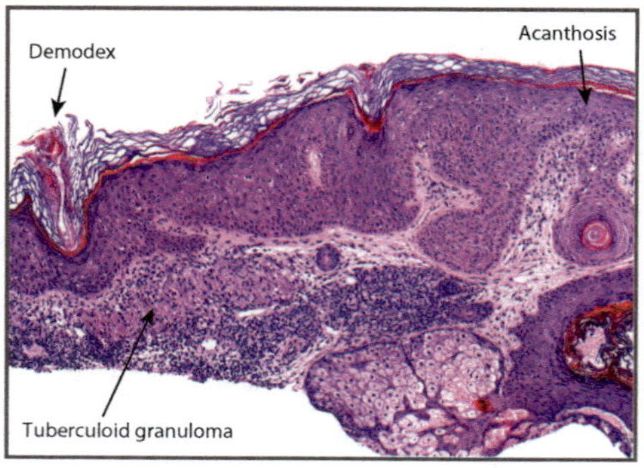

Figure 3.65 Granulomatous rosacea: there is a tuberculoid granuloma in the upper dermis (collection of epithelioid cells surrounded by a mantle of lymphocytes).

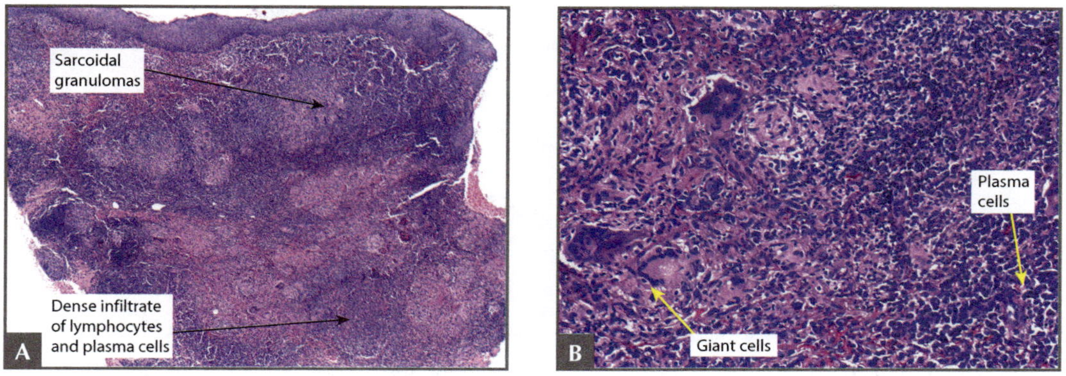

Figure 3.66 Crohn's disease, a metastatic lesion. **A** In Crohn's disease there are sarcoidal granulomas in a sea of dense inflammation which occupy the entire dermis. **B** Note the dense infiltrate of lymphocytes and plasma cells.

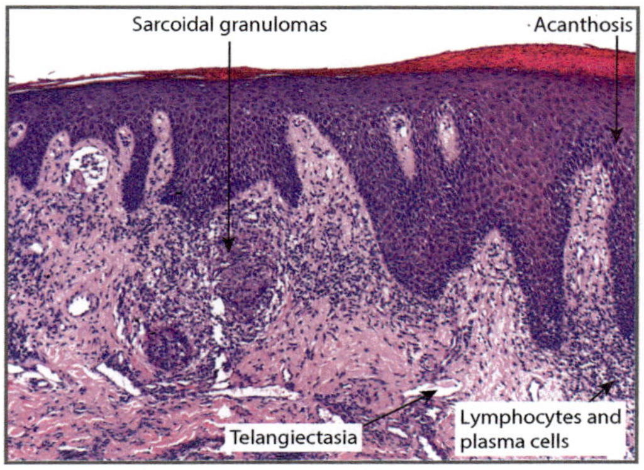

Figure 3.67 Granulomatous cheilitis: there are small sarcoidal granulomas in the dermis and dense infiltrate of lymphocytes and plasma cells.

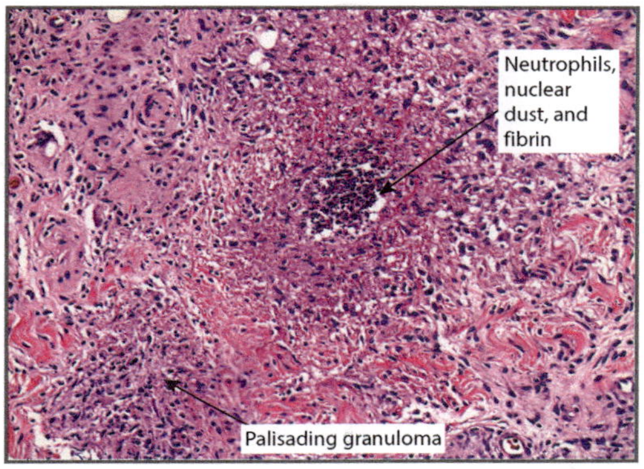

Figure 3.68 Palisaded neutrophilic granulomatous dermatitis (PNGD). The pattern is similar to GA but has a bluish hue due to the presence of neutrophils and fibrin mixed with mucin.

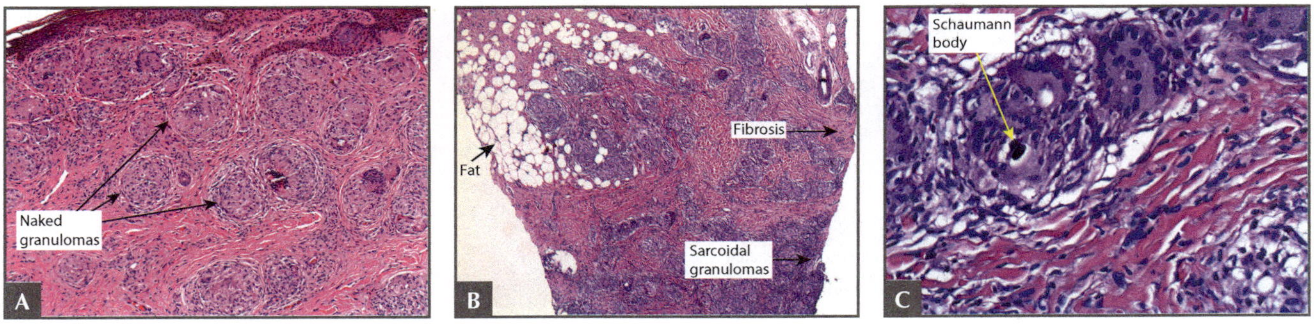

Figure 3.69 Sarcoidosis. **A** Naked granulomas in sarcoidosis. **B** In Darier-Roussy subcutaneous sarcoidosis, the granulomas infiltrate the subcutaneous fat. **C** Schaumann body in sarcoidosis.

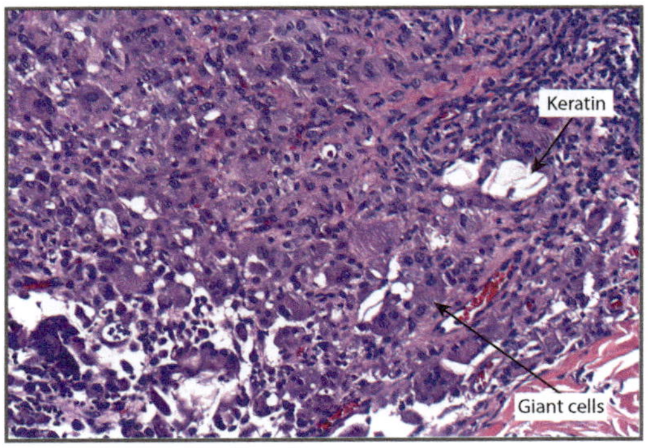

Figure 3.70 Keratin granuloma is a ruptured cyst: note the presence of angulated shaped keratin fragments within the giant cells. There is also a mixed cell infiltrate.

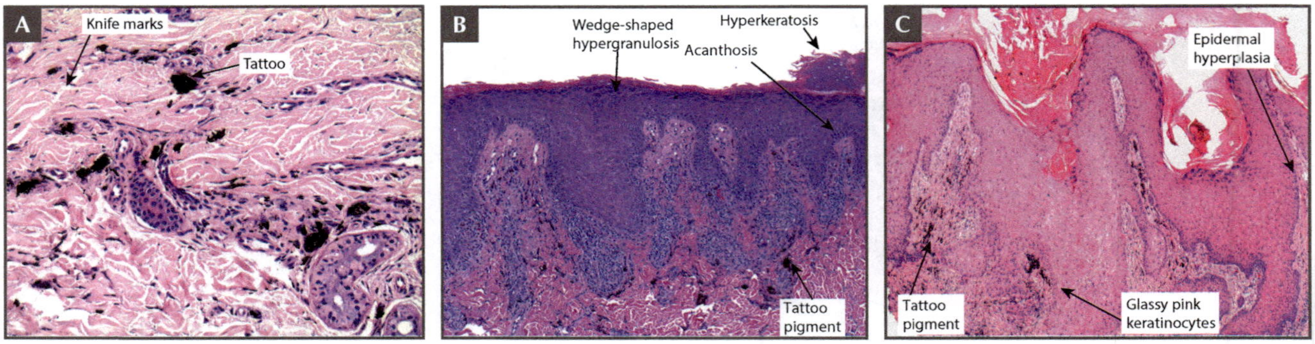

Figure 3.71 Tattoo. **A** Graphite tattoo: note the thick black pigment around the vessels in the dermis. **B** Lichenoid reaction to tattoo. **C** A keratoacanthoma-like reaction to tattoo.

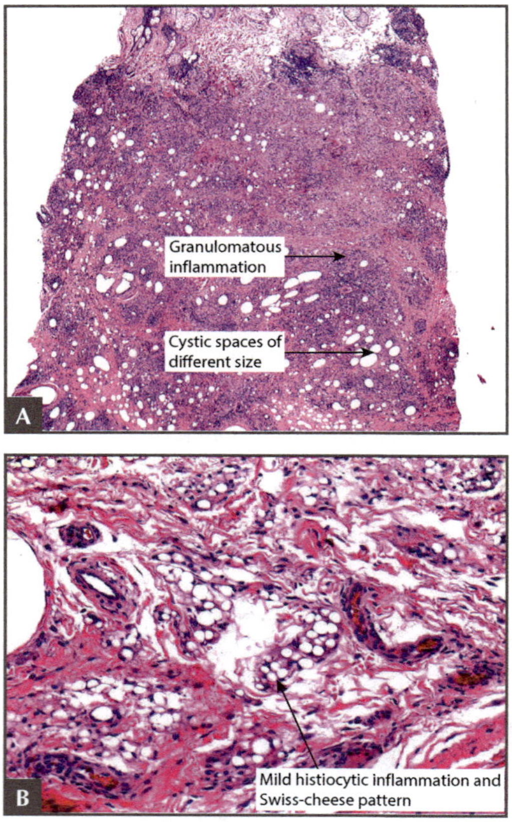

Figure 3.72 Foreign body granuloma. **A** Foreign body reaction to solid silicone elastomers (granuloma). Dense granulomatous inflammation with fibrosis replaces the dermis and subdermis. Note many cystic-shaped spaces which correspond to the silicone material. **B** Foreign body reaction to liquid silicone (siliconoma). Note the sparse histiocytic inflammation around the Swiss cheese-like cystic spaces.

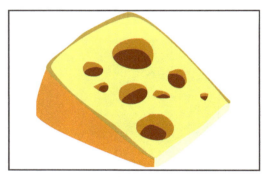

Photomnemonic 3.12 Silicone particles in a foreign body granuloma resemble the holes in Swiss cheese.

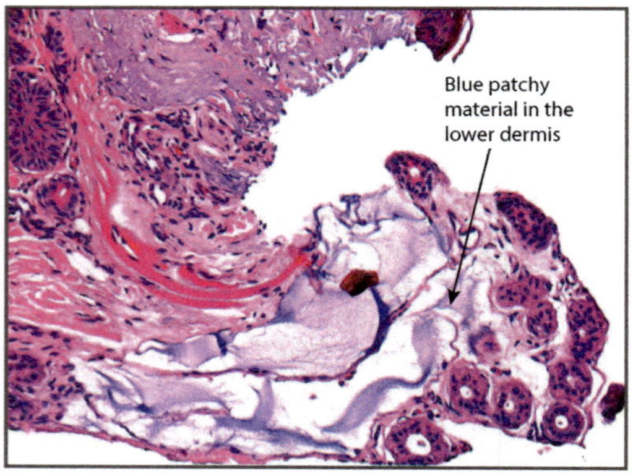

Figure 3.73 Foreign body reaction to hyaluronic acid. The bluish material in the lower dermis is hyaluronic acid. This lesion was biopsied to rule out cystic basal cell carcinoma.

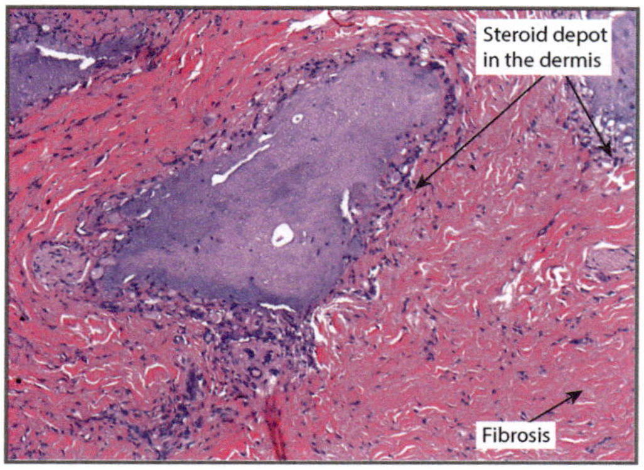

Figure 3.74 Depot steroid material in the dermis. The intralesional injection was done to improve a scar.

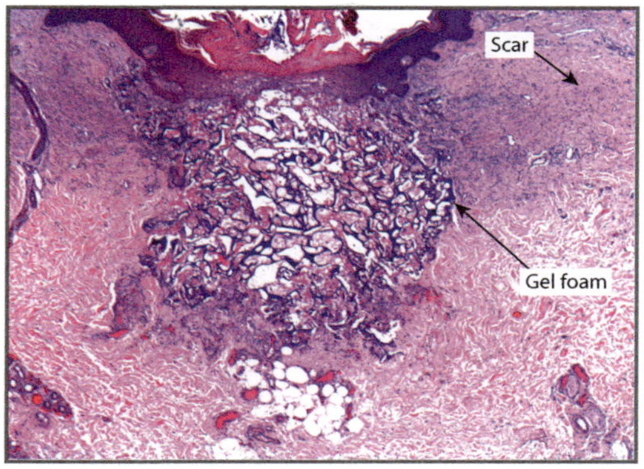

Figure 3.75 The angulated particles of the gel foam are more superficially located within the area of the surgical scar compared to injectable fillers, with angulated particles which are deposited deeper.

VESICULAR AND BULLOUS DISORDERS

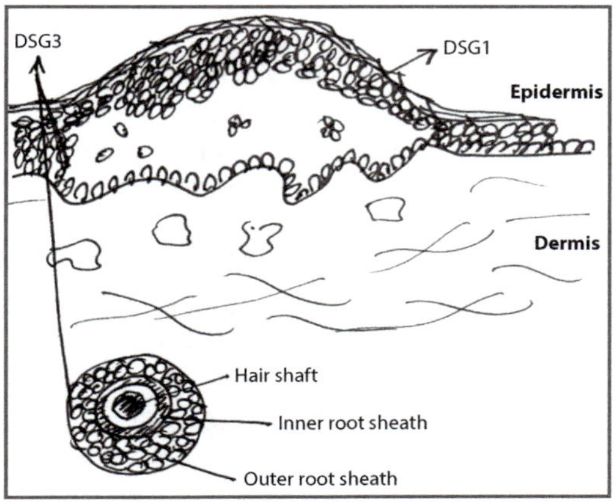

Figure 3.76 In pemphigus vulgaris the acantholysis is intraepidermal and affects also the follicular epithelium following the distribution of the desmogleins in the skin: DSG1 (upper epidermis) and DSG3 (lower epidermis and the outer root sheath of the hair follicles).

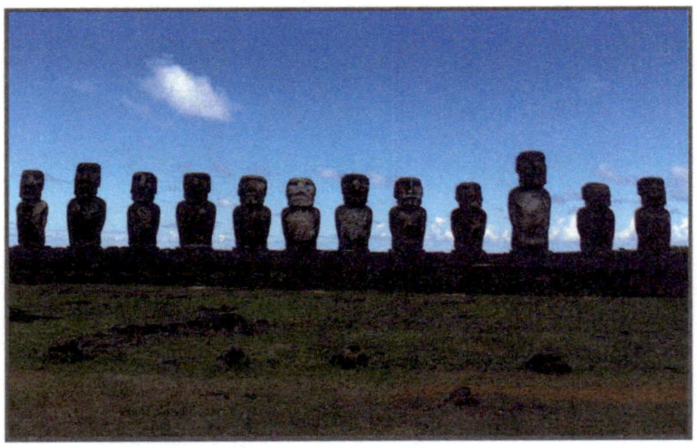

Photomnemonic 3.13 The suprabasal acantholysis combined with the intercellular detachment of the basal cells gives the basal cell layer in pemphigus vulgaris the appearance of a row of individual standing stones (Easter Island).

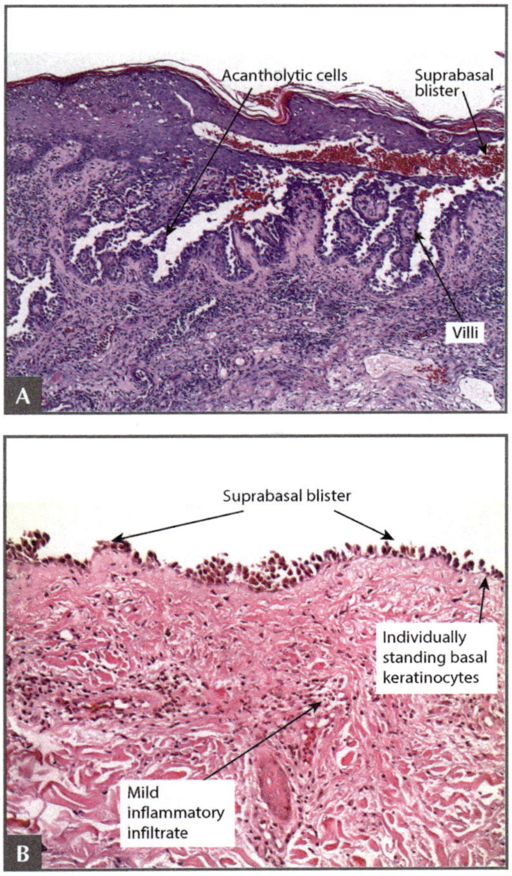

Figure 3.77 Pemphigus vulgaris. **A** Note the suprabasal acantholysis and protruding villi. **B** Note the individual standing basal keratinocytes.

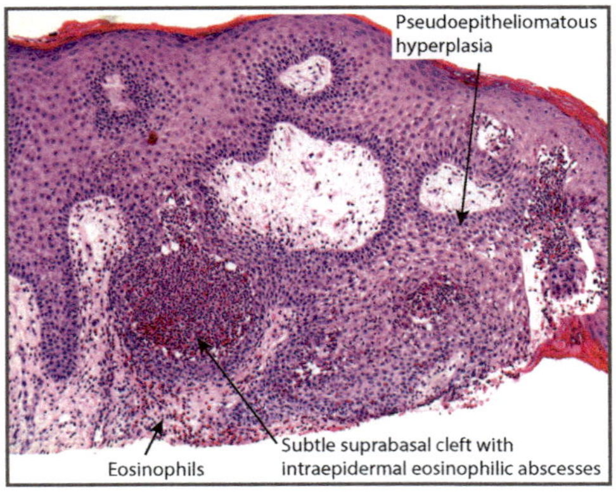

Figure 3.78 Pemphigus vegetans. Note the prominent pseudoepitheliomatous hyperplasia and the subtle suprabasal cleft with prominent eosinophilic abscesses.

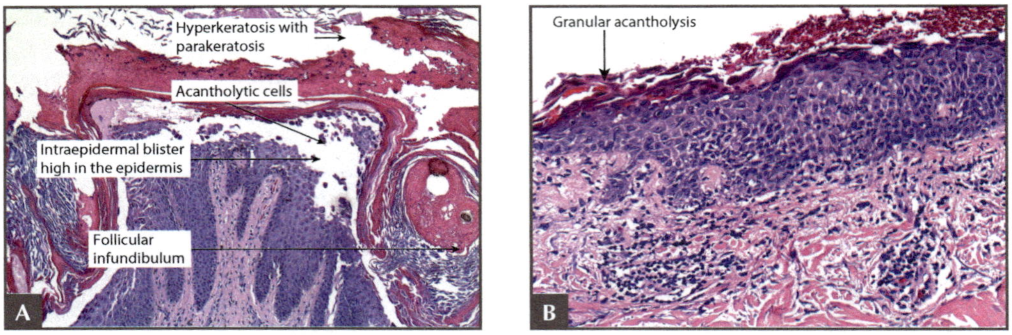

Figure 3.79 Pemphigus foliaceus. **A** An upper epidermal blister that also involves the follicles. Note the thick hyperkeratosis and parakeratosis which corresponds to the clinical features of "cornflakes-like scaling." **B** The acantholysis is through the granular layer; the roof of the blister is missing.

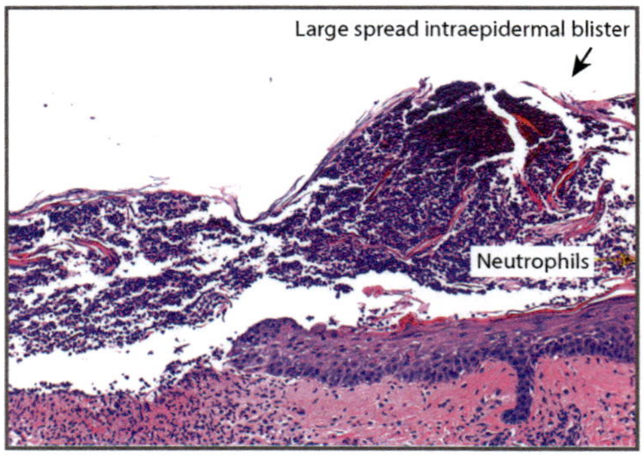

Figure 3.80 IgA pemphigus: there is a large spread epidermal blister containing numerous neutrophils.

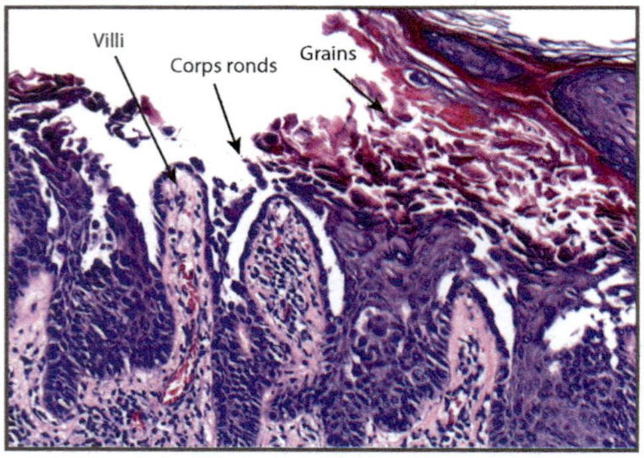

Figure 3.82 Darier's disease: dyskeratotic acantholysis.

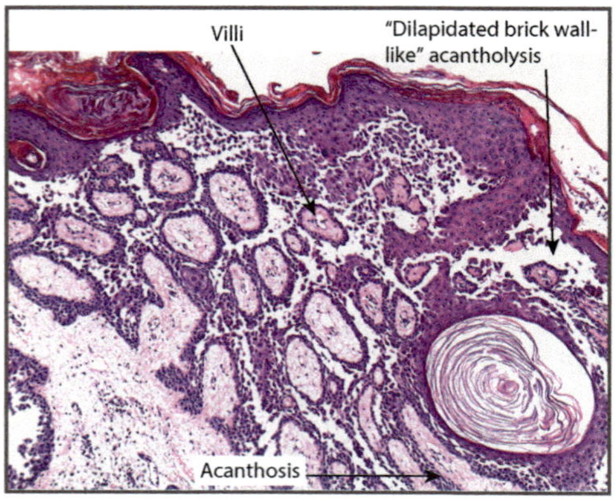

Figure 3.81 Hailey-Hailey disease: the acantholysis is spread along the epidermis and involves at least half of its height.

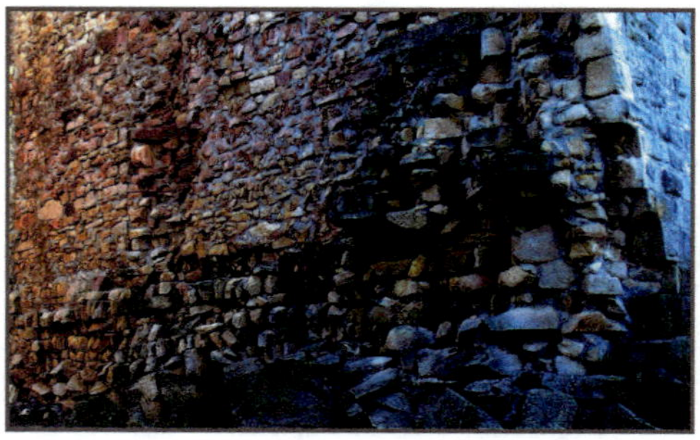

Photomnemonic 3.14 Widespread and full-thickness acantholysis can be compared to a dilapidated brick wall.

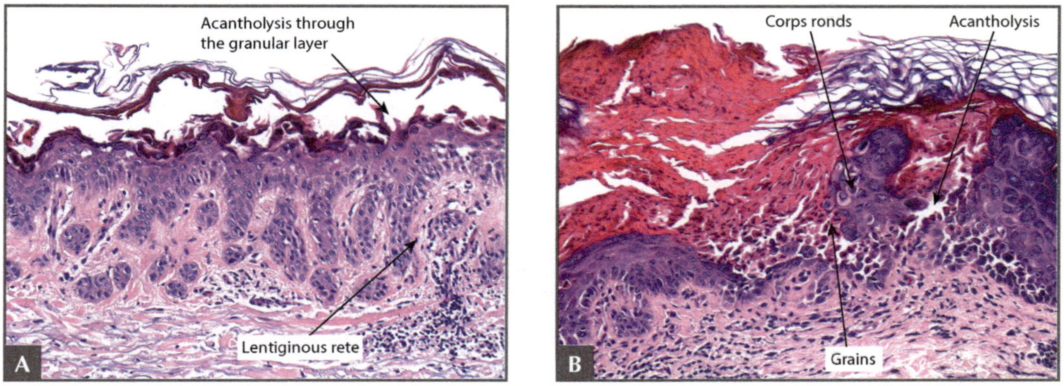

Figure 3.83 Grover's disease. **A** Pemphigus foliaceus type: note the acantholysis through the granular layer. **B** Darier's disease type: there is acantholytic dyskeratosis.

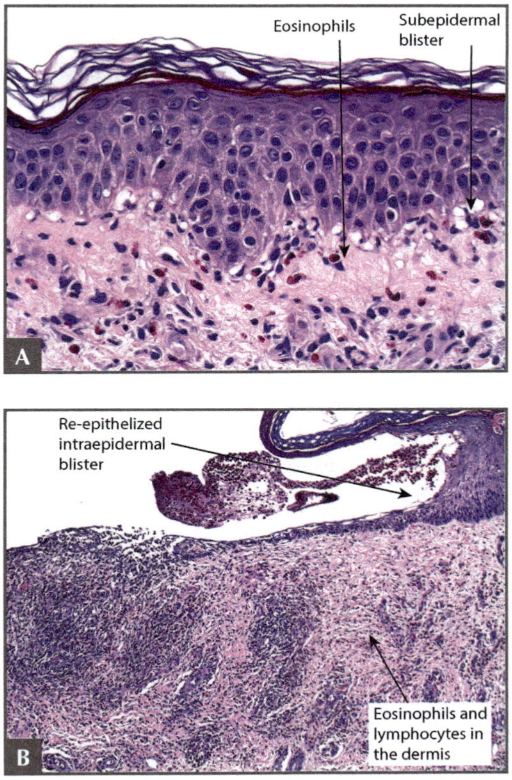

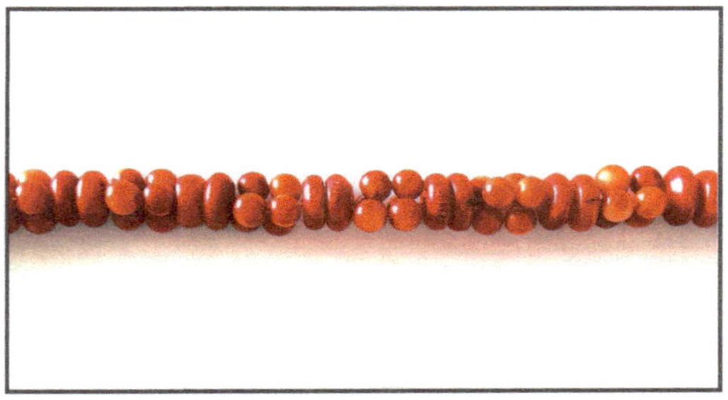

Photomnemonic 3.15 Eosinophils line the subepidermal cleft in bullous pemphigoid, like a string of beads.

Figure 3.84 Bullous pemphigoid. **A** There are initial subepidermal blisters with many eosinophils in the papillary dermis. **B** The regenerating epidermis shows the intraepidermal level of the blister. There is significant inflammation of lymphocytes and eosinophils in the dermis.

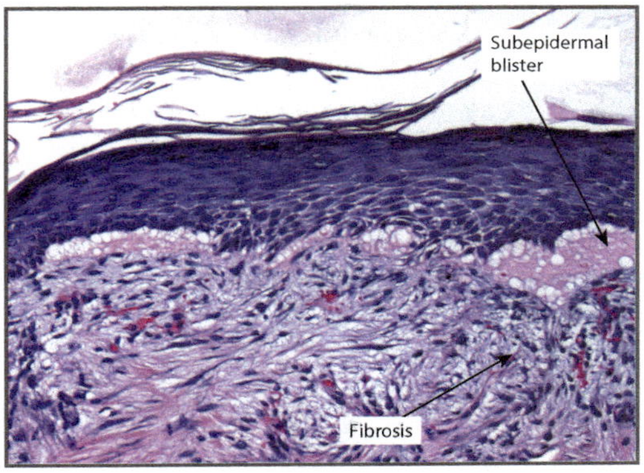

Figure 3.85 Cicatricial pemphigoid of the scalp. There is a subepidermal cleft with a lymphoplasmocytic infiltrate and predominant fibrosis.

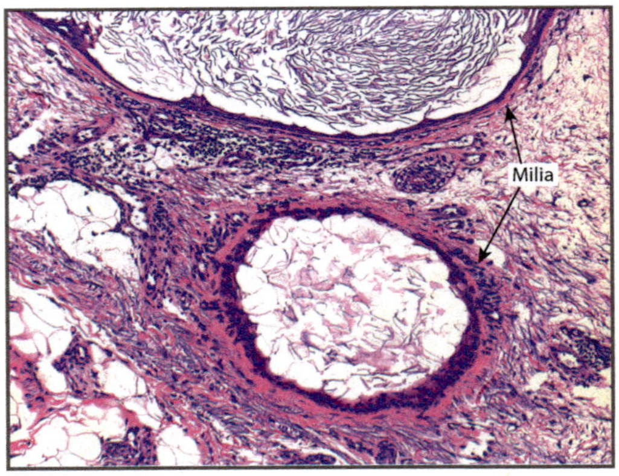

Figure 3.86 Epidermolysis bullosa acquisita: milia.

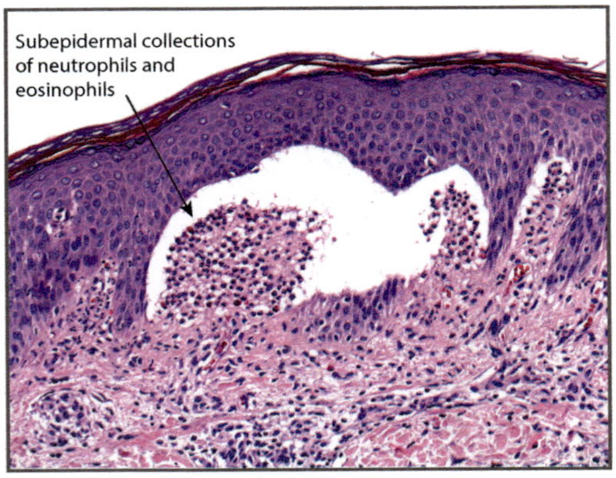

Figure 3.87 Dermatitis herpetiformis: note the preserved rete ridges around the subepidermal microabscesses of neutrophils and eosinophils.

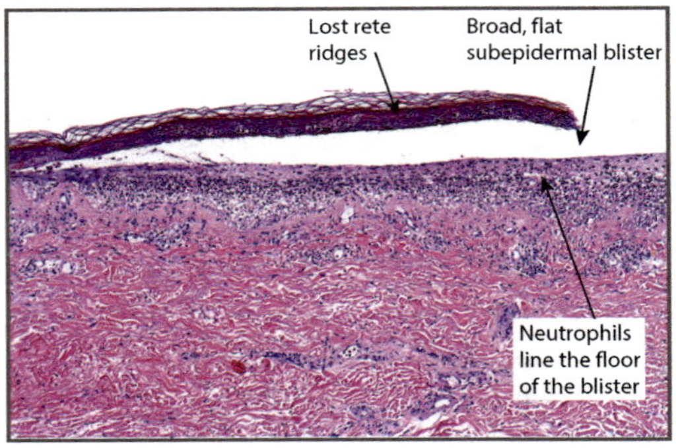

Figure 3.88 Linear IgA dermatosis (LAD) due to vancomycin: the subepidermal blister is broad with a flat floor lined by neutrophils. Note the loss of the rete ridges compared to dermatitis herpetiformis.

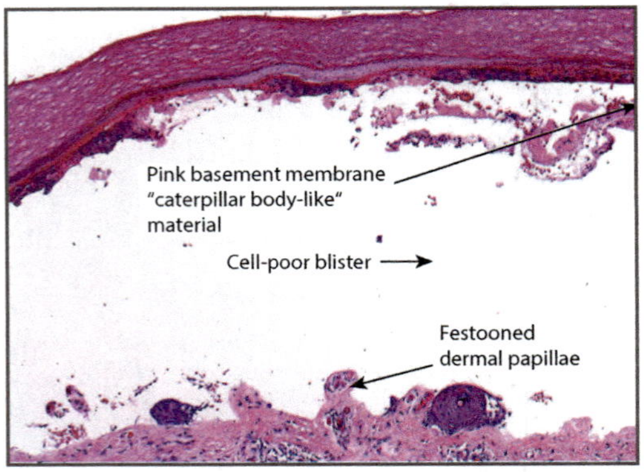

Figure 3.89 Porphyria cutanea tarda (PCT): a cell-poor subepidermal blister on acral skin.

VASCULAR DISEASE

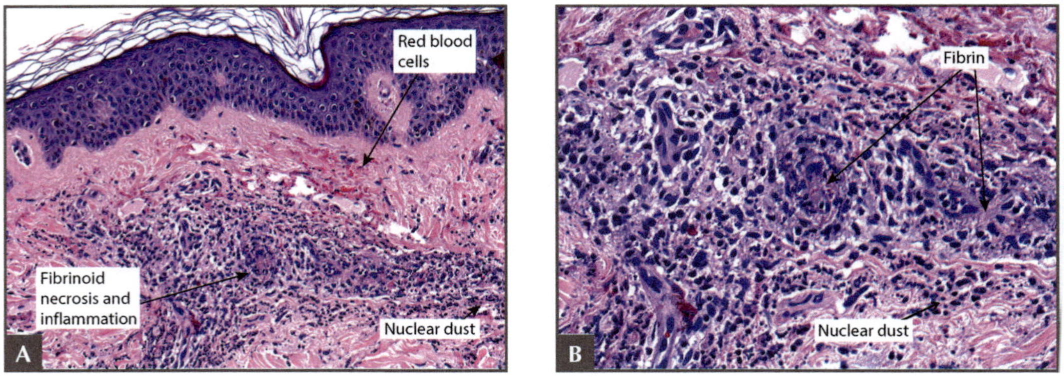

Figure 3.90 Leukocytoclastic vasculitis (LCV). **A** LCV is characterized by fibrinoid necrosis of the vessel wall, intramural neutrophils, and nuclear dust and red blood cells in the dermis. **B** LCV on high power.

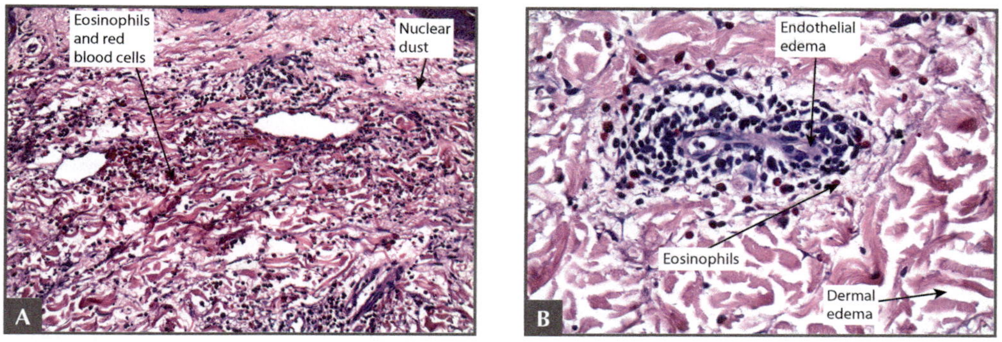

Figure 3.91 Urticarial vasculitis (UV). **A** UV shows less fibrinoid necrosis and occlusion. There is perivascular nuclear dust, eosinophils, and red blood cells. **B** Another case of UV demonstrates the perivascular eosinophils. Note the edema of the endothelial cells as well as the dermal edema in the dermis.

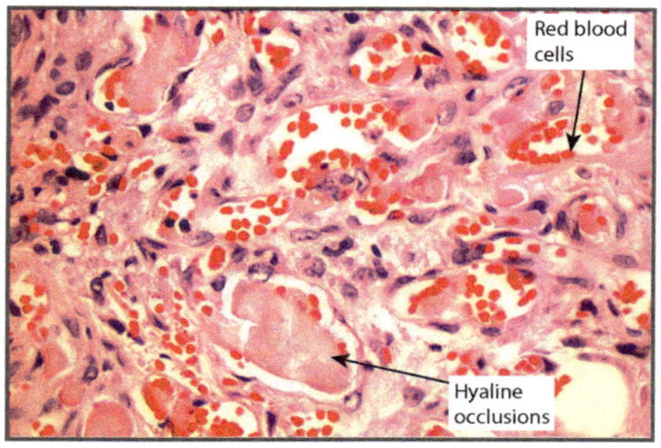

Figure 3.92 Cryoglobulinemia, Type I. There are hyaline occlusions within the lumina of the affected vessels. No vasculitis is present.

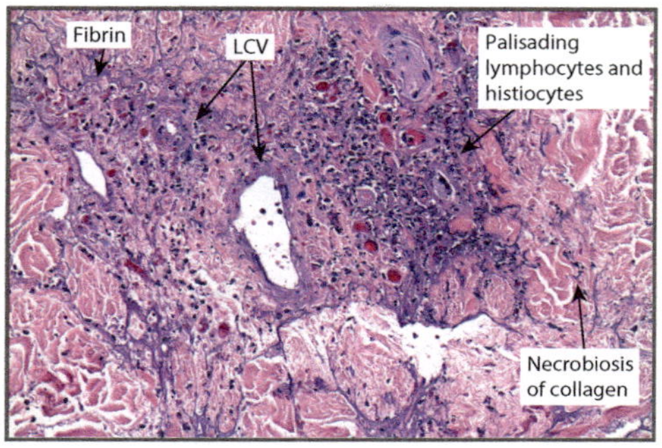

Figure 3.93 Wegener's granulomatosis (granulomatosis with polyangiitis (GPA)). There is LCV and fibrinoid necrosis in the dermis surrounded by lymphocytes and histiocytes ("blue granulomas").

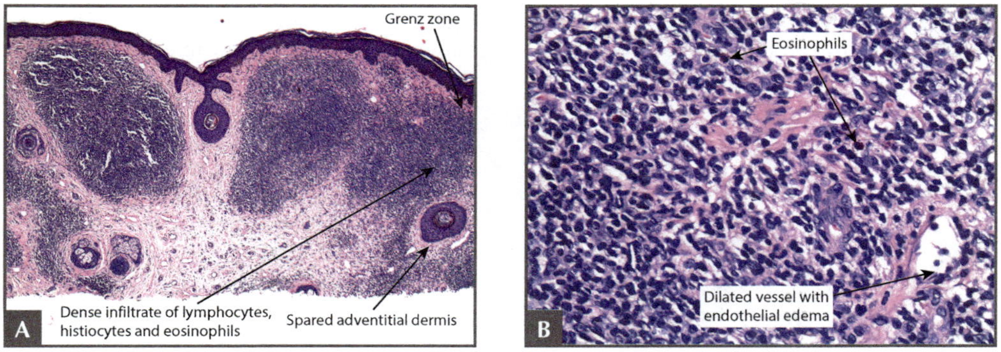

Figure 3.94 Granuloma faciale. **A** Note that the infiltrate spares the epidermis and the adventitial dermis. **B** Eosinophils and dilated vessels with edema of the endothelial lining.

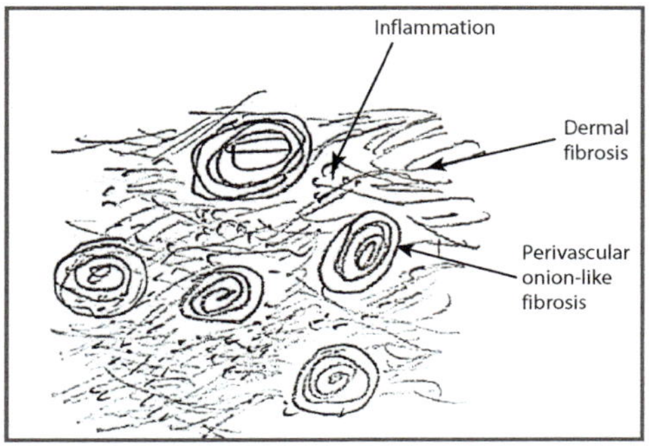

Figure 3.95 Erythema elevatum diutinum. Note the perivascular "onion-like" fibrosis in older lesions.

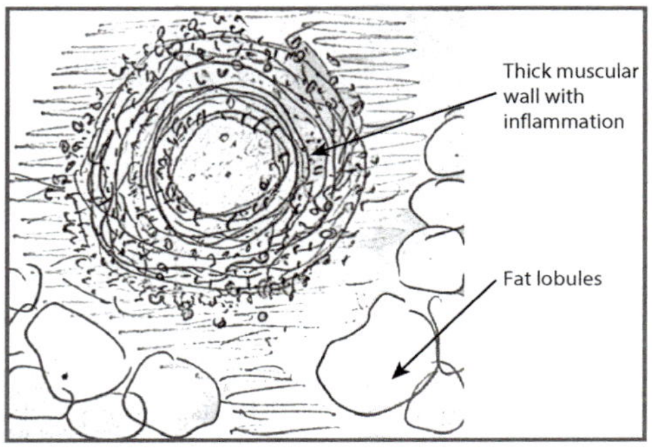

Figure 3.96 PAN. Note the full-thickness inflammation of the vessel wall and the absence of thrombosis.

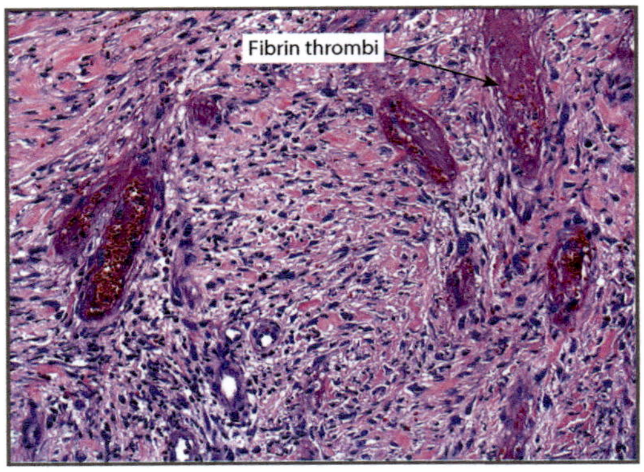

Figure 3.97 Vasculopathy. There is occlusion of the lumina by fibrin thrombi and absence of intramural inflammation.

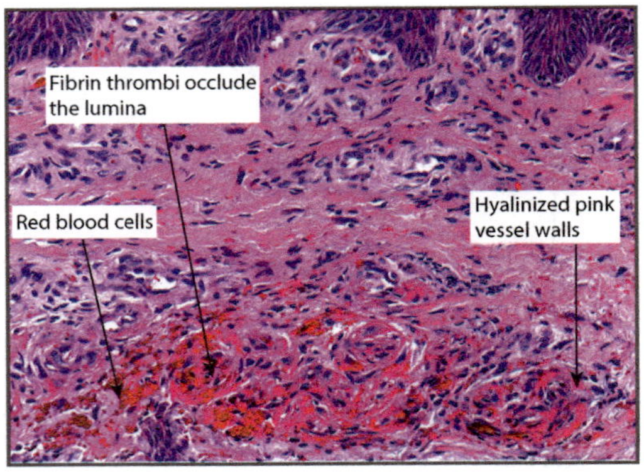

Figure 3.98 Atrophie blanche. There is an increased number of vessels in the upper dermis. The vessels appear pink due to fibrin thrombi in the lumina and hyalinization of the vessel walls.

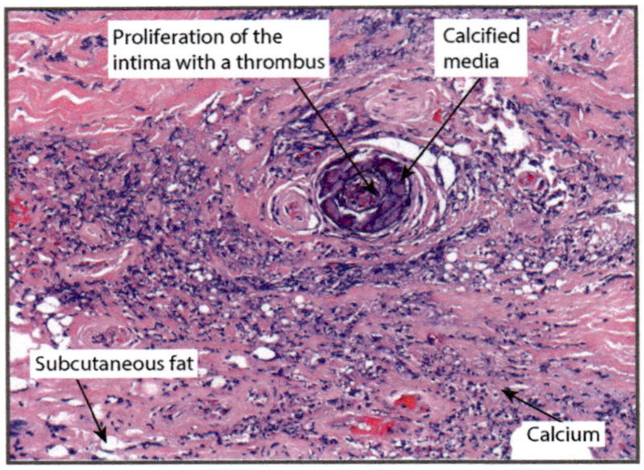

Figure 3.99 Calciphylaxis. This small vessel in the subdermis shows proliferation of the intima with calcification of the media. Note the dispersed calcium salts in the surrounding tissue.

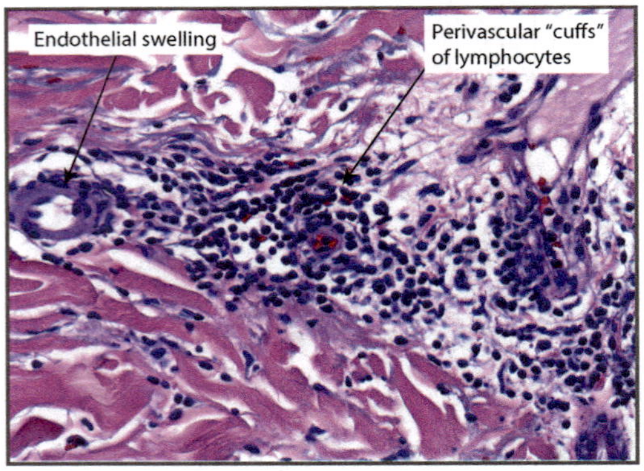

Figure 3.100 Lymphocytic vasculitis. There is minimal vascular injury with endothelial swelling and tight perivascular lymphocytic infiltrates.

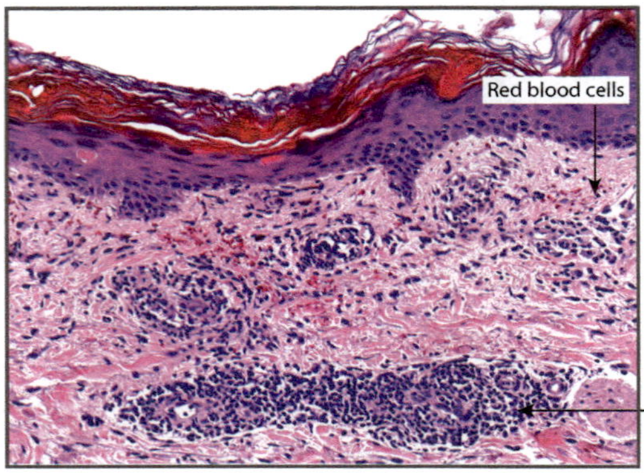

Figure 3.101 Pigmented purpura. Note the absence of vasculitis. There is tight perivascular lymphocytic infiltrate and red blood cell extravasation in the dermis.

PANNICULITIS

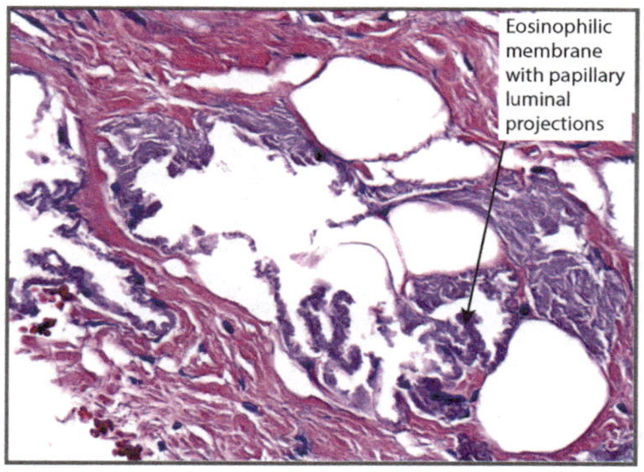

Figure 3.102 Lipodermatosclerosis. The membranous fat necrosis presents with cystic adipocytes showing papillary projections into the lumina.

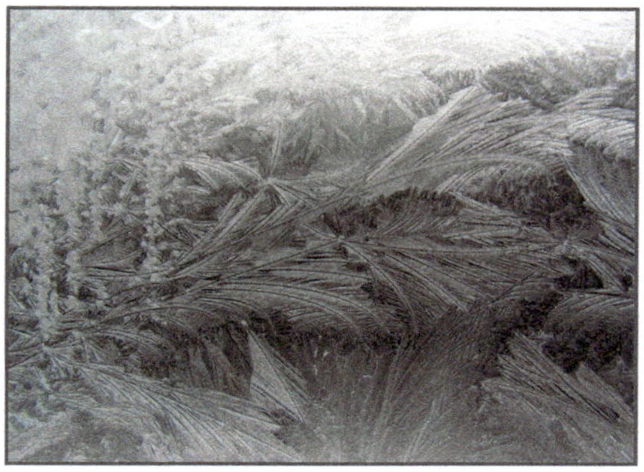

Photomnemonic 3.16 Frost on a window (membranous fat necrosis).

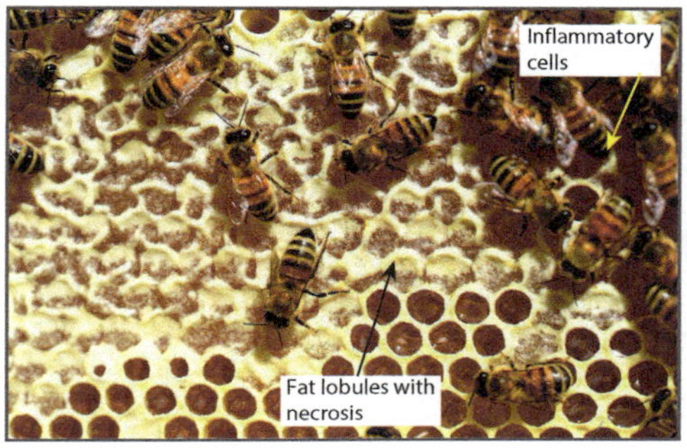

Photomnemonic 3.17 Honeycomb with bees (lobular panniculitis).

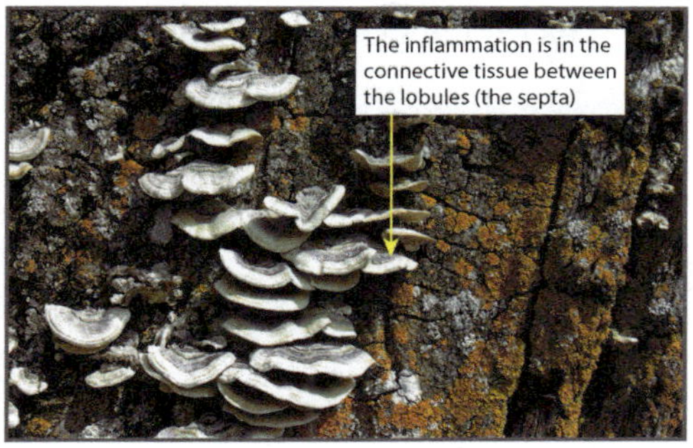
The inflammation is in the connective tissue between the lobules (the septa)

Photomnemonic 3.18 A log with mushrooms (septal panniculitis).

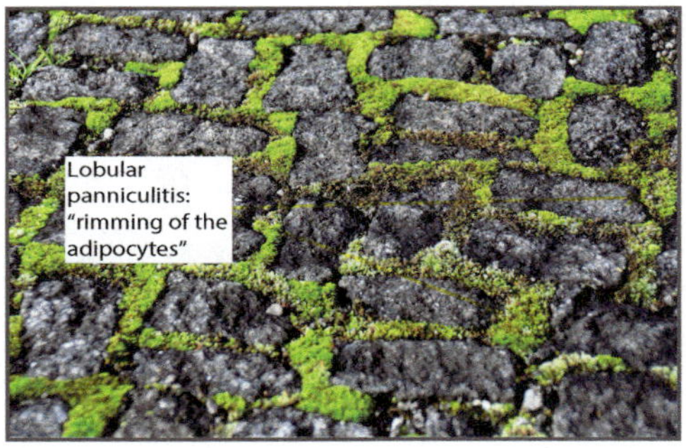
Lobular panniculitis: "rimming of the adipocytes"

Photomnemonic 3.19 Moss on a stone (lupus panniculitis).

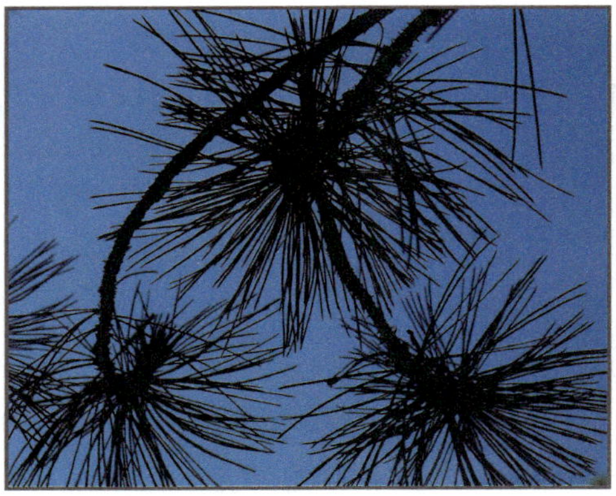

Photomnemonic 3.20 The radially arranged needle-shaped clefts in the adipocytes of sclerema neonatorum and subcutaneous fat necrosis of the newborn resemble pine tree needles.

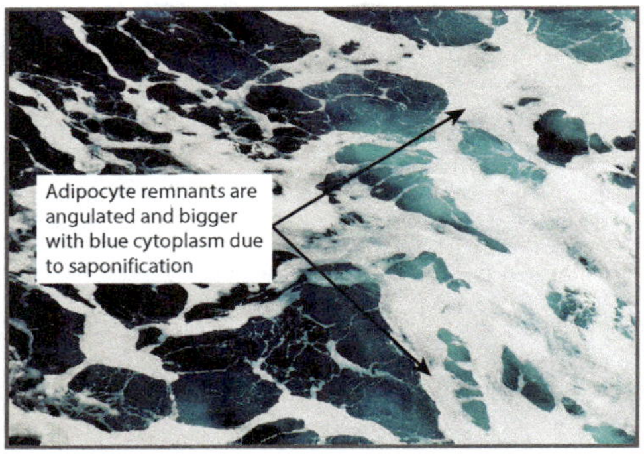
Adipocyte remnants are angulated and bigger with blue cytoplasm due to saponification

Photomnemonic 3.21 Blue foamy water (pancreatic panniculitis).

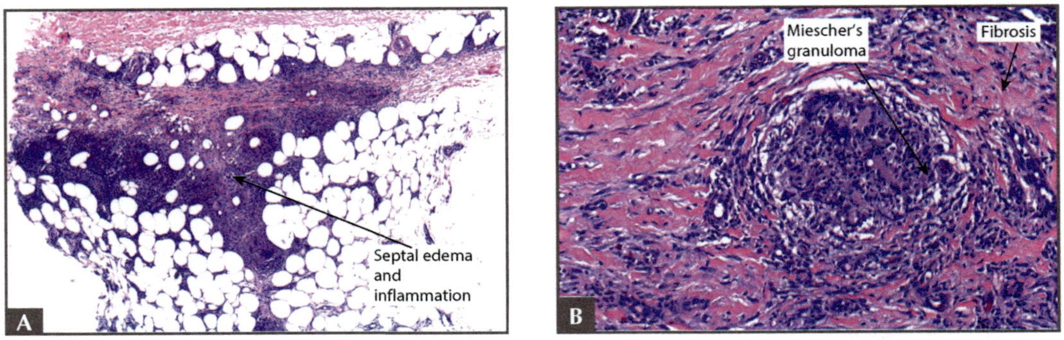

Figure 3.103 Erythema nodosum (EN). **A** Septal edema and inflammation in EN. **B** Miescher's radial granuloma: a small well-defined radial granuloma of palisading histiocytes and giant cells usually around a vessel or a banana-shaped cleft.

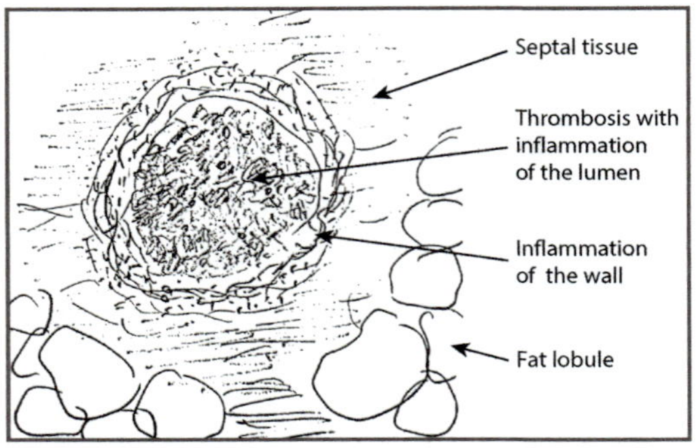

Figure 3.104 Superficial migratory thrombophlebitis: a thrombosed lumen is the distinguishing feature from PAN. Inflammation of the vessel wall is characteristic for both lesions.

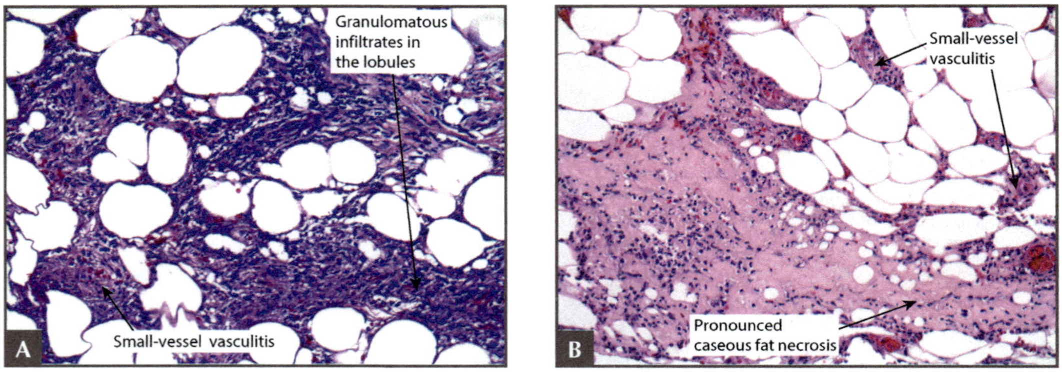

Figure 3.105 Erythema induratum of Bazin. **A** There is lobular panniculitis with small vessel vasculitis. **B** A different case showing pronounced fat necrosis.

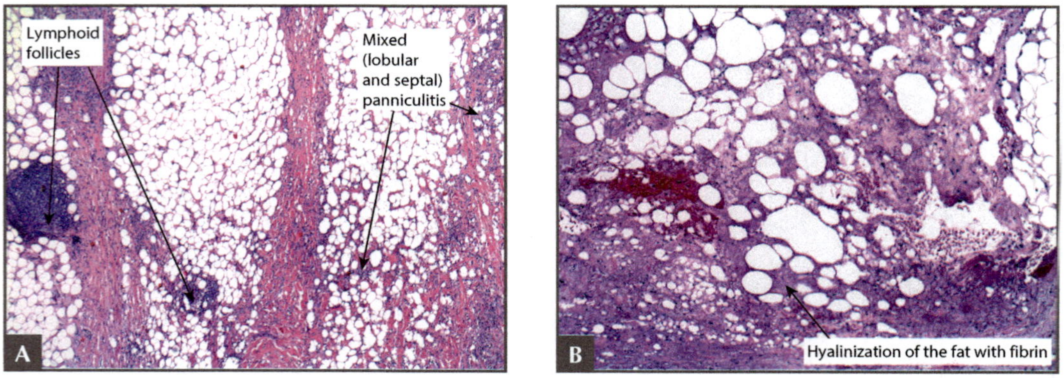

Figure 3.106 Lupus panniculitis. **A** Note the presence of lymphoid follicles in the fat. **B** There is extensive hyaline necrosis of the fat with fibrin deposits.

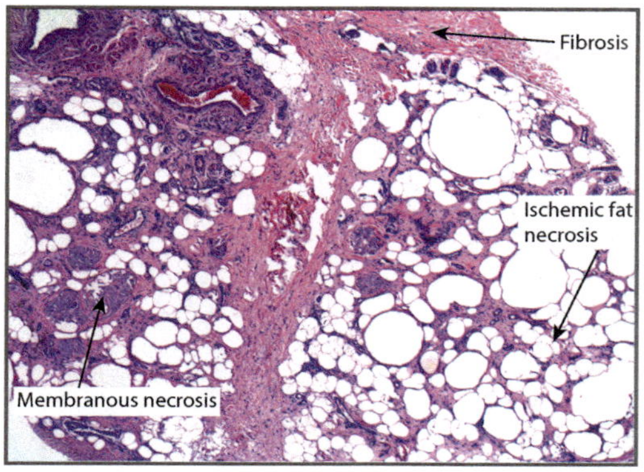

Figure 3.107 Lipodermatosclerosis. Note the membranous and ischemic fat necrosis. The septae are fibrotic.

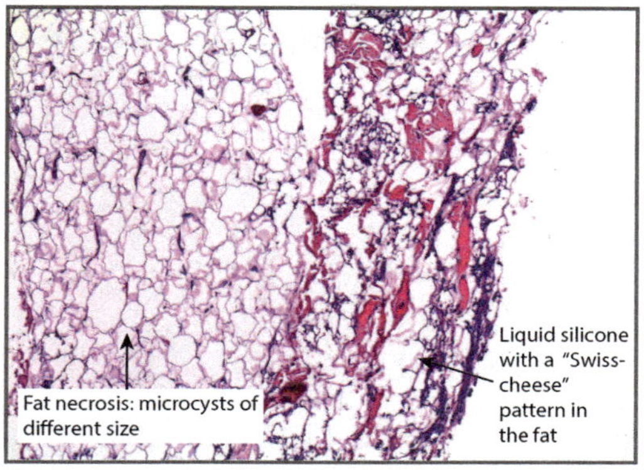

Figure 3.108 Factitial panniculitis after an injection with liquid silicone.

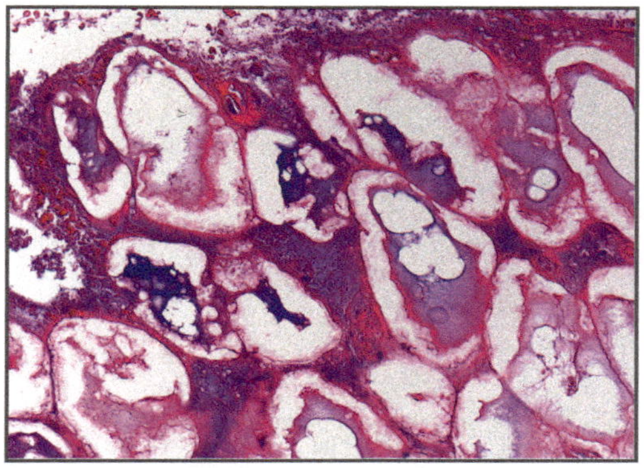

Figure 3.109 Pancreatic panniculitis. Ghost adipocytes. Image courtesy of Luis Requena, MD.

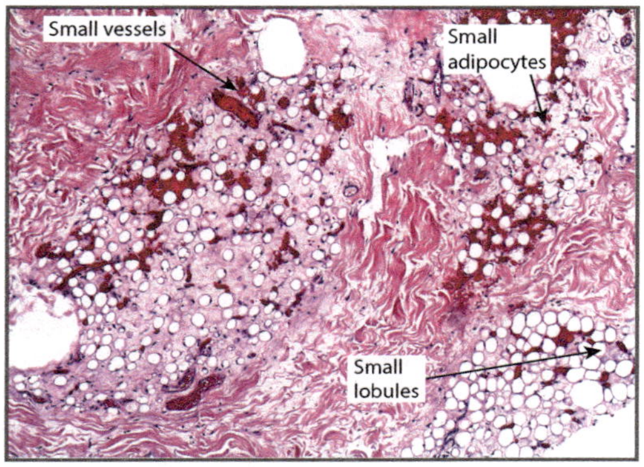

Figure 3.110 Lipoatrophy: small (shrunken) lobules, small adipocytes, increased number of small vessels in the lobules.

NEUTROPHILIC DERMATOSIS *PER SE*

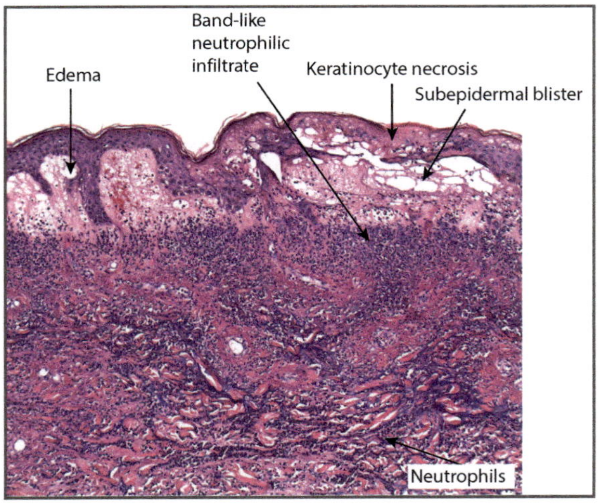

Figure 3.111 Sweet's syndrome. There is prominent edema with a subepidermal blister and a dense band-like and diffuse interstitial neutrophilic infiltrate.

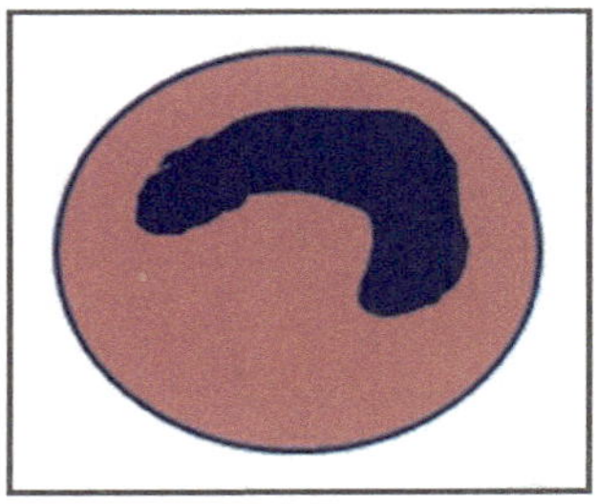

Figure 3.112 A band cell (stab cell) undergoing granulopoiesis. It has a curved nucleus (compare to a mature neutrophil, see Chapter 1).

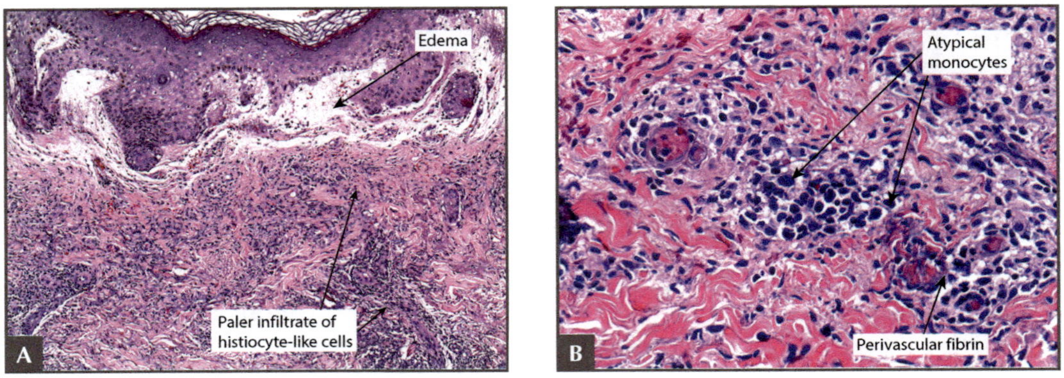

Figure 3.113 Histiocytoid Sweet's syndrome. **A** The pattern is similar to Sweet's syndrome but the infiltrate is paler because it is composed of histiocyte-like cells. **B** Note the presence of atypical cells with blast-like morphology (reniform nuclei). Leukemia cutis must be ruled out.

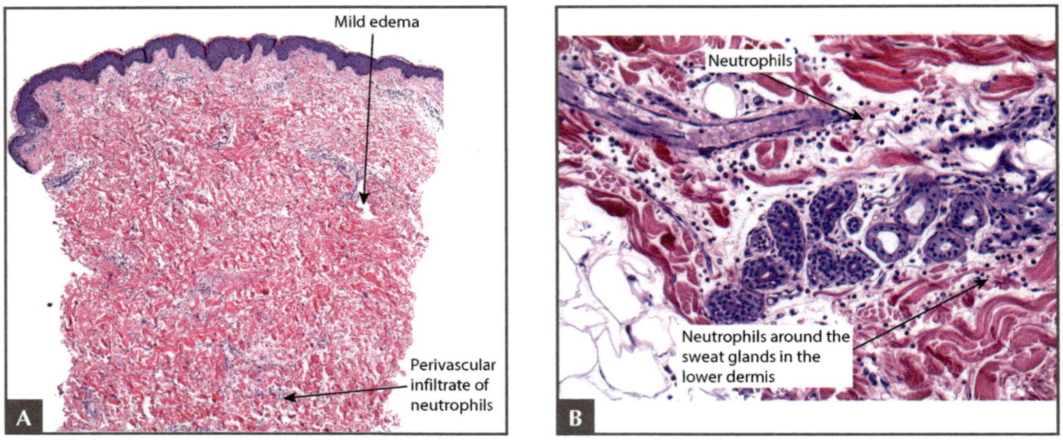

Figure 3.114 Neutrophilic urticarial dermatosis. **A** The features are similar to neutrophilic urticaria but the infiltrate extends throughout the entire specimen into the lower dermis and fat. **B** Note the neutrophils in the deep dermis and subdermis.

4 | Non-inflammatory dermatoses

DEPOSITION DISORDERS

Definition: A group of disorders characterized by abnormal deposition of endogenous material (mucin, hyaline, amyloid, colloid, urate crystals, and calcium) in the skin.

General concepts

- Most deposition disorders are characterized by pink–pale blue amorphous material in the dermis; the epidermis is usually normal.
- The material remains in the skin because it is resistant to proteolytic digestion.
- Inflammation is usually not observed but, if present, is scarce. Look for:
  - Plasma cells in amyloidosis
  - Palisading histiocytes and giant cells in gout and calcinosis
  - Perivascular and periadnexal lymphocytes in some mucinosis
- Special stains and immunostains are useful to identify the type of material:
  - Congo red and crystal violet for amyloid; Igλ and k immunostains for monoclonal versus polyclonal proteins in primary systemic versus secondary systemic amyloid
  - Keratin stain for localized cutaneous amyloidosis
  - Colloidal iron and Alcian blue for mucin
  - PAS for hyaline
  - Polarized microscopy for urate crystals and for Congo red (apple-green positive amyloid and colloid)
  - Von Kossa for calcium

On low power

(Table 4.1)

Table 4.1 Deposition disorders on low power.

On low power H&E	Pale blue "edema"/ space	Dark blue/ purple chunks or powder	Pale blue gray feathery material	Pink gray amorphous material			Brown gold bananas
				Amyloid	Hyaline	Colloid	
Main disorders	**Mucinoses:** • pretibial myxedema • lichen myxedematosus • scleromyxedema • focal mucinosis • reticular erythematous mucinosis • follicular mucinosis • digital mucous cyst	**Calcinosis cutis:** • metastatic calcinosis • dystrophic calcinosis • idiopathic calcinosis • subepidermal calcified nodule	Gout	**Systemic:** • primary systemic amyloidosis • secondary systemic amyloidosis **Cutaneous:** • macular type • lichenoid type • nodular	Lipoid proteinosis	Adult colloid milium Juvenile colloid milium	Ochronosis Alkaptonuria

On high power

MUCINOSES

- Mucin is a protein–hyaluronic acid complex produced by fibroblasts and mast cells (this is why mast cells love to hang around mucin); during processing it shrinks and appears as fine blue granules in the empty spaces.
- Hyaluronic acid holds water and therefore the dermis looks swollen.
- If mucin persists, collagen production and fibrosis are stimulated (scleromyxedema).

NB Older lesions have less mucin than early lesions.

Pretibial myxedema

- Greatly thickened dermis
- Large amounts of mucin, particularly in upper half of the dermis (empty spaces on H&E, blue on the colloidal iron or Alcian blue stain) **(Figure 4.1)**
- The mucin splits the collagen bundles into thinner fibers

NB The stellate fibroblasts (mucoblasts) have receptors for TSH and secrete mucin when stimulated.

Scleredema

- Greatly thickened dermis (up to three times the normal thickness) **(Figure 4.2)**
- Thick hyalinized collagen: looks like "juicy scleroderma" because the collagen bundles are separated (fenestrated) by mucin
- Mucin is more prominent in the lower dermis (vs in the upper dermis in pretibial myxedema)
- No fibroblasts

Scleromyxedema/Lichen myxedematosus

Scleromyxedema is the generalized counterpart of papular mucinosis (lichen myxedematosus), characterized clinically by diffuse indurated skin.

- Focal increased deposition of mucin in upper reticular dermis (in the middle of the specimen)
- Fragmentation of the thickened collagen bundles by mucin **(Figure 4.3)**
- Increased number of fibroblasts

NB Distinguishing from nephrogenic systemic fibrosis (NSF) may be difficult as both demonstrate increased 1) mucin, 2) collagen, and 3) fibrosis, but in NSF the process extends to the septa in the subdermis and the fascia.

(Table 4.2)

Table 4.2 Distinguishing pathologic features among pretibial myxedema, scleredema, and scleromyxedema **(Photomnemonic 4.1)**

Pretibial myxedema	Scleredema	Scleromyxedema
Diffuse mucin in upper dermis	Diffuse mucin in lower dermis	Focal mucin in mid-dermis
+/– some stellate fibroblasts	No fibroblasts	Increased fibroblasts
Collagen bundles are thinner (fibers) and widely separated	Collagen bundles are thicker and separated	Collagen bundles are thicker and separated, with fibroblasts
("juicy dermis")	(thick "juicy dermis")	("thick juicy" and "busy" dermis)

Focal mucinosis

Protruding dome-shaped, well-circumscribed, pale blue lesion full of mucin **(Figure 4.4)**

Follicular mucinosis

See Chapter 3, Spongiotic pattern

Reticular erythematous mucinosis

- Sparse perivascular and periadnexal lymphocytic infiltrate
- Increased dermal mucin

NB A distinguishing feature from lupus erythematosus and dermatomyositis is the absence of vacuolar damage.

AMYLOIDOSES

- Amyloid (abnormal proteinaceous material) is either produced by cells at the deposition site (localized forms) or precipitates in the skin after being produced systemically (systemic forms).
- Two systemic forms exist based on the amyloid type: 1) primary: amyloid AL – monoclonal light-chain immunoglobulins, associated with myeloma; 2) secondary: amyloid AA – non-immunoglobulinemic acute phase proteins, associated with chronic inflammatory conditions.

NB Secondary amyloidosis does not involve the skin; however, a deep biopsy including abdominal fat may be positive for amyloid.

The skin biopsy in systemic amyloidosis:

- Pale, pink–gray amorphous fissured material close to the epidermis **(Photomnemonic 4.2)**
- Amyloid also around adnexae and within the blood vessel walls (hence the extravasated red blood cells manifesting clinically as purpura) **(Figure 4.5)**
- Amyloid around individual fat cells (amyloid rings) **(Figure 4.6)**

Primary localized cutaneous amyloidosis

The amyloid derives from degenerated keratinocytes (due to rubbing) and acts as a sponge which absorbs immunoglobulins and complement.

Macular amyloidosis and lichen amyloidosis

- Dermal papillae filled with globular deposits of amyloid (rounded papillae) (See Photomnemonic 4.2)
- Pigment incontinence (hence the clinical appearance of rippled postinflammatory hyperpigmentation)
- More epidermal changes with acanthosis and hyperkeratosis in lichen amyloidosis **(Figure 4.7)**

NB There is no vascular, adnexal, or fat involvement compared to systemic amyloidosis.

Nodular amyloidosis

This is a "localized systemic form" of AL amyloidosis: local cutaneous plasma cells produce the AL amyloid.

- Large masses of amyloid from the top of the dermis to the bottom of the fat **(Figure 4.8)**
- Amyloid is found within and around the vessels, adnexal structures, and fat cells
- Lymphocytes and plasma cells mostly around the vessels; possible Russell bodies

NB Nodular amyloidosis cannot be distinguished from systemic amyloidosis on a histologic base only.

Table 4.3 Summary of the staining pattern in the amyloidoses group

Stains	Systemic amyloidosis (AL)	Cutaneous amyloidosis	Localized nodular amyloidosis
λ or k	Positive, monoclonal	Negative	Positive, monoclonal
Keratin stain	Negative	Positive	Negative
Collagen IV	Negative	Positive	Negative
CD79a	Positive	Negative	Positive

(Table 4.3)

Colloid milium (adult type)

The colloid is the ultimate degeneration product of elastic fibers in patients with solar damage.

- Grenz zone
- Pale pink fissured material in upper dermis (very similar to amyloid) **(Figure 4.9)**
- Solar elastosis at the base

Colloid milium (juvenile type)

The colloid is the product of degenerated basal layer cells (keratin-derived).

- The epidermis is flat
- The basal cells show transformation into colloid bodies (clumps of pink material)
- Pale pink fissured material in the upper dermis (very similar to amyloid)

- NB There is no solar elastosis and no Grenz zone to distinguish from adult type

Lipoid proteinosis

Hyaline is not a single substance, it is proteinaceous material which can form from duplication of basement membranes or it can be produced by the fibroblasts.

- Thick mantles of pink material around blood vessels and sweat glands ("pink onion rings")
- Pale pink material may fill the dermal papillae and the entire upper dermis (very similar to amyloid)

Gout

Needle-shaped urate crystals are deposited in the skin.

- They appear as pink pale amorphous material with needle-shaped clefts

NB The crystals look pale when the lesion has been preserved in formalin and brown when it has been preserved in 100% alcohol.

- A palisading rim of macrophages and giant cells as well as calcifications may develop (more in older lesions) **(Figure 4.10)**
- The stain for gout is de Galantha

Calcinosis cutis

Calcium deposits in the skin may result from different mechanisms **(Table 4.4)**.

- Compact deep blue–purple masses **(Photomnemonic 4.3, Figure 4.11)**

Ochronosis

Endogenous: Homogentisic acid accumulates in alkaptonuria due to enzymatic defect

Exogenous: Homogentisic acid accumulates from using hydroquinone or antimalarials

- Thickened and bizarre collagen bundles with so-called banana bodies **(Figure 4.12)**
- The "bananas" form because the ochronic pigment impregnates collagen bundles irreversibly and they fracture

Table 4.4 Overview of the most common forms of calcinosis cutis in the skin

Type	Metastatic	Dystrophic	Idiopathic	Subepidermal calcified nodule
Mechanism	Hypercalcemia due to hyperparathyroidism Hypervitaminosis D	Tissue damage Normal serum calcium and phosphorus	No underlying cause Normal serum calcium and phosphorus	No underlying cause Normal serum calcium and phosphorus
Skin involvement	Rare in skin, only in renal insufficiency • white papules or plaques • calciphylaxis	Exclusively in skin • in previously damaged skin due to collagen vascular disorders • in tumors and cysts • in infections	Resembles dystrophic calcinosis but no tissue damage • tumoral calcinosis • idiopathic calcinosis of the scrotum	Resembles dystrophic calcinosis + perforating disorder
Pathology	Granules in the dermis Masses in the subdermis Possible foreign body reaction with histiocytes and giant cells Intravascular calcification (calciphylaxis)	Granules in the dermis Masses in the subdermis Possible foreign body reaction Collagen and fat appear degenerated	Large masses in the subdermis surrounded by foreign body reaction	Hypertrophic epidermis: acanthosis and hyperkeratosis Closely aggregated globules in the upper dermis Foreign body reaction

COLLAGEN AND ELASTIC TISSUE DISORDERS

Definition: Group of disorders affecting the two major components of the dermis (collagen and elastic tissue) mainly in two opposite patterns: excess in amount or deficiency/absence.

General concepts

- Sclerosing disorders are characterized by markedly thickened dermis due to excessive deposition of collagen (sclerosis); scleroderma is their prototype.
- The epidermis is usually normal but may be thinned with lost rete ridges and pigmented basal layer.
- Atrophic collagenoses (aplasia cutis, focal dermal hypoplasia, atrophoderma) are rare and difficult to distinguish from normal skin; they are characterized by a slightly thinned dermis with sclerosis and decreased space among collagen bundles.

- NB Normal elastic fibers are not visible without special stains.

- Increased elastic tissue is characterized by collections of coarse and fragmented fibers usually in the upper dermis; solar elastosis is their prototype.
- Decreased elastic tissue is invisible on H&E; differentiation from normal skin may be difficult without stains.
- Extrusion of collagen and elastic tissue through the skin surface is another pattern, discussed in detail in the section on Perforating disorders.

(Table 4.5)

Table 4.5 A comprehensive classification of the most common connective tissue abnormalities

Feature	Possible disorders
Increased collagen	Scleroderma/morphea Sclerodermoid disorders: • eosinophilic fasciitis • lichen sclerosus and atrophicus • GVHD • scleromyxedema • scleredema • nephrogenic systemic fibrosis • radiation dermatitis Other connective tissue disorders: • keloid • hypertrophic scar • connective tissue nevus
Decreased collagen	Aplasia cutis congenita Focal dermal hypoplasia Atrophoderma of Pasini and Pierini
Increased elastics	Pseudoxanthoma elasticum Solar elastosis Erythema ab igne

(continued)

Table 4.5 ***(continued)***

Feature	Possible disorders
Decreased elastics	Macular atrophy (anetoderma) Cutis laxa Striae distensae Acrokeratoelastoidosis
Perforating connective tissue disorders	Reactive perforating collagenosis Elastosis perforans serpiginosa

On low power

- Elastic disorders may be indistinguishable from normal skin on H&E.
- Biopsies from sclerosing disorders have a rectangular shape and look pink from the top to the bottom; the dermis may have diminished/lost adnexal structures.
- Solar elastosis "paints" the upper dermis in a light blue-grayish color.

On high power

Scleroderma (systemic sclerosis) and morphea

Early lesions: Increased interstitial as well as perivascular and perieccrine lymphocytes with variable plasma cells, eosinophils, and less sclerosis

Developed lesions: Decreased inflammation and increased sclerosis:

- Thickened and homogenized, pink "acellular" collagen fills the entire dermis **(Figure 4.13A)**
- The collagen extends down the subcutaneous septa (like thick columns) and may replace large portions of the fat
- Entrapment of the eccrine coils by collagen with loss of the surrounding fat pad is a clue **(Figure 4.13B)**
- Adnexal structures may be completely lost in advanced sclerosis
- "Floating sign": histiocytes surround individual collagen fibers in morphea **(Figure 4.14)**

Differential diagnosis:

- Decreased CD34 expression (acellular sclerosis with decreased number of fibroblasts) and preserved elastic fibers in morphea vs lost elastic fibers in LSA
- Perineural inflammation and more vascular changes (hyalinization of the vessel walls with narrowing of the lumina) in scleroderma vs morphea

Lichen sclerosus et atrophicus

See Lichenoid pattern.

Eosinophilic fasciitis

NB Incisional biopsy including the fascia is required for the diagnosis.

- The epidermis and large part of the reticular dermis are unaffected
- The adnexal structures are preserved (vs absent in scleroderma)
- The fascia and the entire subdermis are replaced by layers of hyalinized thick collagen **(Figure 4.15)**
- Perivascular and periadnexal infiltrate of lymphocytes, plasma cells, and eosinophils with possible lymphoid follicles
- Increased mucin (vs absent in scleroderma)

Nephrogenic systemic fibrosis

NB Incisional biopsy including the fascia is required.

Early lesions: May be subtle on pathology, with subtly increased number of large epithelioid or stellate fibroblasts

Developed lesions:

- Thick collagen bundles and spindled CD34-positive fibroblasts in the dermis extend through the subcutaneous fat and the fascia
- The fibroblasts as bipolar cells with dendrites extend along both sides of the elastic fibers and have been described as "tram track sign" **(Figure 4.16, Photomnemonic 4.4)**
- Cleft-like spaces with mucin

NB Differential diagnosis: Compared to scleroderma, NSF shows "cellular" sclerosis involving also the fascia with diffusely distributed stellate and multinucleated fibroblasts; there is also mucin.

Pseudoxanthoma elasticum

- Middle third of reticular dermis is involved (compare to upper dermis in solar elastosis)
- Numerous short wavy fragmented purple–blue fibers (these are fragmented elastic fibers impregnated with calcium deposits) **(Figure 4.17A)**
- The fragmented fibers stain black with VVG (for elastic) **(Figure 4.17B)** and von Kossa (for calcium)

Solar elastosis

- A thin Grenz zone
- Gray–blue to light blue deposits in the upper dermis (these are abnormal thick and tangled elastic fibers in a matrix of ground substance-like colloid) **(Figure 4.18)**
- Amount ranges from individual fibers to thick clumps in the dermis

Erythema ab igne (EAI)

See Cutaneous reactions to exogenous factors.

Striae distensae

Early lesions:
- Fragmented thin collagen bundles
- Short and fragmented elastic fibers
- Edema with possible mild lymphocytic infiltrate around dilated blood vessels

Chronic lesions:
- Collagen bundles arranged parallel to the skin surface
- Increased elastic fibers on the VVG stain

Anetoderma

Primary, inflammatory type: Interstitial lymphocytes, plasma cells, and neutrophils
Chronic, non-inflammatory type: Absence of elastic fibers in the papillary and upper reticular dermis on the VVG stain **(Figure 4.19)**

Cutis laxa

Two patterns are recognized on the VVG stain:
- Elastic fibers regularly diminished throughout entire dermis
- Elastic fibers completely absent from upper or lower dermis and fragmented in the rest of the dermis

Mild infiltrate of lymphocytes, neutrophils, or histiocytes may be present.

Acrokeratoelastoidosis

NB Thick stratum corneum is a clue to the site.

- Hyperkeratosis
- Epidermal cells with diminished and fragmented elastic fibers

CUTANEOUS REACTIONS TO EXOGENOUS FACTORS

Definition: Various skin conditions resulting from direct injury to the skin by physical factors: UV light, heat, cold, trauma, and radiation.

General concepts

- Light, heat, and cold induce dermal edema.
- Radiation effaces the cutaneous structures but may preserve the eccrine glands.
- Trauma causes epidermal hemorrhage and/or blisters.
- The stratum corneum is a dead layer and is not sensitive to injury.

On low power

- **Photodermatoses:** Epidermal involvement with spongiosis; dermal edema
- **Radiation dermatitis:** Massive necrosis but the eccrine glands may be preserved;

NB In thermal burn the adnexal structures are destroyed.

- **Bizarre fibroblasts + satellite cell necrosis:** Think radiation dermatitis
- **Perniosis:** Acral skin with edema and blue patches of inflammation around vessels and eccrine glands

On high power

PHOTOSENSITIVITY DERMATOSES

Phototoxic and photoallergic dermatitis

Phototoxic dermatitis is a sunburn reaction which shows an irritant contact dermatitis pattern.
- Changes can be very subtle
- Epidermal apoptosis (sunburn cells) and necrosis **(Figure 4.20)**
- Intraepidermal or subepidermal blisters
- Neutrophils may be prominent

Photoallergic dermatitis is a delayed type hypersensitivity reaction to UV and visible light and therefore shows an acute allergic dermatitis pattern.
- Acanthosis with spongiosis and vesiculation **(Figure 4.21)**
- Lymphocytic exocytosis
- Edema
- Superficial perivascular infiltrate of lymphocytes with/without eosinophils

Polymorphous light eruption

Early lesions show subtle changes:
- Mild spongiosis with lymphocytic exocytosis
- Superficial and deep "patchy" perivascular lymphocytic infiltrate with occasional eosinophils

Established lesions show also:
- Edema **(Figure 4.22)**
- More pronounced inflammation
- Focal vacuolar interface change

Differential diagnosis:
- Erythema multiforme: necrotic keratinocytes at all levels of the epidermis, vacuolar change
- Lupus erythematosus: less edema, mucin and the interface changes affect the adnexal structures
- Actinic prurigo (rare disease in Native Americans): more marked hyperkeratosis and acanthosis, large lymphoid germinal centers

Chronic actinic dermatitis (CAD)

Early lesions are indistinguishable from other forms of spongiotic dermatitis.
Established lesions:

> NB Lichen simplex chronicus with Pautrier's-like microabscesses on sun-damaged skin: think CAD.

- Infundibular acanthosis
- Signs of excoriations: epidermal necrosis, serum crust, fibrin at the dermoepidermal junction
- Pautrier's-like microabscesses of Langerhans cells (similar to those seen in contact dermatitis)
- Increased fibroblasts in the papillary dermis with small Montgomery giant cells (angulated multinucleated cells, common in other chronic inflammatory disorders such as lichen simplex chronicus and prurigo nodularis)
- CD8+ lymphocytic inflammation may be prominent and difficult to distinguish from lymphoma (look for atypia)

HEAT-INDUCED DERMATOSES

Extreme heat results in thermal burns. These are very rarely biopsied and will not be discussed. Less intense heat results in erythema ab igne.
Non-specific pathology with mild features:
- Thin epidermis with hyperpigmented basal layer
- Mild vacuolar dermatitis
- Increased and fragmented elastic fibers (visible only with the VVG stain)

COLD-INDUCED DERMATOSES

Pernio

The acute form is self-resolving and rarely biopsied. The features below describe the chronic form.

> NB Busy "bluish slide" – this is a clinically and histologically blue lesion **(Figure 4.23A)**.

- Bluish thick stratum corneum (acral site)
- Acanthosis, spongiosis, and scattered necrotic keratinocytes (to frank necrosis) are variable
- Edema in the papillary dermis
- Blue patchy lymphocytic infiltrate (lymphocytic vasculitis) around congested small vessels
- Deep blue patchy infiltrate around eccrine glands **(Figure 4.23B)**

PHYSICAL TRAUMA

Friction blister

- Usually on acral skin
- Pale keratinocytes with lost membrane outlines ("fading away appearance")
- Intraepidermal blister with jagged outlines underneath the granular layer
- The necrotic blister extends throughout the epidermis **(Figure 4.24)**
- No inflammation (cell-poor)

Talon noir (black heel)

- Acral skin
- Red blood cells in the stratum corneum with/without serum (hemorrhagic blister) **(Figure 4.25)**
- Parakeratosis

> - NB Iron stains for hemosiderin are negative

Acanthoma fissuratum

- Nose and ear location

> NB Look for vellus hairs with increased capillaries as a clue to ear site and vellus hairs with sebaceous glands as a clue to nose site.

- Irregular bulbous acanthosis with a central dell (attenuation of the rete ridges) **(Figure 4.26)**
- Hyperkeratosis and hypergranulosis

RADIATION-INDUCED ALTERATIONS

Radiation dermatitis

Acute radiation dermatitis is rarely biopsied.
Subacute radiation dermatitis:
- May be indistinguishable from other interface dermatitides (GVHD)
- Look for satellite cell necrosis (lymphocyte adjacent to necrotic keratinocyte) (see Chapter 3, Interface dermatitis)
- Inflammatory lymphocytic infiltrate in the upper dermis

> - NB There is no collagen alteration.

Chronic radiation dermatitis shows poikiloderma-like changes **(Figure 4.27A)**:
- Striking pink homogenous sclerosis of the collagen in the dermis
- Bizarre fibroblasts (atypical large fibroblasts)

- Hyperkeratosis overlying a thin epidermis with effaced rete ridges and slightly atypical keratinocytes and/or necrotic keratinocytes
- Superficial vessels: dilated (telangiectasias); deep vessels: thick and thrombosed

- NB The pilosebaceous units are gone but eccrine glands may be preserved; in radiation-induced chronic ulcers the eccrine ducts may show features for squamous eccrine syringometaplasia **(Figure 4.27B)**.

SELECTED GENODERMATOSES

ICHTHYOSES

Definition: Genetic disorders of keratinization characterized clinically by thick and scaly skin. The pathologic features are usually non-specific and include thick stratum corneum due to hyperkeratosis or parakeratosis.

(Figure 4.28, Table 4.6)

EPIDERMOLYSIS BULLOSA (EB)

Definition: A group of genetic disorders caused by mutations in the keratin family or the structural proteins of the basement-membrane zone.

Bullous lesions arise from minor trauma (due to cytolysis in EB simplex **(Figure 4.29)** and cleavage through the basement membrane in junctional and dystrophic EB); associated with hair, nail, and other abnormalities resulting from the defective keratinization.
(Table 4.7)

Table 4.6 Main pathologic characteristics in the ichthyoses group

Disorder	Mode of inheritance	Stratum corneum	Stratum granulosum	Other features
Ichthyosis vulgaris	AD	Hyperkeratosis	*Absent* granular layer	Large keratotic plugs (hyperkeratosis of the follicular ostia) Atrophic sebaceous glands
X-linked ichthyosis	XR	Hyperkeratosis Occasional parakeratosis	Normal or thickened granular layer	Perivascular lymphoid infiltrates
Epidermolytic hyperkeratosis (EHK)	AD	Hyperkeratosis	Large keratohyaline granules Vacuolization (clear spaces around the nuclei of the cells)	Acanthosis Bullae (form through separation of the edematous cells)
Erythrokeratoderma variabilis (EKV) Progressive symmetric erythrokeratoderma (PSEK)	AD	Hyperkeratosis	Normal granular layer	Moderate acanthosis
Ichthyosis linearis circumflexa	AR	Parakeratosis ("double-edged scale" clinically)	Normal granular layer	Psoriasiform acanthosis Spongiosis

Table 4.7 Main pathologic characteristics in the epidermolysis bullosa group

Disorder	Mode of inheritance	Mutation	Level of separation	Pathology
EB simplex	AD	K5 and 14	*Basal cell layer* and/or spinous layer	Separation between cells in the basal and suprabasal layer Focal dyskeratosis is possible
Junctional EB	AR	Laminin 5; alpha-3 and GAMMA 2	Dissolution through the *lamina lucida*	The basal layer is separated from the basement membrane (collagen IV stain for basement membrane is positive on the blister floor)
Dystrophic EB	AD/AR	Collagen VII	Dissolution through the anchoring fibrils of *lamina densa*	The entire epidermis is separated from the dermis (collagen IV stain for basement membrane is positive on the blister roof)

MASTOCYTOSES

Definition: A group of disorders characterized by an increased number of mast cells and variety of clinical presentations (see below).

NB See Chapter 1 for more on mast cells.

Clinical types:
- Maculopapular lesions with urtication (urticaria pigmentosa in children) **(Figure 4.30A)**
- Brownish-red macules with fine telangiectasia, no urtication (telangiectasia macularis eruptive perstans (TMEP) in adults)
- Solitary nodule with urtication, possible bullae (mastocytoma) **(Figure 4.30B)**
- Diffuse erythroderma

NB Special stains highlight the mast cells, which may not be easily identified on H&E only (Giemsa, toluidine blue, and Leder stain).

(Table 4.8)

POROKERATOSES

Definition: A group of keratinization disorders inherited in AD mode and presenting clinically with a peripheral keratotic ridge (the optimal site for the biopsy).

Clinical types:
- Plaque-type (Mibelli porokeratosis)
- Linear porokeratosis (resembles ILVEN and has a risk for squamous cell carcinoma)
- Disseminated actinic porokeratosis (DSAP)
- Porokeratosis palmaris, plantaris, and disseminata
- Punctate porokeratosis
- Porokeratotic eccrine ostial and dermal duct nevus (PEODDN)

On low power:
- Wedge-shaped invagination of the epidermis extending downward at an angle
- The invagination is filled with a layered column of parakeratosis (cornoid lamella) **(Figure 4.31A)**
- In the epidermis underneath the lamella there are: 1) a decreased granular layer, and 2) disorganized keratinocytes and dyskeratotic cells
- DSAP can show thin and disorganized keratinocytes in the lower third of the epidermis (actinic changes) **(Figure 4.31B)**
- PEODDN: the cornoid lamella fills dilated infundibular ostia of eccrine ducts (acrosyringia)

INCONTINENTIA PIGMENTI (IP)

Definition: An XD-inherited disorder due to mutation in the NEMO gene.

1. **Vesicular stage:**
   - Spongiosis in the epidermis associated with eosinophils (eosinophilic spongiosis) **(Figure 4.32)**
   - Dyskeratotic cells and swirls of squamoid cells with glassy cytoplasm
2. **Verrucous stage:**
   - Hyperkeratosis, acanthosis, and papillomatosis
   - Dyskeratotic cells and swirls of squamoid cells with glassy cytoplasm
3. **Hyperpigmentation stage:**
   - Vacuolization and degeneration of the basal cell layer
   - Prominent melanophages in the dermis

NB Subungual keratoacanthoma can be a complication in later IP.

Table 4.8 Main pathologic characteristics in the mastocytoses group

Disorder	Morphology of mast cells	Distribution of mast cells	Other pathologic features
Urticaria pigmentosa and TMEP	Spindle nuclei (mimic fibroblasts)	Loose infiltrate of mast cells in the upper third of the dermis Perivascular	Increased pigmentation of the basal layer Melanophages Absent eosinophils in TMEP
Mastocytoma	Round/oval cells with ample cytoplasm Cuboidal nuclei, mimic nevus cells or histiocytes	Sheets of tightly packed cells (tumor-like aggregates) Extend throughout the entire dermis including the fat	Pale pink tumor on low power which may resemble a dermal nevus but has many eosinophils
Diffuse erythroderma	Oval nuclei	Band-like infiltrate	Dilated vessels, eosinophils

PERFORATING DISORDERS

Definition: Disorders characterized by elimination of normal dermal components through the epidermis (transepidermal elimination (TEE)).

General concepts

- **Primary perforating disorders:** Kyrle's disease, perforating folliculitis, elastosis perforans serpiginosa (EPS) and reactive perforating collagenosis

NB The acquired perforating dermatosis (APD) may resemble any of these disorders.

- **Secondary perforating disorders** (TEE occurs as a secondary phenomenon): Granuloma annulare, chondrodermatitis nodularis helicis; elastic fibers may be eliminated in diabetic ulcers (mal perforans), collagen may be eliminated in keratoacanthomas **(Table 4.9)**

On low power

- The epidermis has "a small blue cap" (the crust overlying a perforating channel is blue due to the degenerated collagen mixed with the nuclear debris from neutrophils) in reactive perforating collagenosis.
- The epidermis has "a small blue cap and a blue beard" (elastic fibers at the bottom of the perforating channel with fibrin) in elastosis perforans serpiginosa.
- There is a "pink trash bag" in the epidermis (degenerated material, parakeratosis, and dyskeratotic cells) in Kyrle's disease.
- There is a "blue trash bag" (degenerated blue material) in the follicular infundibulum in perforating folliculitis.

On high power

Kyrle's disease (hyperkeratosis follicularis et parafollicularis in cutem penetrans)

- A large keratotic plug fills an epidermal invagination
- The plug is busy: parakeratosis, dyskeratotic cells, blue debris from acellular keratinization
- Irregular epidermal hyperplasia **(Figure 4.33)**
- Granulomatous infiltrate in the dermis (think of the plug as an abnormal keratotic body which needs to be expelled)
- Elastic and collagen stains are negative

Perforating folliculitis

- Dilated infundibulum with compact orthokeratosis and parakeratosis

NB Follicular involvement is a clue.

- Degenerated blue material (from degenerated collagen and nuclear debris from neutrophils) and fragmented red fibers (collagen) and elastic fibers in the infundibulum **(Figure 4.34)**
- Elastic and collagen stains are positive in the TEE

Elastosis perforans serpiginosa (EPS)

- The hyperplastic epidermis forms a longer wavy or straight channel for TEE (like "a clutch")
- A crust of blue material over the channel of perforation and a collection of blue-like material at the bottom of the channel (degenerated elastic fibers with granular fibrin material)

Table 4.9 Patterns of transepidermal elimination (TEE)

Perforating disorder	Mechanisms of transepidermal elimination	Perforating elastics (VVG stain)	Perforating collagen (Masson trichrome)
Kyrle's disease	Abnormal keratinization in a non-follicular epidermis/follicular unit	–	–
Perforating folliculitis	Abnormal keratinization in a follicular unit	+	+
Elastosis perforans serpiginosa	Abnormal coarse elastics	+	–
Reactive perforating collagenosis	Abnormal collagen bundles	–	+
Acquired perforating dermatosis in renal disease and diabetes	Dermal necrosis due to pruritus, trauma, and diabetic microangiopathy alter the connective tissue	+/–	+
Chondrodermatitis nodularis helicis	Ischemic alteration of the collagen due to chronic trauma	–	+

- Mixed inflammatory infiltrate in the dermis
- Elastic stain highlights the degenerated elastic fibers in the channel of TEE and the abnormal thick elastic fibers close to it

Reactive perforating collagenosis

- The hyperplastic epidermis forms a short, straight channel for TEE
- A crust of blue material in the channel (degenerated collagen fibers, neutrophilic debris, and fibrin) **(Figure 4.35)**
- Vertically oriented fragmented bundles of red collagen
- Collagen stain highlights the abnormal fibers in the channel

Chondrodermatitis nodularis helicis (CDNH)

Vascular compromise (ischemia) of collagen → necrobiotic collagen → wedge-shaped epidermal defect for TEE

NB An increased number of capillaries and vellus hairs in a loose stroma underlying a papillomatous undulating epidermis is a clue to the ear location. A portion of perichondrium is a clue to the helix location.

- Epidermal ulceration with a crust (exudate, parakeratosis, and dermal debris) **(Figure 4.36)**
- Pink (eosinophilic) necrosis of the collagen in the dermis
- Dermal inflammation with lymphocytes, neutrophils, and plasma cells may be present

INFECTIONS

Definition: A wide range of disorders caused by viruses, bacteria, fungi, and other organisms affecting the skin primarily or secondarily

VIRAL INFECTIONS

General concepts

- Viruses replicate in the epidermal cells at the sites of inoculation.
- Intraepidermal viruses can be identified as inclusion bodies in the nuclei surrounded by a halo (papilloma virus, herpes virus) or in the cytoplasm (poxvirus); the inclusions are usually the size of an erythrocyte.
- Intraepidermal viral replication leads to spongiosis, focal necrosis, acantholysis, and ballooning/reticular degeneration of the epidermis (see Chapter 3, Spongiotic pattern).
- Immunohistochemical stains distinguish between HSV and VZV; HPV in situ hybridization (ISH) is helpful to distinguish the type of papilloma virus.

On low power

- Papilloma and poxvirus infections form exophytic/papillomatous (warts) and endophytic (molluscum) lesions
- Look for the thicker granular layer.
- Papillomatous lesion on a mucosal surface with bad mitoses: think Bowenoid papulosis.
- Herpes infection and orf: ballooning and reticular degeneration

On high power

HUMAN PAPILLOMAVIRUS (HPV) INFECTION GROUP

Verruca vulgaris

- Papillomatosis (undulated "wavy" surface) with a church spire-like elongated exophytic growth **(Figure 4.37, Photomnemonic 4.5)**
- Hyperkeratosis alternating with tiers of parakeratosis with rounded/plump nuclei
- Red blood cells in the hyperkeratosis and small blood vessels in the papillary dermis
- Granular layer shows hypergranulosis and so-called koilocytotic cells with raisin-like nuclei surrounded by a clear halo due to pyknosis (nuclear shrinkage) (see Condyloma acuminatum below)

Verruca plana

Similar to verruca vulgaris except:

- No papillomatosis
- Normal basket-weave stratum corneum
- Vacuolated cells in the granular layer with round, centrally located nuclei: "bird eye" **(Figure 4.38)**

Plantar wart

Superficial wart

Similar to verruca vulgaris

Deep plantar wart (myrmecia)

- Endophytic growth with flat surface covered by thick hyperkeratosis
- Epidermal cells contain pink/red cytoplasmic inclusions composed of keratin filaments; they form ring-like structures around the nuclei **(Figure 4.39)**
- Blue dots (viral inclusions) in the nuclei

Condyloma acuminatum

NB The absence of granular and cornified layers is a clue to mucosal location.

- Exo-endophytic growth of bulbous papillomatous acanthosis (compare to the more "slender" silhouette of warts) **(Figure 4.40, Photomnemonic 4.6)**
- Koilocytes: pale cells with central hyperchromatic (dark) pycnotic (shrunken or raisin-like) nuclei
- Occasional mitoses

NB Vacuolization is normal in the upper mucosal epidermis but in condyloma it extends to full thickness.

Bowenoid papulosis

NB Bowenoid papulosis has the silhouette of a condyloma with "the windblown look" of Bowen's disease.

NB The absence of granular and cornified layers is a clue to the mucosal location.

- Disordered maturation
- Crowded atypical nuclei
- Many metaphase mitoses above the basal layer (in metaphase the chromosomes align in the middle of the cell) **(Figure 4.41)**

Epidermodysplasia verruciformis

- Similar to plane warts
- Swollen blue–gray pale cells in the upper epidermis
- Large cells in nests in the granular and spinous layer: the cells have bluish cytoplasm and "empty nuclei" surrounded by a halo **(Figure 4.42)**

POXVIRUS INFECTIONS

Orf/Milker's nodule

- Acanthosis with finger-like projections in the dermis, which shows prominent edema
- Balloon-like degeneration/reticular degeneration of the epidermis
- Focal necrotic keratinocytes or more pronounced necrosis
- Look for inclusion bodies: intracytoplasmic red granules
- Older lesion show lichenoid reaction, CD30+ large lymphocytes, and eosinophils

Molluscum contagiosum

- Endophytic proliferation of bulbous acanthosis
- Hypergranulosis
- Crateriform epidermal invagination filled by keratinocytes loaded with red intracytoplasmic inclusions (Henderson bodies) reminiscent of a "basket with cherries" **(Figure 4.43, Photomnemonic 4.7)**
- Ruptured lesions may show dense inflammation with CD30+ lymphocytes

HERPES INFECTION GROUP

Herpes simplex virus (HSV)

NB Note the preserved stratum corneum with basket-weave pattern or slight hyperkeratosis.

Ballooning degeneration of keratinocytes (cytoplasmic swelling) begins at the basal layer and moves upwards through the epidermis.

- Necrosis ranging from individual necrotic keratinocytes to frank necrosis
- Striking peculiar nuclear findings (cytopathic viral findings in the affected keratinocytes) **(Figure 4.44)**:
  - Slate-gray nuclei
  - Nuclear molding
  - Multinucleated acantholytic keratinocytes; look for inclusion bodies which are ground-glass nuclear inclusions

Reticular degeneration (multilocular vesicles) evolves due to the rupture of the balloon cells.

NB In ulcerated HSV lesions: look at the margins of the specimen for cytopathic findings.

NB The differential diagnosis of reticular degeneration is contact dermatitis.

Varicella zoster virus (VZV)

Changes are similar to HSV lesions and in many instances immunohistochemistry is needed to distinguish both.

Additional features:

- Perivascular or diffuse infiltrate of lymphocytes and neutrophils which may also surround cutaneous nerves
- Leukocytoclastic vasculitis

- NB Necrosis of the pilosebaceous units in the dermis: the VZV reaches the dermatome through the myelinated nerves which end around the isthmus of the hair follicles where the sebaceous gland enters.

BACTERIAL INFECTIONS

General concepts

- Gram-positive cocci (staphylococci and corynebacteria) on the skin surface and in serum crusts over eroded and ulcerated skin are considered normal flora.
- Gram-positive cocci in the dermis and subdermis are always pathogenic (cellulitis, infective panniculitis, and fasciitis).
- Biopsies from immunosuppressed individuals (AIDS) may contain more than one microorganism.
- Special stains are helpful in the identification of the microorganisms: Brown-Brenn stain is a modified Gram stain which picks up the Gram-positive bacteria better.

On low power

- **Subcorneal pustules:** Impetigo; candidiasis
- **Neutrophils in the dermis:** Ecthyma; infectious cellulitis, infectious folliculitis; bacillary angiomatosis; septic/pustular vasculitis: meningococcemia and gonococcemia
- **Plasma cell collections:** Syphilis, Lyme disease, HIV infection; leprosy; leishmaniasis; deep fungal infections
- **Granulomatous infiltrates:** Mycobacterial infections; deep fungal infections; syphilis
- **Pale dermis due to foamy histiocyte collections:** Leprosy; leishmaniasis

On high power

Impetigo

- Serum crust with bacteria and fibrin
- Subcorneal cleft through stratum granulosum forming a neutrophil-rich bulla with Gram-positive cocci **(Figure 4.45)**

> NB A biopsy from the edge of the bulla may not show organisms.

- No acantholysis or only single acantholytic cells (compare to pemphigus foliaceus)
- Superficial inflammation in the dermis

Ecthyma (ulcerated impetigo)

- Well-circumscribed ulcer with a serum crust
- Dense infiltrate of neutrophils in the upper dermis

Staphylococcal scalded skin syndrome (4S)

Same features as bullous impetigo except:
- No cocci in the blister
- No inflammation in the dermis

Erysipelas, cellulitis and necrotizing fasciitis

- Marked edema in the dermis
- Dilated vessels, especially dilated lymphatics
- Diffuse infiltrate of neutrophils dissect the collagen in the dermis in erysipelas and also invade the subdermis in cellulitis **(Figure 4.46)**
- Severe necrosis of the subdermis and fascia with fibrin, neutrophils, and very high amounts of Brown-Brenn-positive bacteria in necrotizing fasciitis

> NB Bacteria are so numerous that they can be seen without special stains in necrotizing fasciitis.

> NB Other infectious entities presenting with cellulitis pattern are erysipeloid and anthrax.

Erythrasma and pitted keratolysis

- Short Brown-Brenn-positive and Giemsa-positive coccobacilli and filamentous bacteria (*Corynebacteria* spp.) in the stratum corneum
- In pitted keratolysis the bacteria dig out crateriform defects

> NB Thick stratum corneum and no pilosebaceous follicles are clues to the acral location.

Folliculitis

- A subcorneal pustule in the infundibulum
- Distension and disruption of the follicular canal
- Dense mixed-cell inflammation (lymphocytes, neutrophils, histiocytes, plasma cells, and eosinophils) fills the canal and the surrounding perifollicular tissue **(Figure 4.47)**
- Ruptured follicles form granulomatous infiltrate with foreign body and Langhans giant cells

> NB Deep folliculitis, furuncle, and carbuncle show tissue necrosis with abscess formation.

Dissecting cellulitis of the scalp

See Hair and nail disorders

Bacillary angiomatosis (BA)

> NB Pyogenic granuloma with dense neutrophils and clumps of bacteria: think bacillary angiomatosis (BA).

- A polypoid lesion which may be ulcerated
- A lobular proliferation of capillaries which are ectatic
- Edema in the stroma
- Dense infiltration of neutrophils with/without karyorrhexis
- Purple clumps of bacteria on H&E; black clumps of *Bartonella* on Warthin–Starry stain

Lyme disease

Erythema chronicum migrans

- Normal epidermis
- Biopsy from the center of lesion shows necrotizing granulomatous vasculitis (differential diagnosis: Churg–Strauss syndrome)
- Biopsy from the periphery shows lymphocytic vasculitis with many plasma cells
- Steiner stain can highlight the spirochetes; immunohistochemistry for anti-Borrelia antibody can be used too

Lymphocytoma (pseudolymphoma)

See Chapter 5, Cutaneous lymphoid neoplasms

- Dense mixed-cell infiltrate of lymphocytes, histiocytes, plasma cells, and eosinophils
- Reactive germinal centers ("blue balls" in the dermis)
- Immunohistochemistry: polyclonal expression for T- and B-cells

MYCOBACTERIAL INFECTIONS

General concepts

- Mycobacteria are intracellular bacilli which are either rapid growers or slow growers (*M. tuberculosum*).

> NB *M. leprae* cannot be cultured.

- The non-tuberculous mycobacteria are also known as atypical mycobacteria.
- All mycobacteria are resistant to decoloration by acid stains (therefore are called acid-fast bacilli or AFB) and stain with the Ziehl–Neelsen stain in red (except for *M. leprae*) and its modified version, the Wade Fite stain.
- The main pathologic pattern is the formation of caseating tuberculoid granulomas which show: 1) caseation infarct-like necrosis in the center (these are dead macrophages with dead bacilli); 2) rim of epithelioid macrophages and Langhans giant cells; and 3) mantle of lymphocytes **(Figure 4.48)**.
- In patients with impaired cellular immunity the mycobacterial infections are less granulomatous and with higher density of bacilli due to their inability to restrain the infection.
- Tuberculids (immunologic skin reactions to dead bacilli or fragmented antigens in patients with occult tuberculosis): the AFB stains and the cultures are negative.

Cutaneous tuberculosis

M. tuberculosum is more virulent than the atypical mycobacteria.

Lupus vulgaris

- The epidermis is atrophic with epidermal hyperplasia at the borders
- Non-caseating granulomas in the upper dermis

> NB If necrosis is present, reconsider the diagnosis.

- Epithelioid macrophages in the center and a mantle of lymphocytes: the macrophages are able to phagocytize the bacilli and limit the infection in people with a good cellular immunity
- Negative AFB stains

Tuberculosis verrucosa cutis

- Verrucous surface (pseudoepitheliomatous hyperplasia with hyperkeratosis)
- Abscess with tuberculoid caseating granulomas in the dermis
- Positive AFB stains

Atypical mycobacteria (AMB)

- *M. marinum* and *M. ulcerans* (slow growers) cause the most common AMB infections of skin
- *M. chelonei*, *M. fortuitum*, and *M. abscessus* (rapid growers) are most commonly acquired through contaminated cannulas and injectable materials; also reported to cause furunculosis in women's legs after pedicure
- AMB infections mostly occur in immunocompromised individuals but can occur in immunocompetent patients after skin trauma

Swimming pool granuloma (M. marinum)

- Elbows are a common location and sporotrichoid pattern can develop
- Pseudoepitheliomatous hyperplasia
- Early lesions: non-specific abscess-like inflammation in the dermis

> NB AFB stains are positive early.

- Later lesions (older than 6 months): tuberculoid granulomas form without necrosis or occasional necrosis

> NB AFB are usually negative later.

Buruli ulcer (M. ulcerans)

- Painless ulcers in children/young adults on the extremities and the buttocks
- Extensive deep dermal and subcutaneous fat necrosis down to the fascia ("ghost"/ischemic type of necrosis caused by the released mycolactone exotoxin) **(Figure 4.49A)**
- Subtle inflammation contrasts the marked necrosis

- Infectious panniculitis with numerous extracellular clusters of AFB-positive bacteria **(Figure 4.49B)**
- Late lesions show tuberculoid granulomas and no bacteria

Leprosy

- *M. leprae* is a weakly acid-fast Gram-positive intracellular organism which can be found in three cell types:
  - Macrophages
  - Schwann cells
  - Endothelial cells

> - NB Clues to distinguish from other granulomatous infections (deep fungal infections and mycobacterial infections):
>   - The epidermis is flat and normal
>   - The granulomas are tight and vertically oriented following the sweat glands and the nerves
>   - Necrosis is absent

- *Stains:*
  - Wade-Fite (a modified Ziehl–Neelsen stain) and GMS (more rarely used)

> NB 1000 bacilli/cm^3 must be present to detect a single bacillus in a section and at least six sections should be examined; treated lesions may be negative.

  - Even one bacillus makes the diagnosis
  - Solid-staining, slightly curved filaments or rods mean the organisms are capable of multiplication
  - Fragmented and granular bacilli in clumps (globi) mean dead bacilli
  - Immunohistochemistry: Polyclonal BCG antibody

> NB It takes years to clear the antigen from the skin so the immunohistochemical stain may remain positive.

Early indeterminate leprosy

- Mild infiltrates of lymphohistiocytes and macrophages around the neurovascular bundles, the sweat glands, and the arrector pili muscle of the hair follicles

Tuberculoid leprosy ("vertical granulomas")

- Large epithelioid cells in tight "stretched-out" granulomas: the neurovascular bundles and sweat glands are enveloped by tight "muff"-like granulomas **(Figure 4.50A)**
- Dense peripheral lymphocytic infiltrate

> - NB No giant cells, just epithelioid macrophages.

> - NB The nerves may be absent/obliterated or eroded – the S100 stain helps to detect them.

- *Stains:* Negative

Lepromatous leprosy ("pale and foamy dermis")

- Flattened epidermis
- Grenz zone
- Extensive dense pale collections and sheets of heavily parasitized macrophages with sparse lymphocytes in the dermis extending to the subdermis; in older lesions the macrophages are foamy ("lepra/xanthomatous cells" because they contain lipids) **(Figure 4.50B)**

> - NB The appendages are basically absent because they have been destroyed by the heavy infiltrate

- Numerous Fite-positive solid ("cigars pack") or fragmented bacilli are found in the endothelial cells, macrophages, nerves, and sweat glands **(Figure 4.50C)**

> - NB No granulomas

- Even if the nerves contain a high number of bacilli, they remain preserved (compare to erosion and disappearance of the nerves in tuberculoid leprosy)
  - *Histoid variant:* spindled macrophages form a storiform dermatofibroma-like tumor in the deep dermis due to incomplete treatment or drug resistance

> NB Histoid variant has the highest load of bacilli.

  - *Erythema nodosum leprosum:* background of lepromatous leprosy (pale dermis of foamy macrophages) + abscess-like inflammation of neutrophils, eosinophils, plasma cells in the dermis and subdermis + leukocytoclastic vasculitis
  - *Lucio's phenomenon:* "endarteritis obliterans pattern" of endothelial swelling (endothelial cells are loaded with bacilli) and thrombosis leading to luminal obliteration and ischemic necrosis

FUNGAL INFECTIONS

General concepts

Hyphae: Septate filamentous fungi which form a tangled mass called mycelium
Yeasts: Single cells of rounded fungi which reproduce by budding
Conidia (budding yeasts): Asexually reproductive spores produced by fragmentation of the hyphae and attached at their tips; they detach when mature

Pseudohyphae: Chains of yeast cells formed by repeated budding (budding yeast cells with their progeny) **(Figure 4.51)**, followed by nodular granulomatous perifolliculitis
Arthrospores: Small, usually single-celled bodies which allow fungi to reproduce asexually; they are highly resistant to heat and desiccation
Chlamydospores: Fungi can reproduce sexually when two haploid (containing one copy of each chromosome) mycelia of the same species meet. When their haploid nuclei fuse, they form chlamydospores
Dematiaceous fungi: Fungi which contain melanin in their walls (*Phaehyphomycosis* and *Alternariosis*, *Tinea nigra*, and *Chromomycosis*)
Dimorphic fungi: Fungi which grow in different forms: mold, yeast, sulfur grains

NB Special stains: PAS stains fungi because their walls contain neutral polysaccharides; other stains include GMS and Fontana-Masson.

On low power

- **Superficial fungal infections** may present as "invisible dermatoses" on H&E or with a slight spongiotic or psoriasiform pattern with or without pustules and mild dermal infiltrate
- **Clues to dermatophytosis** in the stratum corneum:
  - The sandwich sign: "orthokeratosis–fungi–parakeratosis"
  - Collections of neutrophils
  - Clear round spaces in parakeratosis more visible by lowering the microscope condenser (these are created by the retractile fungal walls)
- **Deep fungal infections** show epidermal hyperplasia with neutrophilic microabscesses and mixed dermal granulomatous inflammation with or without fibrosis (suppurative granulomas)

NB Lobomycosis and histoplasmosis show epidermal thinning.

- **Disseminated candidiasis, mucormycosis, and aspergillosis** present with vascular invasion of hyphae

On high power

SUPERFICIAL FUNGAL INFECTIONS

NB Organisms causing superficial fungal infections are not found in the dermis except for cases of follicular rupture.

(Table 4.10)

Table 4.10 Superficial fungal infections of the skin

Superficial fungal infections	Fungal species
Piedra	Black piedra: *Piedraia hortae* White piedra: *Trichosporon beigelii*
Dermatophytosis classified according to anatomic site: • scalp: tinea capitis (non-inflammatory and inflammatory (kerion)) • face: tinea barbae and tinea faciei • trunk: tinea corporis • inguinal folds: tinea cruris • fungal folliculitis (Majocchi's granuloma) • acral sites: tinea manuum and tinea pedis • nails: tinea unguium (onychomycosis)	*Microsporum* spp. *Trichophyton* spp. *Epidermophyton* spp.
Tinea versicolor Pityrosoporum folliculitis	*Malassezia* spp.
Candidiasis • acute mucocutaneous candidiasis • chronic mucocutaneous candidiasis • disseminated candidiasis	*Candida* spp.

Dermatophytosis

Dermatophytes parasitize the keratinized tissues: stratum corneum, hair shafts, and nail plate.

- Invade and consume dead keratin by generating proteases
- Dermatophyte hyphae are slender and uniform, 1–2 μm

NB Compare to thick, plump 2–4 μm pseudohyphae of *Candida* (see Figure 4.51).

Tinea of glabrous skin

NB Clear spaces within a hyperkeratotic stratum corneum: think tinea! The hyphae remain within the stratum corneum and do not invade hairs.

- Acanthosis, parakeratosis, spongiosis with/without a sandwich sign **(Figure 4.52)**
- Neutrophils in the stratum corneum: PAS stain must be performed to exclude tinea

Majocchi's granuloma *(fungal folliculitis)*

- Hyphae and spores within hair shafts and hair follicles

- Inflammatory mixed-cell infiltrate and granulomatous infiltrate in the dermis (abscess or suppurative granulomas), followed by nodular granulomatous perifolliculitis
- The fungal organisms break the follicular wall and invade the dermis **(Figure 4.53)**

NB Agminate folliculitis is when the fungi remain within the hair follicles without invading the dermis (grouped pustular folliculitis).

Tinea capitis

- Hyphae invade the hair follicle from the interfollicular scalp surface
  - *Ectothrix infection:* Hyphae and spores cover the outside surface of the hair shaft, which results in destruction of the cuticle (*M. canis* from the *Microsporum* spp. causes the "gray patch" tinea capitis) **(Figure 4.54A, B)**

    Remember: *Ecto* means "out" and *canis* means "dog": the dog stays outside the house
  - *Endothrix infection:* invasion to the inside of the hair shaft only by rounded and box-like arthrospores and not by hyphae! (*T. tonsurans* (TT) from the *Trichophyton* spp. causes "black dots" tinea capitis; *T. mentagrophytes* (TM) and *T. verrucosum* (TV) cause kerion, which is a type of inflammatory tinea capitis, and *T. shoenleinii* causes favus);
  - Remember: *Endo* means inside: **T**T, T**M**, and TV: the table, the mirror, and the TV are inside the house

  NB In kerion there is dense mixed-cell inflammation with giant cells involving the follicles and extending from the upper dermis to the fat (suppurative granulomatous folliculitis) **(Figure 4.54C)**.

- In kerion, half of the cases the fungal stains may be falsely negative due to the dense inflammation; numerous step sections as well as a fungal culture are therefore necessary for the diagnosis

Onychomycosis *(Tinea unguium)*

T. rubrum is the most common agent.

- Hyphae and spores in the superficial nail plate layers (in superficial onychomycosis) or within lower layers and/or invading from underneath the nail plate (distal onychomycosis) **(Figure 4.55)**
- Parakeratosis in the nail plate and subungual hyperkeratosis with neutrophilic debris
- Lacunae filled with PAS-positive serum (artifacts)

Tinea versicolor

- Hyperkeratosis
- Slight acanthosis
- Numerous hyphae and spores in the stratum corneum: "spaghetti and meatballs" on PAS **(Figure 4.56)**

Pityrosporum folliculitis (*malassezia folliculitis*)

- Dilated infundibulum plugged with keratinous material
- Numerous spores within the infundibulum **(Figure 4.57)**

  NB Hyphae are very rare.

- Intra- and perifollicular inflammation (lymphocytes, histiocytes, neutrophils)

Candidiasis

Candida spp. belong to the dimorphic fungi (grow as both yeast and filamentous forms).

Acute mucocutaneous candidiasis

Clinically presents with vesicles and pustules

- Collections of neutrophils and neutrophilic debris of two types: 1) broad pustule (as found in impetigo), or 2) spongiform pustule of Kogoj (as seen in pustular psoriasis)
- Spores and pseudohyphae branching at 90° angle and constricted at site of branching **(Figure 4.58)**

NB Chronic mucocutaneous candidiasis: epidermal papillomatosis with *Candida* granulomas in the dermis.

Disseminated candidiasis

Variable clinical presentation from macular–papular to ulcerated and eschar-like lesions in immunocompromised

- Microabscesses in the dermis
- Aggregates of hyphae and spores in the dermis close to the blood vessels
- Edema in the vessel walls
- In kerion, in half of the cases LCV may be present

Candida onychomycosis

Clinically presents as onycholysis, except for the cases of chronic mucocutaneous candidiasis

- NB No nail plate invasion compared to tinea unguium in which the nail plate invasion is diagnostic

- Spores and bulbous pseudohyphae along the undersurface of the nail plate (compare to the thin and uniform septate dermatophyte hyphae within the nail plate) **(Figure 4.59)**

DEEP FUNGAL INFECTIONS

NB Deep fungal infections are a group of mycoses which affect the deep structures of the skin (dermis and subdermis) usually at the portal of traumatic inoculation. There may also be visceral involvement.

(Table 4.11)

Table 4.11 Deep fungal infections: an overview with clues to the diagnosis

Clues	Deep fungal infections
Dimorphic fungi (transform from filamentous mold at 25°C to unicellular yeast at 37°C in the host)	North American blastomycosis Coccidioidomycosis Paracoccidioidomycosis Histoplasmosis
Pseudoepitheliomatous hyperplasia with lichenoid granulomas	North American blastomycosis Chromoblastomycosis Coccidioidomycosis
Pseudoepitheliomatous hyperplasia with dermal abscess	Phaeohyphomycosis Sporotrichosis Coccidioidomycosis Paracoccidioidomycosis Fungal mycetoma
No pseudoepitheliomatous hyperplasia	Lobomycosis Aspergillosis
Minimal inflammation in loose gelatinous stroma	Cryptoccocosis
Presenting with hyphae (the rest present with spores)	Aspergillosis Mucormycosis Phaeohyphomycosis
Septate hyphae branching at 45 degrees ("broom-like" hyphae) 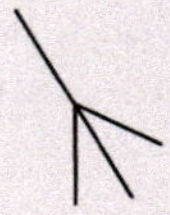	Aspergillosis
Non-septate plump hyphae branching at 90° (like a baseball bat) with ring-like (collapsed) hyphae (like a baseball ball) NB *Candida* spp. are also branching at 90° but they are septate and have a septum at the site of branching.	Mucormycosis
Angioinvasive fungi • cause thrombosis, necrosis and infarcts NB *Candida* spp. can also be angioinvasive in disseminated candidiasis.	Aspergillosis Mucormycosis
Largest hyphae (7–30 µm)	Mucormycosis
Smallest hyphae (2–4 µm)	Aspergillosis
Pigmented fungi (the melanin in their walls binds the hydrolytic enzymes and scavenges the free radicals produced by the macrophages to kill the fungi) • brown hyphae • brown spores	Phaeohyphomycosis (Alternariosis) Chromoblastomycosis
Spores are almost never identified, even with the help of special stains	Sporotrichosis
Smallest spores (2–4 µm) *The size of an erythrocyte is about 7 µm	Histoplasmosis

(continued)

Table 4.11 *(continued)*

Clues	Deep fungal infections
Largest spores (10–80 µm) *Sporangium (a cluster of many individual spores) (300–500 µm)	Coccidioidomycosis Rhinosporidiosis
Double-contoured spores 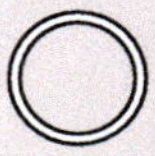	North American blastomycosis
Spores in the cytoplasm of giant cells ("punched-out cytoplasm")	North American blastomycosis
Spores within macrophages *Compared to leishmaniasis, the spores in histoplasmosis are bigger, with clear halo and can be seen outside the macrophages	Histoplasmosis
Spores with narrow-based budding	Histoplasmosis Paracoccidioidomycosis
Spores with broad-based budding	North American blastomycosis
Sieve-like spores (large spores containing endospores) (40 µm)	Coccidioidomycosis
Copper pennies (thick-walled brown spores in clusters)	Chromoblastomycosis
Lemon-shaped spores	Lobomycosis
Marine-wheel spores (with multiple narrow-based buds)	Paracoccidioidomycosis
Red fish eggs (spores hang loose in a gelatinous stroma)	Cryptococcosis
Large pomegranate-like sporangia in the dermis	Rhinosporidiosis

Aspergillosis (*Aspergillus fumigates, A. flavus, A. niger*)

- No pseudoepitheliomatous hyperplasia
- Dermal necrosis prevails over inflammation
- Small septate "broom-like " hyphae branching at 45° in a radiate fashion within blood vessels and in areas of ischemic necrosis in the dermis (the word *aspergillum* means an implement which resembles a broom used to sprinkle holy water)

- NB Spores are absent

Zygomycosis (*Mucor, Rhizopus, Absidia*)

- Occurs 1) in burns, 2) in ketotic diabetics and other immunosuppressed patients, especially neutropenic, and 3) on the face in healthy people in tropical climates
- Ulcerated epidermis
- Sparse inflammation or granulomatous inflammation
- Vascular invasion by 1) large plump hyphae branching at 90°, and 2) ring-like hyphae (collapsed hyphae due to thin wall) **(Photomnemonic 4.8)**

- NB Spores are absent

Phaeohyphomycosis (*Phialophora, Exophiala, Alternaria*)

- In immunocompetent patients is due to trauma (splinter); alternariosis (a variant of phaeohyphomycosis) is prevalent in immunocompromised patients
- Suppurative granulomatous inflammation
- "Cystic" abscess in the dermis with central cavity and fibrous capsule may form (phaeohyphomycotic cyst)
- Irregular brown hyphae which have constrictions at the sites of branching similar to yeasts

NB Search for the hyphae in the center of the abscess or cystic cavity, or at the edges of the specimen **(Figure 4.60)**.

- Pigment is not always obvious and may be highlighted by Fontana-Masson stain

NB Chromoblastomycosis shows only brown spores without budding and no hyphae.

Chromoblastomycosis (*Fonsecaea pedrosoi*)

- A localized cutaneous infection on the lower extremities after trauma (splinter)

- Pseudoepitheliomatous hyperplasia with lichenoid granulomatous and mixed-cell inflammation (very similar to North American blastomycosis) **(Figure 4.61A)**
- Dark brown, thick-walled round spores (copper pennies), individual or in clusters **(Figure 4.61B)**
- No budding; reproduction occurs by fusion

North American blastomycosis (*Blastomyces dermatidis*)

- Occurs in three forms: 1) primary (very rare) or secondary cutaneous (70%), 2) systemic, and 3) pulmonary
- Pseudoepitheliomatous hyperplasia with lichenoid granulomatous and mixed-cell inflammation
- Intraepidermal abscesses **(Figure 4.62A)**
- The giant cells usually lie individually without forming granulomas
- Small round, double-contoured, thick-walled spores with a single broad-based bud **(Figure 4.62B)**

NB Look for spores in the cytoplasm of the giant cells (punched-out cytoplasm) or within the abscess foci.

Coccidioidomycosis (*Coccidioides immitis*)

- Occurs in three clinical forms in the same way as North American blastomycosis
- Pseudoepitheliomatous hyperplasia with *lichenoid* granulomatous and mixed-cell inflammation but less tendency for abscess formation
- Big spores can be seen on H&E within giant cells or free in the dermis **(Figure 4.63)**; the large spores reproduce through forming endospores at 37 °C in the affected host; the endospores are released in the tissue through rupture of the cell wall and are very contagious

NB **Dangerous to culture.**

Differential diagnosis: Rhinosporidiosis: numerous much larger sporangia of various shapes, forming clusters

Paracoccidioidomycosis (*Paracoccidioides brasiliensis*)

- The primary infection is pulmonary and the skin is secondarily involved
- Pseudoepitheliomatous hyperplasia with lichenoid granulomatous and mixed-cell inflammation
- Large thick-walled yeasts with usually single narrow-based bud; rarely, buds are distributed in chains or cover concentrically the entire surface of the yeast as a "marine wheel" **(Figure 4.64)**

Lobomycosis (*Loboa loboi*)

- The infection is limited to skin only
- Atrophic epidermis with a Grenz zone
- Scattered lymphocytes and plasma cells as well as giant cells, but no neutrophils
- Thick-walled, ovoid "lemon"-like spores with single budding **(Figure 4.65)**

Histoplasmosis (*Histoplasma capsulatum*)

- Occurs in three clinical forms in the same way as North American blastomycosis and coccidioidomycosis
- In acute cutaneous lesions there is little inflammation
- In chronic cutaneous lesions there is suppurative granulomatous inflammation with/without necrosis
- Small spores within the cytoplasm of histiocytes (rarely in giant cells) or in clusters free in the dermis like a "flock of fish" **(Figure 4.66A)**
- The spores have a pseudocapsule (a clear surrounding space – halo) and form narrow buds

Stains: PAS, GMS, Giemsa, and Gram stain **(Figure 4.66B)**

Differential diagnosis:
- From *Leishmania*: the histoplasma spores highlight with fungal stains and have a pseudocapsule
- From *Cryptococcus*: the histoplasma spores are smaller with a pseudocapsule (no true capsule)

Cryptococcosis (*Cryptoccocus neoformans*)

The spores spread by aerosol and cause a pulmonary and rarely a secondary skin infection; meningitis can occur.
Three pathologic types:
- **Granulomatous** (in high immunity):
  - Pseudoepitheliomatous hyperplasia with granulomas (has the classic deep fungal infection look)
  - Small number of organisms, found usually in giant cells
- **Gelatinous** (in low immunity):
  - Very little tissue reaction", "vacuolated or sponge-like dermis" **(Figure 4.67A)**
  - Numerous organisms resembling red fish eggs (caviar)
  - The spores are a little bigger than in histoplasmosis (PAS, GMS and Fontana-Masson(+) with a true capsule which is PAS(-) and mucicarmine(+) **(Figure 4.67B)**
- **Suppurative**

Sporotrichosis (*Sporothrix schenckii*)

- Affects the cooler parts of the body: skin, joints, and lungs
- Three clinical forms: lymphocutaneous, fixed cutaneous, and systemic

NB A culture must be performed since the microorganism is rarely identified on histology; results from the culture are ready in 3–5 days.

- Pseudoepitheliomatous hyperplasia with suppurative diffuse granulomatous inflammation in the majority of cases: 1) neutrophils in the middle, 2) rim of histiocytes, and 3) outer cuff of lymphocytes and plasma cells
- Small cigar-shaped spores are detected in only 35% of specimens
- Asteroid bodies

Rhinosporidiosis (*Rhinosporidium seeberi*)

- Clinically a "strawberry nose" appearance
- Pseudoepitheliomatous hyperplasia with granulomatous mixed-cell inflammation
- Swiss-cheese pattern due to large cystic spaces in the dermis (sporangia)
- Sporangia: very large globular cystic spores with endospores, the size of an erythrocyte; resemble a bisected pomegranate **(Photomnemonic 4.9)**

NB The spores are 10 times larger than in coccidioidomycosis.

Eumycetoma/fungal mycetoma (*Madurella mycetomatis, Pseudallescheria boydii*)

NB Actinomycetoma is caused by the bacteria *Actinomyces, Nocardia,* and *Streptomyces* spp.; eumycetoma is caused by fungi producing colored granules (grains): *Madurella mycetomatis* (most common etiologic agent worldwide), *Pseudallescheria boydii* (most common etiologic agent in the USA).

- Extensive granulation tissue with abscesses and sinuses in the dermis
- Sulfur granules in the dermis (very large up to 2 mm, tightly knit clusters of septate hyphae)
- Black sulfur granules in eumycetoma **(Figure 4.68)**
- The organisms may be surrounded by eosinophilic material (immunoglobulin and fibrin): Splendore-Hoeppli phenomenon

NB The granules are PAS(+) and GMS(+) but Gram(−) in eumycetoma and PAS(−) and GMS(−) but Gram(+) in actinomycetoma.

OTHER INFECTIONS

Leishmaniasis

Leishmaniasis is a protozoan infection acquired through a bite by the sandfly, which is the vector for the *Leishmania* spp. (*L. major* and *L. tropica* cause Old World leishmaniasis; *L. braziliensis* and *L. mexicana* cause New World leishmaniasis (*L. braziliensis* causes mucocutaneous leishmaniasis too) and *L. donovanum infantum* causes Mediterranean leishmaniasis).

NB The optimal biopsy specimen is obtained from the active border of an ulcerated lesion.

NB The *Leishmania* spp. parasite inside the macrophages inhibit their lysosomal phosphatase and protein kinase C synthesis as well as the production of proinflammatory cytokines.

Acute lesions: "pale" dermis

- Epidermis may show no specific changes but epidermal hyperplasia and/or ulceration
- Dense diffuse infiltrate of histiocytes (this gives the pale look), lymphocytes, plasma cells, eosinophils, and neutrophils is mostly present in ulcerated lesions
- Look on high power in the histiocytes for *Leishmania* bodies (amastigotes): dull blue–gray, round, non-motile structures of 2–4 μm diameter **(Figure 4.69)**
- If the number of microorganisms is too high, the *Leishmania* bodies can also be seen extracellularly

Stains: The *Leishmania* bodies stain positive with Giemsa and remain negative with the fungal stains because they lack a capsule.

NB In histoplasmosis the fungal stains are positive.

Immunohistochemistry: *Leishmania*-specific antibodies. With time, the number of *Leishmania* bodies decreases but the number of plasma cells increases.
Chronic lesions:

- Absent *Leishmania* bodies
- Tuberculoid granulomas
- Fibrosis (new lesions arise over scars)

Protothecosis

- Very rare cutaneous infection in humans, caused by *Prototheca* spp. algae
- The epidermis is ulcerated or shows hyperplasia
- Dermal necrosis with mixed cell infiltrate, giant cells
- Sporangia: a morula-like structure enclosing clusters of endospores **(Figure 4.70)**; stain with Giemsa; PAS
- Transepidermal elimination of the sporangia can be seen

Syphilis

- *Treponema pallidum* is usually identified by dark-field microscopic examination of mucosal or skin lesions and by serology
- The silver stains Warthin–Starry or Steinert can be helpful in skin biopsies: the *Treponema* is found in the epidermis at the dermoepidermal junction and in the dermis within the blood vessels

NB All these methods are not specific and non-sensitive.

- Immunohistochemical stain for *Treponema pallidum* is 70–90% sensitive **(Figure 4.71A)**
- The *Treponema* induces mononuclear cell infiltrates of lymphocytes and plasma cells
- These infiltrates may surround small arteries and arterioles, leading to arteritis and to endarteritis obliterans (inflamed arteries with swollen endothelial cells which narrow the lumen as well as periarterial onion-like fibrosis)

Primary syphilis *(chancre)*

- Ulcerated genital epithelium with epithelial hyperplasia
- Dense mixed-cell infiltrate in the dermis with predominant plasma cells
- Endarteritis obliterans
- Necrotizing vasculitic changes (secondary to the ulceration)

Secondary syphilis

- Macules: non-specific changes
- Papules:
  - Psoriasiform + spongiotic + lichenoid pattern

  NB Psoriasis with edema and lichenoid infiltrate of plasma cells: think syphilis.

  - Edema
  - Top-heavy infiltrate (perivascular and periadnexal)
  - Endarteritis obliterans with angiocentric plasma cells **(Figure 4.71B)**
- Nodules: similar to papules but may show sarcoidal granulomas or pseudolymphoma-like features

Tertiary syphilis *(gumma)*

- Central caseous necrosis surrounded by dense mixed inflammation with plasma cells

Scabies

- The diagnosis can be made for sure only if *Sarcoptes scabei* or its eggs or feces (scybala) are found in the stratum corneum **(Figure 4.72)**
- Otherwise, the epidermis and dermis show features characteristic for arthropod bite reaction (see Chapter 3, Spongiotic pattern)
- **Postscabietic nodules:** Delayed hypersensitivity reaction to the female mite, its eggs and scybala deposited in the stratum corneum

NB The mite is no longer present in the skin.

Larva migrans

Hookworm infection: larva migrans is caused by *Ancylostoma braziliense*; larva currens is caused by *Strongyloides.*

NB The biopsy should be obtained from a site ahead of the visible track because the latter is just an inflammatory reaction to the migrating larva.

- Small cavities in the epidermis for larva migrans; larva currens moves in the dermis

- NB The larva itself is not identified in skin biopsies and they may be non-specific

- Eosinophilic spongiosis and eosinophilic folliculitis are possible
- Mixed-cell infiltrate in the dermis

HAIR AND NAIL DISORDERS

HAIR DISORDERS

Definition: Hair disorders are characterized by hair loss (alopecia). There are two main categories based on the findings and the prognosis: 1) non-scarring alopecia (preserved follicular structures), and 2) scarring alopecia (loss of follicular structures and fibrosis).

General concepts

Hair disorders can be diagnosed under the microscope in both horizontal and vertical sections. Horizontal sections are created by bisecting the specimen at the level of the isthmus and are evaluated at several levels (bulbar level in the fat, lower follicular level where the sweat coils are, the isthmus where the sebaceous gland enters the follicle, and the infundibulum where the hair emerges in the surface (see Chapter 1, Hair follicle and Figure 1.43). Horizontal sections demonstrate better the follicular architecture and can identify even focal areas of scarring alopecia.

On low power

- The diagnosis of **non-scarring alopecia** is based on preserved follicular architecture including regularly distributed 12–14 follicular units which

contain 3–5 terminal follicles, 1 vellus follicle, and the sebaceous lobules.
  - Non-scarring alopecias present on horizontal sections with a "flower" pattern. At the level of the fat, this resembles "a lawn of daisies" **(Figure 4.73 and Photomnemonic 4.10)**; at the level of the isthmus "a pond with water lilies" **(Figure 4.74 and Photomnemonic 4.11)**; and at the level of the infundibulum "skeleton/monkey faces" **(Figure 4.75 and Photomnemonic 4.12)**.
  - The follicular counts (terminal anagen, telogen, and vellus follicles) and the follicular ratios (terminal : vellus and anagen : telogen) are crucial for diagnosing non-scarring alopecia (see also Figures 1.44 and 1.45).
- The diagnosis of **scarring alopecia** is based on the altered follicular architecture: the follicular units disappear and are replaced by scar tissue (follicular drop-out) **(Figure 4.76)**; the perifollicular inflammation and fibrosis are more pronounced at the level of the isthmus; the sebaceous glands disappear too (they enter the follicles at the level of the isthmus).
  - In *lymphocytic scarring alopecia* the affected follicles are usually grouped in pairs resembling "owl's eyes or goggles" at the isthmus level and/or below.
  - In *neutrophilic scarring alopecia* (such as folliculitis decalvans) the affected follicles are usually grouped as more than 2, usually 4–6 follicles.

> – NB *Traction alopecia* has preserved sebaceous glands.

On high power

Alopecia areata (AA)

1. **Acute stage** (new onset of patches with hair breakage):
   - There is preserved follicular architecture with decreased follicular count
   - In the fat the bulbs of the follicles show intra- and peribulbar follicular infiltrate of closely arranged lymphocytes like "swarm of bees" **(Figure 4.77A)**
2. **Subacute stage** (active patches with broken hairs):
   - Increased number of telogen follicles and telogen germinal units (usually more than 50%) resembling a field of clovers **(Figure 4.77B)**
3. **Chronic stage** (alopecia totalis, long-standing AA):
   - Increased number of vellus follicles and "nanogen" follicles with very thin (pencil-like) hair shafts which may show intermediate features of anagen (hair shaft) and telogen (serrated epithelial borders) **(Figure 4.77C)**

The terminal : vellus ratio is less than 1 : 1.

Trichotillomania

- Decreased follicular density with predominant number of catagen follicles (up to 75%)
- Groups of catagen follicles (due to simultaneous plucking of bunch of hairs which involute together into catagen) **(Figure 4.78A)**
- Trichomalacia: distorted hair shafts **(Figure 4.78B)**
- Pigmented casts: chunks of melanin with irregular shape observed at different levels of the hair canal which result from traumatized matrix cells (because matrix is pigmented) and/or disrupted hair cortex melanization
- Infundibular ostia filled with blood and hair shafts may split into two halves (hamburger sign)

Telogen effluvium

- Normal or slightly decreased follicular density. The biopsy at the level of the bulbs in the fat looks like normal scalp **(Figure 4.79)**
- Normal telogen count. (In acute telogen effluvium, which is very rarely biopsied, it can be increased)
- No follicular miniaturization (terminal : vellus ratio > 4 : 1)

Androgenetic alopecia

- Decreased follicular density. The biopsy at the level of the bulbs in the fat looks "empty" as large number of follicles have miniaturized and their bulbs are situated in the mid and upper dermis
- Follicular miniaturization (terminal:vellus ratio < 4 : 1, usually < 2.2 : 1) **(Figure 4.80)**
- Normal or slightly increased up to 20% telogen count

Lichen planopilaris and frontal fibrosing alopecia (FFA)

- Follicular drop-out
- Most pronounced at the isthmus level: affected follicles show perifollicular fibrosis and lichenoid inflammation
- Often eyes and goggles present **(Figure 4.81A and Photomnemonic 4.13A; Figure 4.81B and Photomnemonic 4.13B)**

> NB FFA more often shows necrotic keratinocytes in the outer root sheath.

Traction alopecia

- Focal or large area of follicular drop-out
- Vellus follicles are the predominant follicular type left after prolonged years of traction of the terminal hairs (decreased terminal:vellus ratio)
- Sebaceous glands are preserved **(Figure 4.82)**

> NB No perifollicular fibrosis and lichenoid inflammation – compare to lymphocytic scarring alopecia.

Discoid lupus erythematosus (DLE)

- Less follicular drop-out and less perifollicular fibrosis
- At the level of the bulbs: collections of lymphocytes and plasma cells (plasmocytoid dendritic cells) forming lymphoid follicles around dilated vessels and around sweat glands **(Figure 4.83A)**
- At the level of the infundibulum: dilated ostia plugged by keratin and interface changes: vacuolar damage in the basal layer of the outer root sheath with pigment incontinence **(Figure 4.83B)**

Dissecting cellulitis of the scalp (DCS, perifolliculitis capitis abscedens et suffodiens)

- Dense mixed-cell infiltrate with edema and granulation tissue in the lower dermis (sea of inflammation), hence the clinical presentation of a boggy scalp **(Figure 4.84)**
- Epithelium-lined sinuses in the lower dermis may be found
- Increased number of telogen follicles

> NB Early DCS shows non-scarring pattern with preserved sebaceous glands.

> NB The upper dermis may look normal or have increased telogen count; make sure the lower dermis and the subdermis are available for assessment.

Differential diagnosis: Inflammatory tinea capitis (kerion)

Folliculitis decalvans (FD)

- There are packs of 4–6 follicles (tufts of hairs or doll's hairs clinically) surrounded by perifollicular fibrosis and a lichenoid mixed-cell inflammation, including eosinophils and plasma cells **(Figure 4.85)**
- The inflammation can be spread diffusely throughout the entire dermis

> NB In FD the inflammation is more follicular-bound and mostly pronounced in the upper dermis whereas in DCS it is more stromal, granulation-like, and diffuse, affecting the lower dermis.

Tinea capitis

See Infections

NAIL DISORDERS

> **Definition:** Nail disorders are characterized by abnormalities in the nails most commonly caused by trauma, tumor or infection or in association with a systemic disease.

General concepts

The nail plate is most commonly evaluated on nail clippings for onychomycosis. The inflammatory and neoplastic diseases in the nail bed and nail matrix are studied in shave biopsies (shave biopsy of the nail matrix in melanonychia), punch biopsies, and longitudinal excisions. The anatomy of the nail unit is reviewed in Chapter 1.

Onychomycosis

See Infections

Nail lichen planus

If the proximal nail matrix is affected, this results clinically in longitudinal grooves and ridges (onychorrhexis) and postinflammatory scarring (pterygium).

- Acanthosis with hypergranulosis of the nail matrix with band-like infiltrate

If the nail bed is affected, this results in proximal onycholysis (in psoriasis the onycholysis is distal), papular lesions, koilonychia, or complete shedding.

- Acanthosis and hypergranulosis of the nail bed with band-like dermal infiltrate **(Figure 4.86)**

Nail psoriasis

> NB Nail psoriasis is indistinguishable from onychomycosis in nail clippings on H&E.

- Foci of parakeratosis in the nail plate (corresponds to nail pitting)
- Hyperkeratosis with parakeratosis
- In punch biopsies and excisional specimens there is uniform hyperplasia of the nail bed with collections of neutrophils (spongiotic pustules)

Onychomatricoma (OM)

A nail clipping can be helpful to diagnose OM as this is the only nail tumor which grows in the nail plate.

- A thickened and dystrophic nail plate with cavities lined by parakeratosis and filled with a PAS-positive serum (the tumor infiltrates the nail plate and creates these defects) **(Figure 4.87A)**
- Epithelial digitate projections of matrix epithelium

The excisional specimen shows the digitate proliferations of the nail matrix within the nail plate and within the underlying stroma, which can be myxoid and has an increased number of vessels and mast cells **(Figure 4.87B)**.

Onychopapilloma

- In the excisional specimen there is thick acanthosis (papillomatosis) of the nail bed **(Figure 4.88)**
- Distal subungual hyperkeratosis
- In its lower part the hyperkeratosis is reminiscent of the keratogenous zone of the nail matrix

MELANONYCHIA

GENERAL CONCEPTS

The pigmented streak forms due to the increased production of melanin and its retention in the nail bed and/or in the nail plate.

NB Normal melanocytic density in the nail unit: 4–9 melanocytes (mean 7.7) per 1 mm segment in the nail matrix; **the nail bed is devoid of melanocytes!**

NB Most pigmented lesions arise from the distal matrix and therefore are linear; pigmented lesions arising from the nail bed present as amelanotic. Pigmented lesions may form also due to hyperproduction of melanin by activated but otherwise normal melanocytes.

NB S100 is the least helpful immunostain and should never be used alone: MART-1, HMB-45, and MITF are the markers of choice.

Melanocytic activation (hypermelanosis) corresponds to ephelides in the skin.

- Heavily melanized keratinocytes in the basal layer of the matrix
- Scattered melanophages

Lentigo (melanocytic hyperplasia) corresponds to a lentigo in the skin.

- Slight to moderate increase of single melanocytes in the matrix (10–31 melanocytes/1 mm interval appreciated with the MART-1 immunostain) **(Figure 4.89)**
- No confluence of melanocytes, no or very limited suprabasal scatter

Melanocytic nevus

NB This is the most common cause of melanonychia in children.

- Lentiginous pattern of increased number of melanocytes forming nests at the junction (junctional nevus) and less often in the dermis (compound nevus)
- Melanocytes are not present in the suprabasal matrix
- Possible melanin granules in the nail plate

Nail unit melanoma

Most arise from the nail matrix in the thumb and great toe. It may involve the proximal nail fold and hyponychium.

NB The Hutchinson's sign often corresponds to melanoma in situ.

Nail unit melanoma in situ

- Lentiginous proliferation of atypical large, irregular, and hyperchromatic melanocytes with dendrites which may predominate over nests **(Figure 4.90)**
- The number of melanocytes is between 39 and 136 (mean 59.8) per 1 mm interval (compared with up to 31 in lentigo)
- Confluence of melanocytes

NB Suprabasal scatter of melanocytes in the matrix is always a concern.

Invasive nail unit melanoma

In addition to the findings for nail unit melanoma in situ:

- Irregular distributed nests in the dermis without maturation
- Neurotropism and lymphovascular invasion are possible

NB Breslow's depth is measured from the most superficial visible epithelial layer. The granular layer is missing in the normal nail unit; however, it is often present in nail tumors, including melanoma.

DEPOSITION DISORDERS

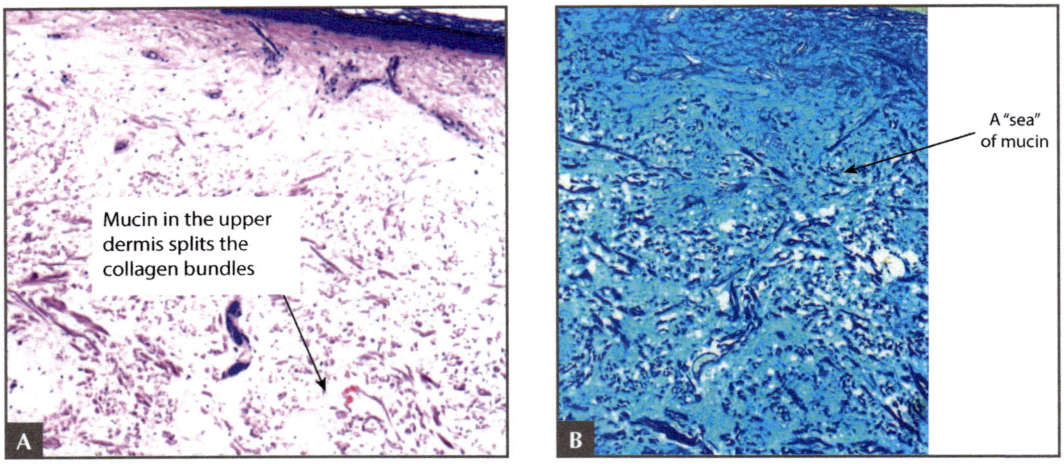

Figure 4.1 Pretibial myxedema. **A** Large amount of mucin (the bluish empty spaces) predominantly in the upper dermis). **B** Pretibial myxedema stained by colloidal iron.

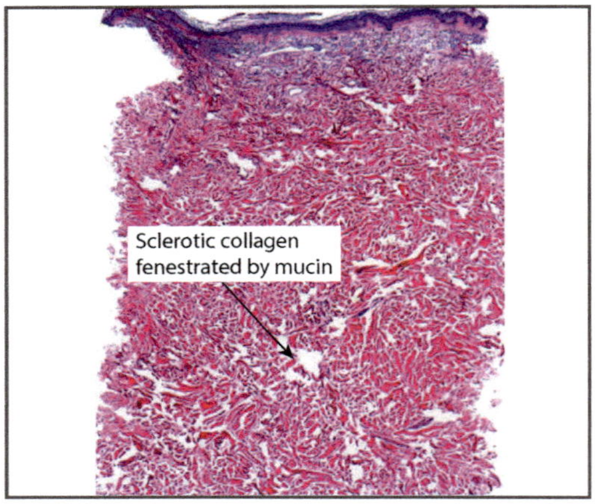

Figure 4.2 Scleredema. Note the rectangular shape of the biopsy due to the sclerotic dermis. The collagen is acellular and is fenestrated by white spaces, mostly in the lower dermis (mucin on colloidal iron stain).

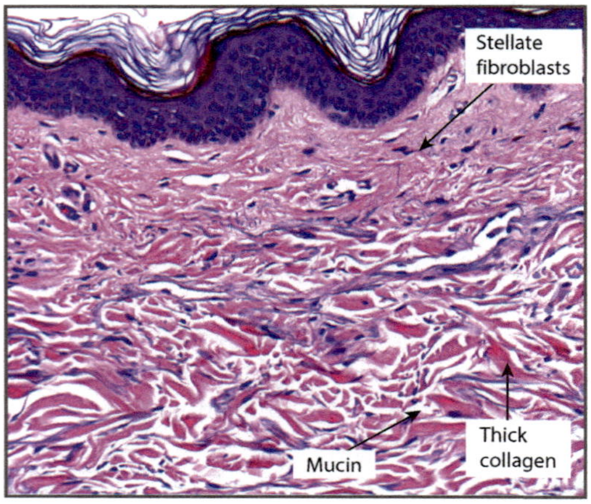

Figure 4.3 Scleromyxedema. Note the presence of mucin in the mid dermis with thickened collagen bundles but also busy look compared to scleredema and pretibial myxedema by the presence of fibroblasts.

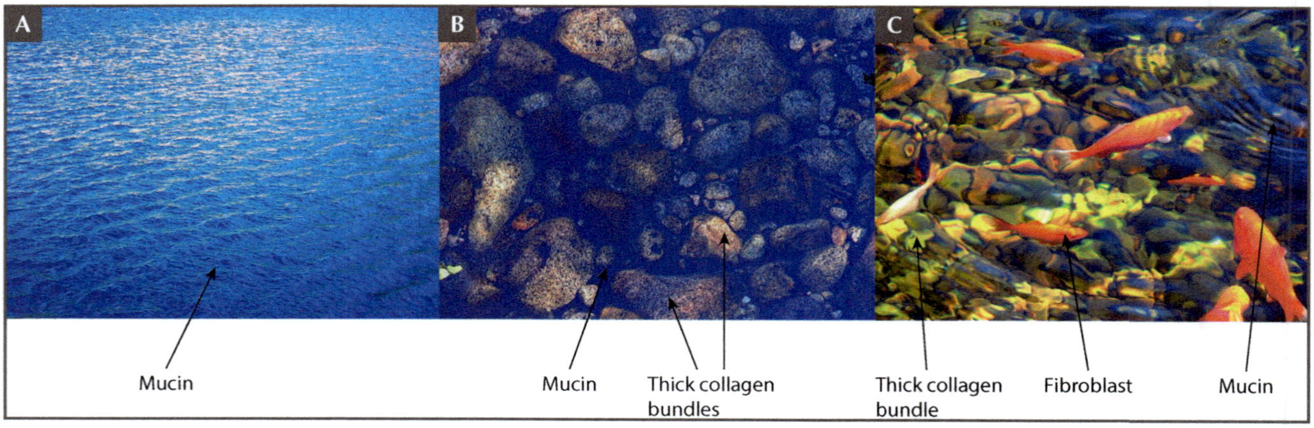

Photomnemonic 4.1 A Pretibial myxedema resembles a blue sea; **B** scleredema resembles a blue sea with stones; and **C** scleromyxedema resembles a blue sea with stones and fish.

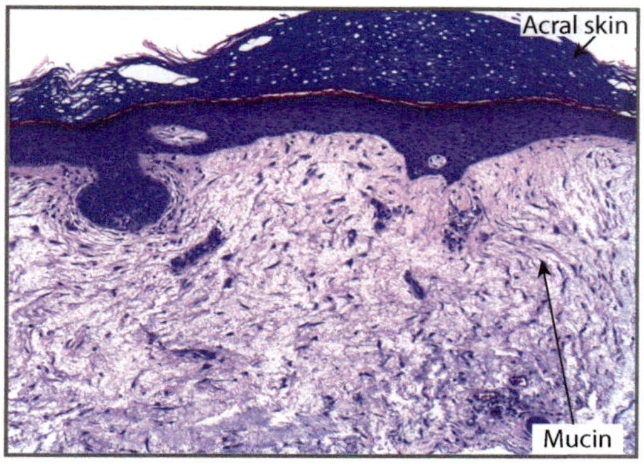

Figure 4.4 Focal acral mucinosis.

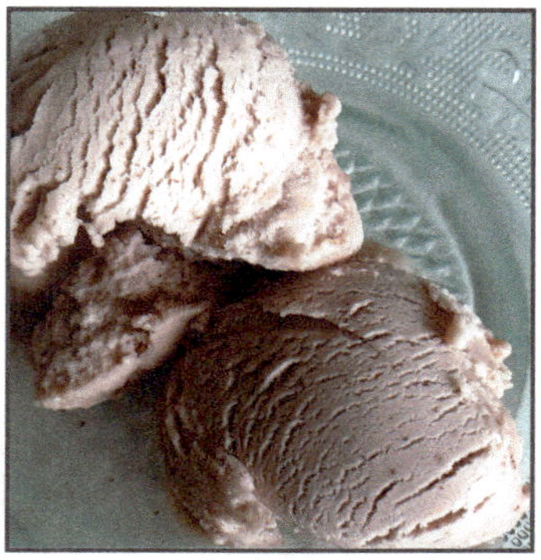

Photomnemonic 4.2 The pink and slightly fissured amyloid material resembles a scoop of pink ice cream.

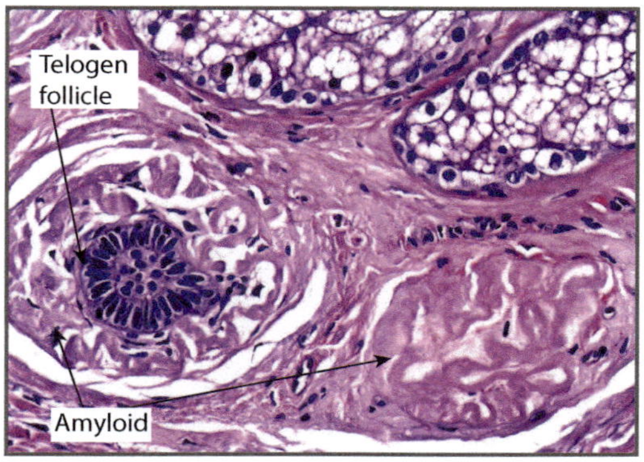

Figure 4.5 Scalp biopsy from a case of systemic amyloidosis with diffuse alopecia. There is a mantle of amyloid around the follicular structures and also lying freely in the dermis.

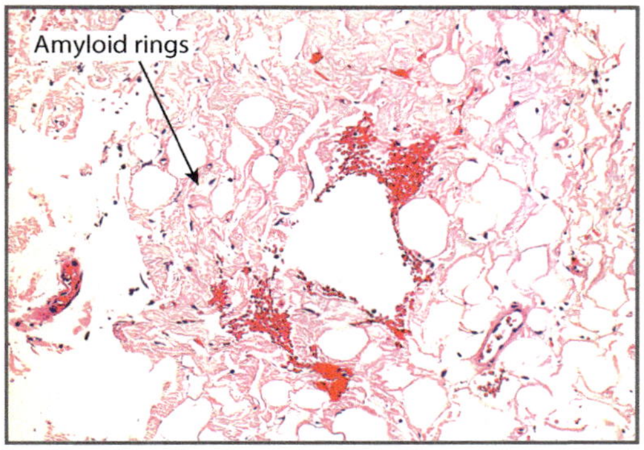

Figure 4.6 A case of systemic amyloidosis involving the subcutaneous fat.

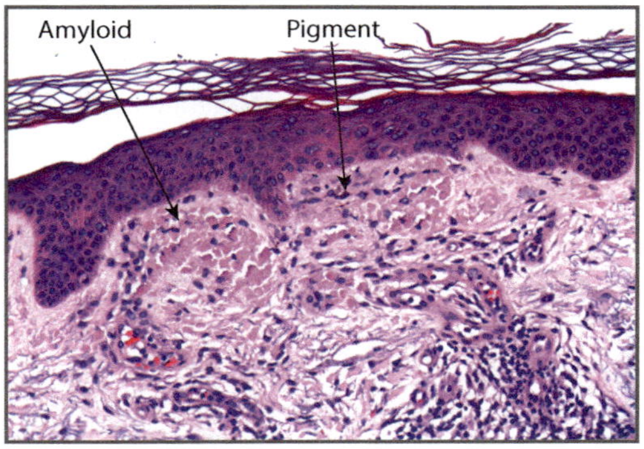

Figure 4.7 Lichen amyloidosis. The amyloid is in the papillary dermis.

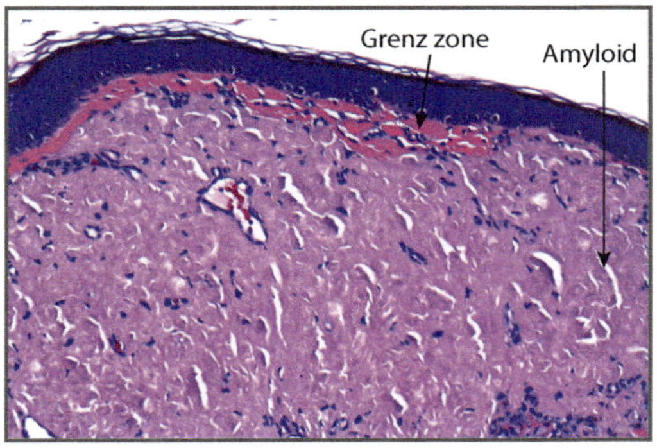

Figure 4.8 Nodular amyloidosis.

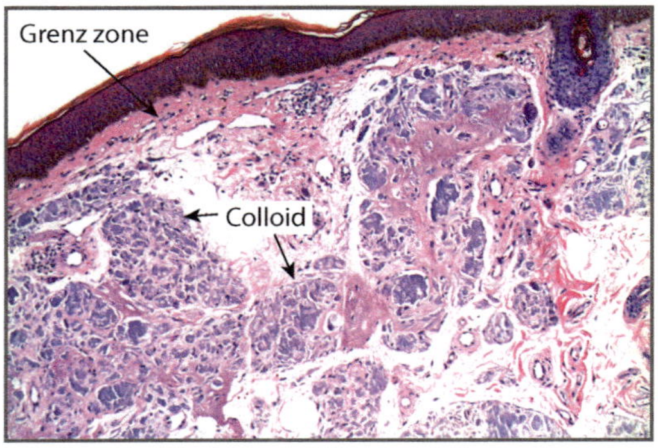

Figure 4.9 Colloid milium (adult type): the colloid is pink grayish fissured material derived from degenerated elastic fibers in solar elastosis.

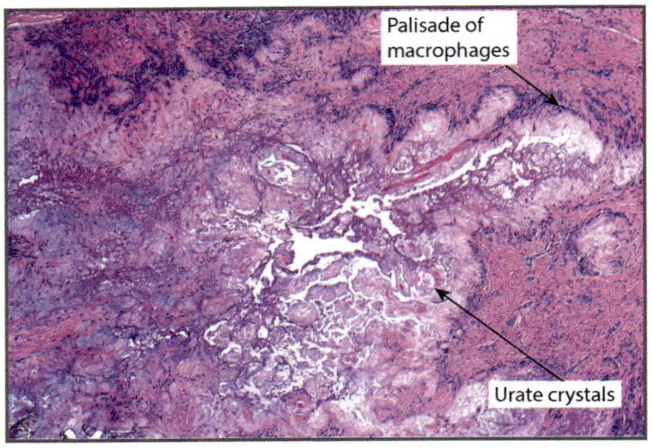

Figure 4.10 Gout. Note the large amorphous pink deposition in the dermis, surrounded by a palisading rim of histiocytes and giant cells.

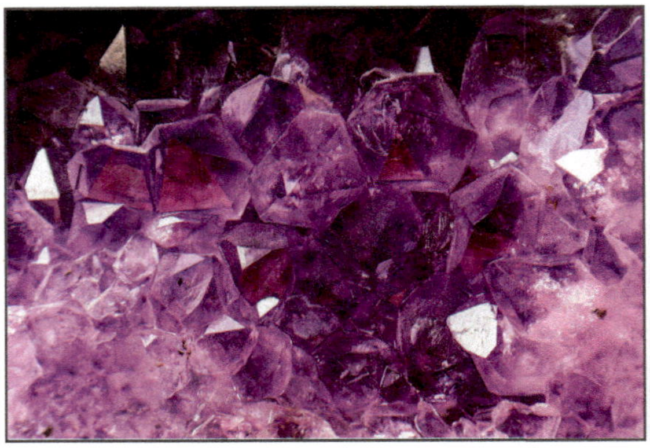

Photomnemonic 4.3 The compact deep blue–purple calcium masses in the skin in gout resemble purple amethyst crystals.

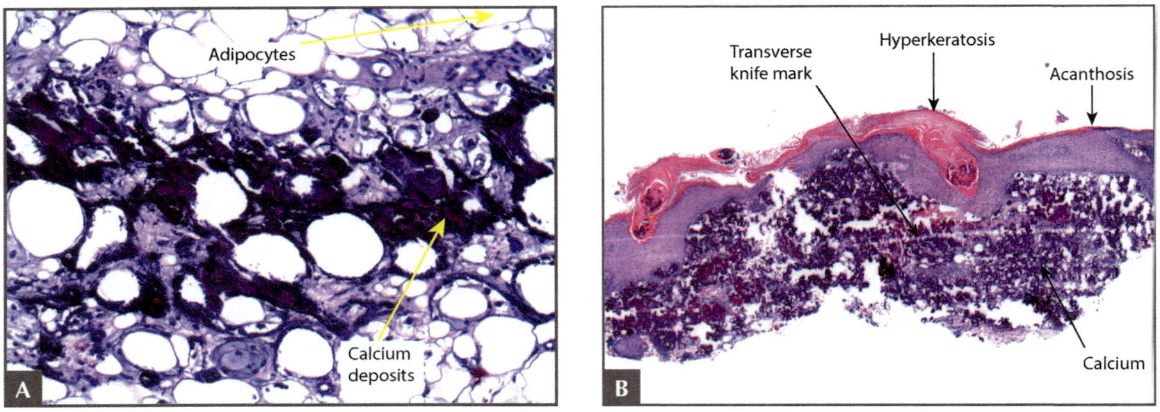

Figure 4.11 Calcinosis cutis. **A** An example of metastatic calcification in the skin (in the subcutaneous fat). **B** Subepidermal calcified nodule. Note the hyperplastic epidermis overlying the aggregation of purple calcium globules in the dermis.

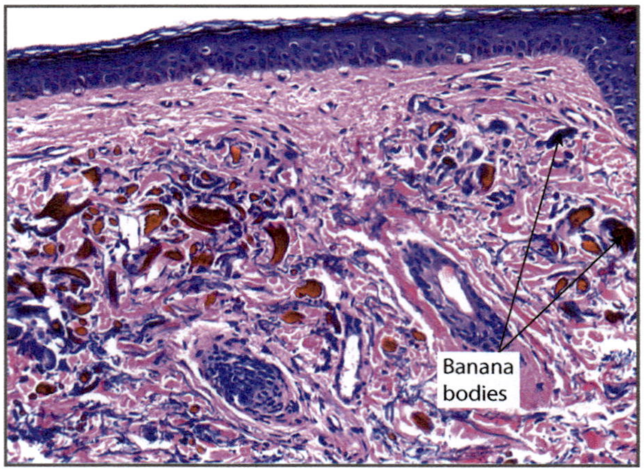

Figure 4.12 Ochronosis, exogenous type.

COLLAGEN AND ELASTIC TISSUE DISORDERS

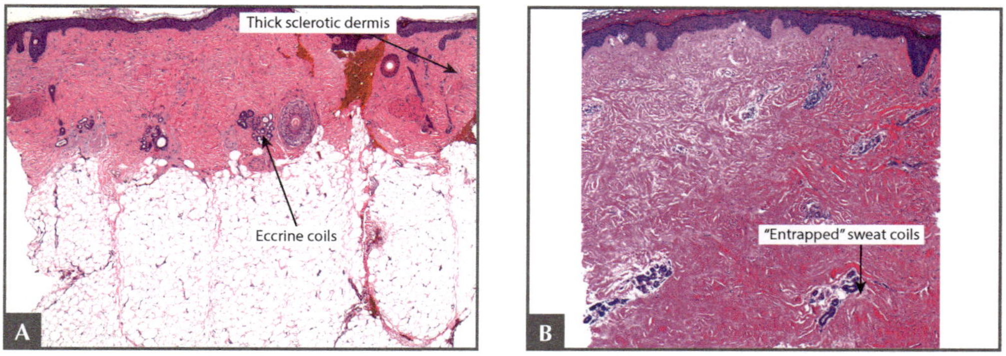

Figure 4.13 Scleroderma and morphea. **A** Morphea The specimen is rectangular because of the sclerotic dermis. Note that the eccrine coils are in the lower dermis. **B** Scleroderma. There is sclerosis of the dermis with entrapped sweat coils. Note the absence of follicles.

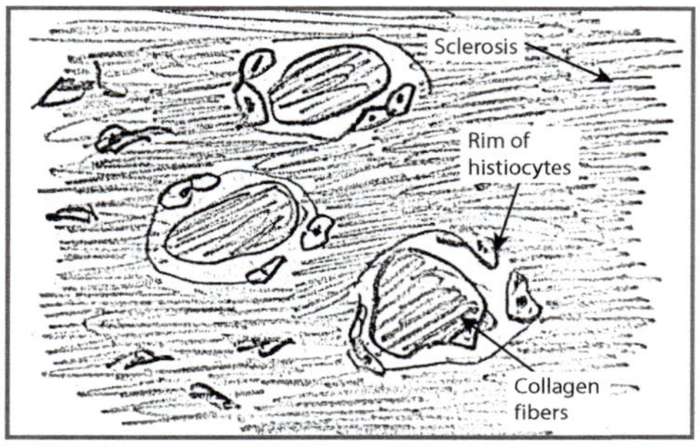

Figure 4.14 The "floating sign" in morphea.

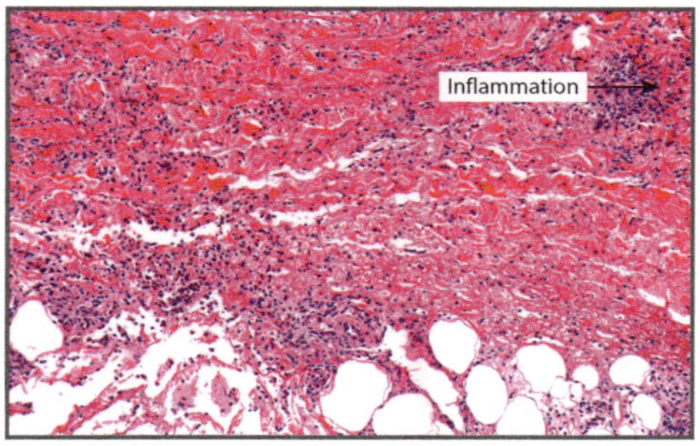

Figure 4.15 Eosinophilic fasciitis. Note the thick collagen replacing the fascia and that the fat tissue is infiltrated with inflammatory cells.

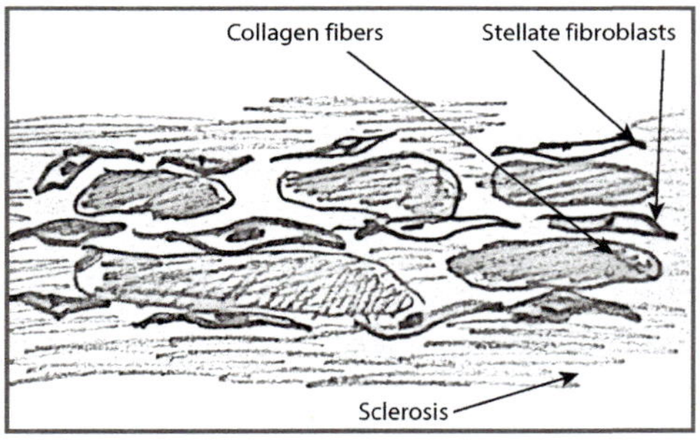

Figure 4.16 The tram track sign of nephrogenic systemic fibrosis: stellate fibroblasts lie with their dendrites along the collagen bundles.

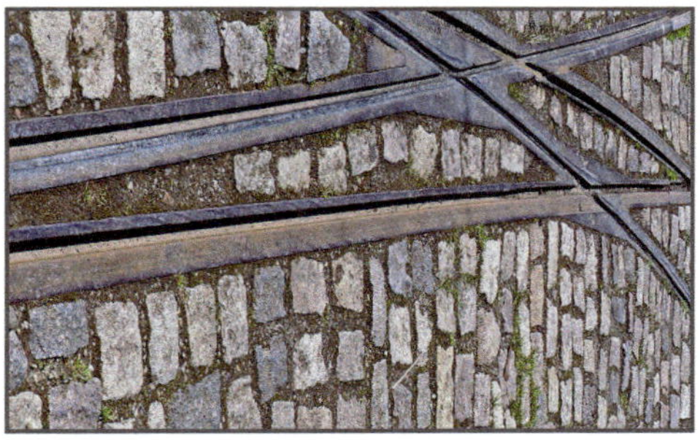

Photomnemonic 4.4 Nephrogenic systemic fibrosis: tram track.

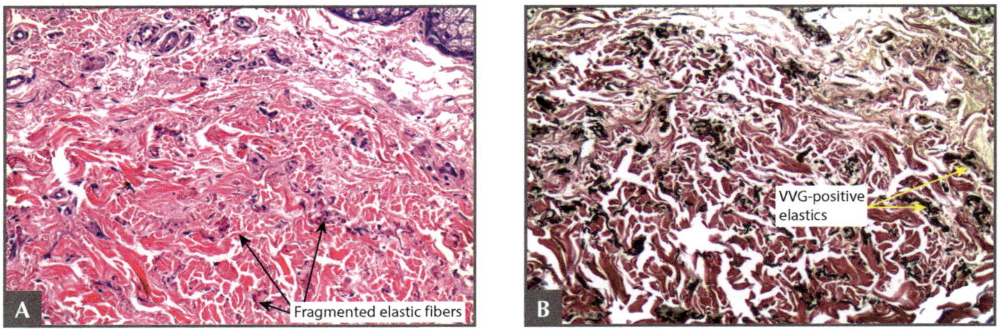

Figure 4.17 Pseudoxanthoma elasticum. **A** Note the purple fragmented elastic fibers in mid dermis. **B** VVG stain highlights in black the fragmented elastic tissue.

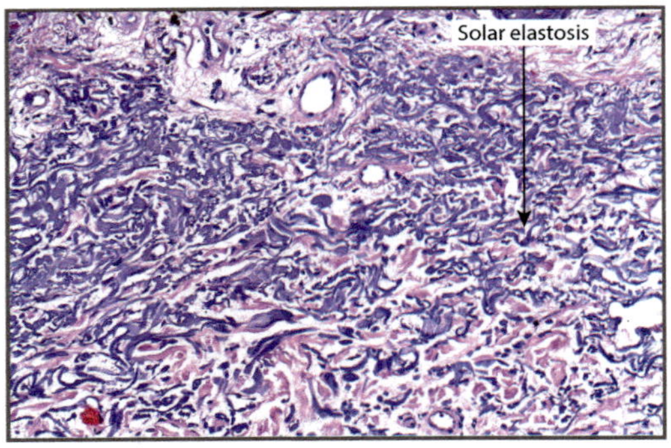

Figure 4.18 Blue–grayish thick and compact elastic deposition in the upper dermis in solar elastosis.

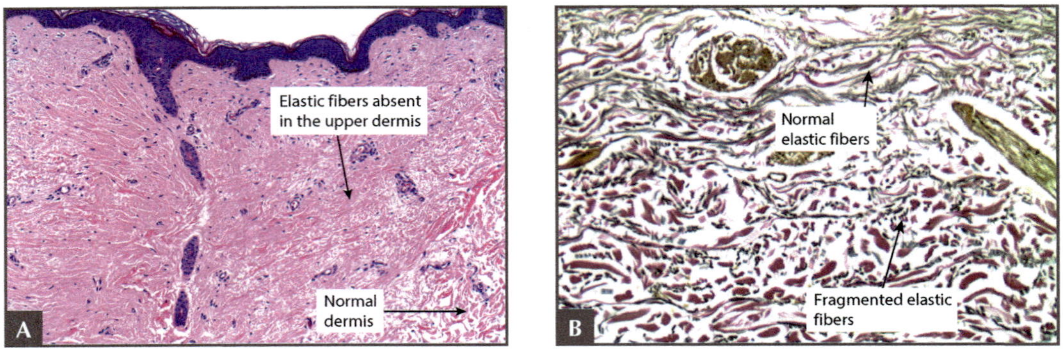

Figure 4.19 Anetoderma. **A** The absence of elastic fibers in the upper dermis gives the appearance of a pink fine scar tissue. **B** VVG stain highlights the fragmented elastic fibers in black.

CUTANEOUS REACTIONS TO EXOGENOUS FACTORS

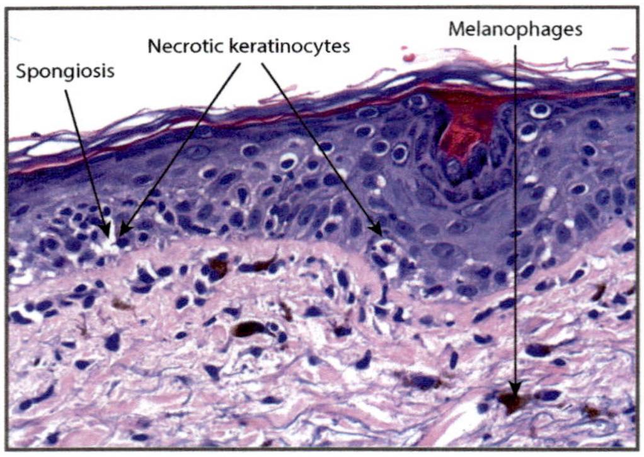

Figure 4.20 Phototoxic dermatitis. There are subtle changes of necrotic keratinocytes, spongiosis, and melanophages in the upper dermis. This corresponds clinically to postinflammatory hyperpigmentation.

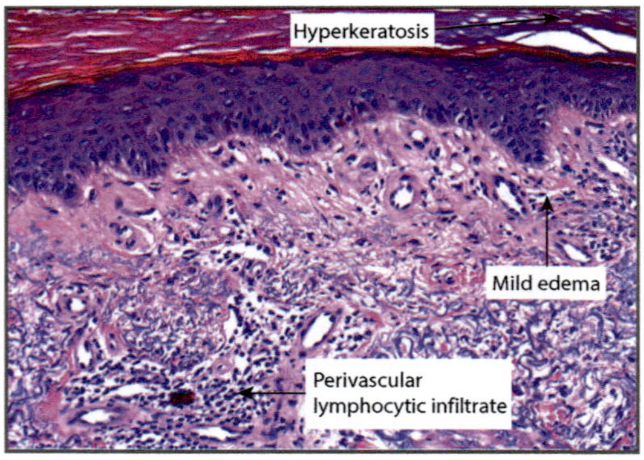

Figure 4.21 Photoallergic dermatitis. Note there are no necrotic keratinocytes but there are hyperkeratosis, mild edema, and perivascular infiltrates.

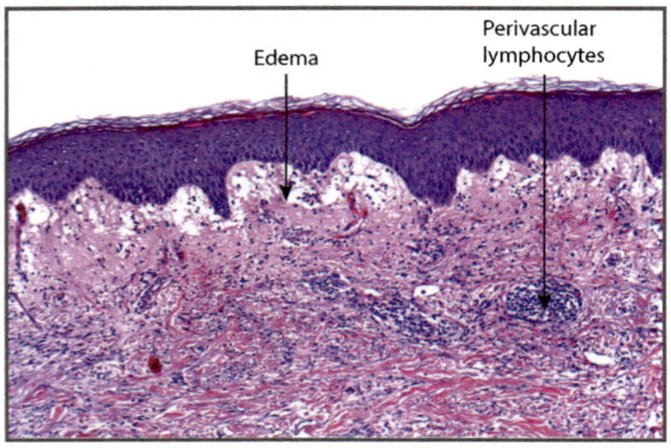

Figure 4.22 PMLE. Note the subepidermal edema and perivascular infiltrates.

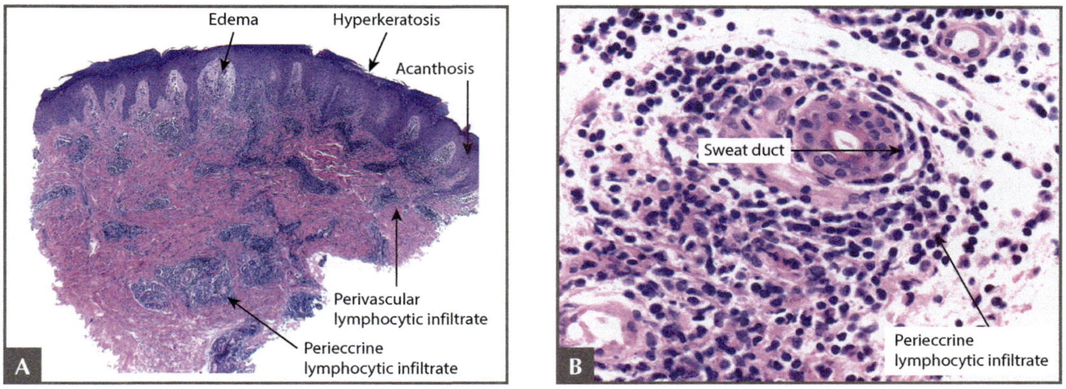

Figure 4.23 Pernio. **A** Note the "bluish color of the specimen. **B** Note the patchy lymphocytic infiltrates around the eccrine glands. (Images courtesy of Rossitza Lazova, MD.)

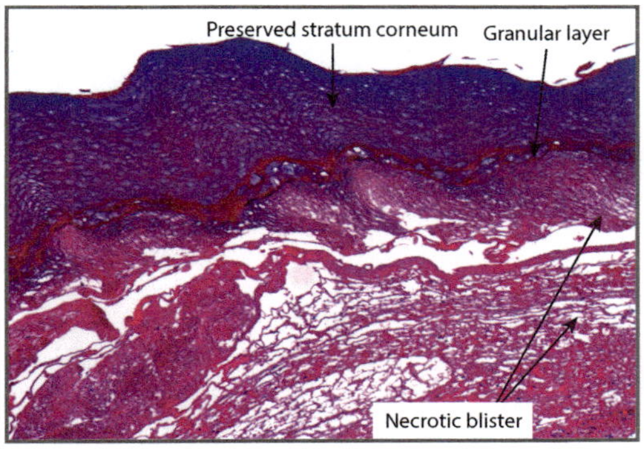

Figure 4.24 Traumatic (friction) blister: the thick stratum corneum of acral skin overlies necrotic epidermis and dermis.

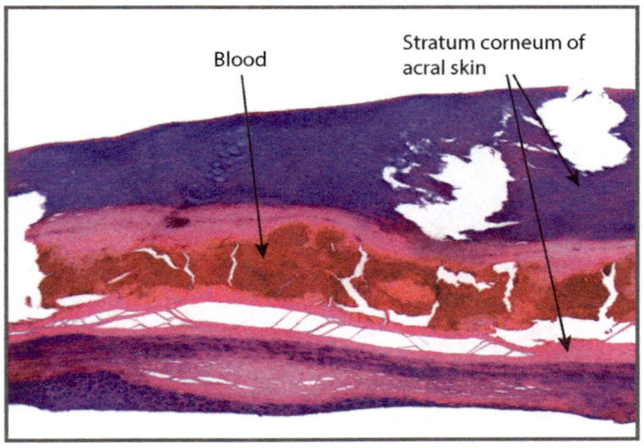

Figure 4.25 Talon noir.

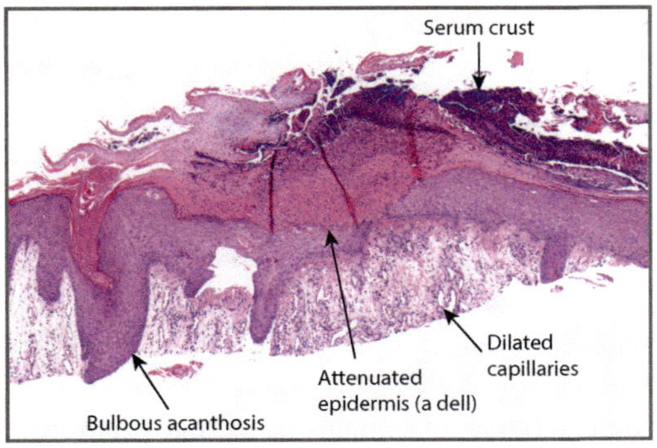

Figure 4.26 Acanthoma fissuratum on the ear (the increased number of capillaries is a clue to the location).

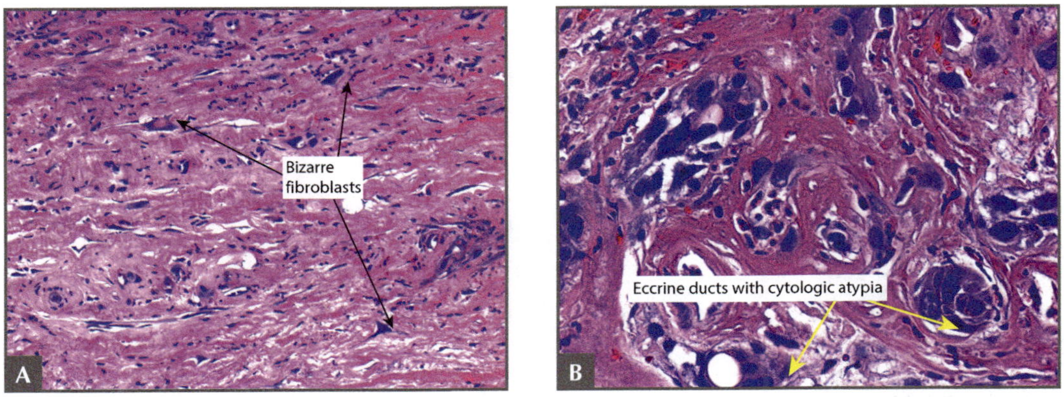

Figure 4.27 Radiation-induced alterations. **A** Bizarre angulated fibroblasts in radiation dermatitis; note the thick fibrotic dermis. **B** Squamous syringometaplasia of the sweat glands in a chronic radiation ulcer.

SELECTED GENODERMATOSES

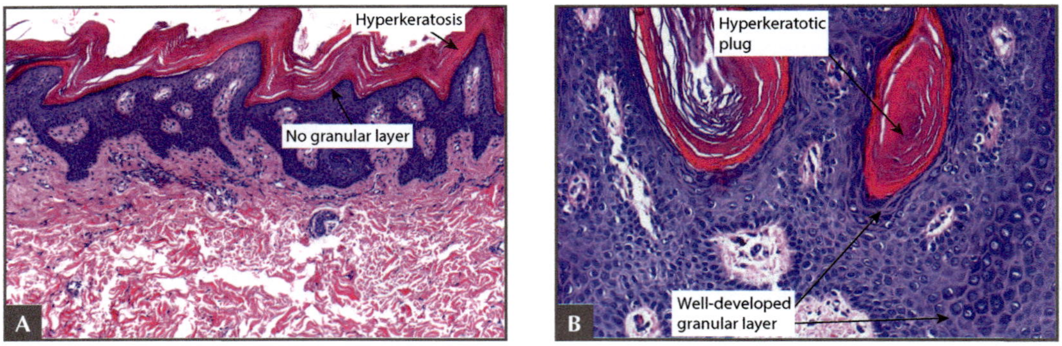

Figure 4.28 Ichthyoses. **A** Ichthyosis vulgaris. The hyperkeratosis covers the epidermis tightly, like with a pink carpet. Note the absence of the granular layer. **B** A case of progressive symmetric erythrokeratoderma (PSEK). Note the presence of the granular layer, in contrast to ichthyosis vulgaris.

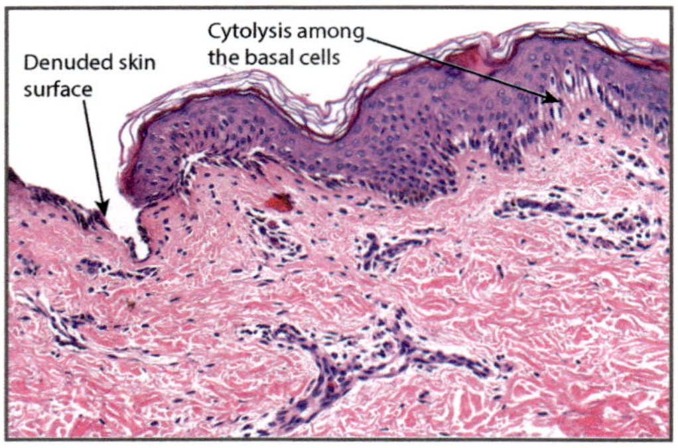

Figure 4.29 Epidermolysis bullosa simplex. Note the separation between the basal cells.

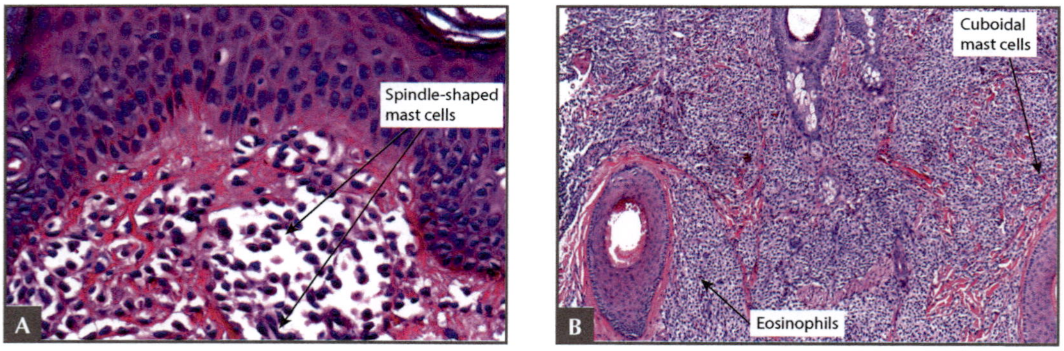

Figure 4.30 Mastocytoses. **A** Urticaria pigmentosa. Note the infiltrate of spindle-shaped mast cells in the papillary dermis. **B** Mastocytoma. There is a pale-looking lesion in the dermis with cuboidal-shaped mast cells. The numerous cells with the red cytoplasm are eosinophils.

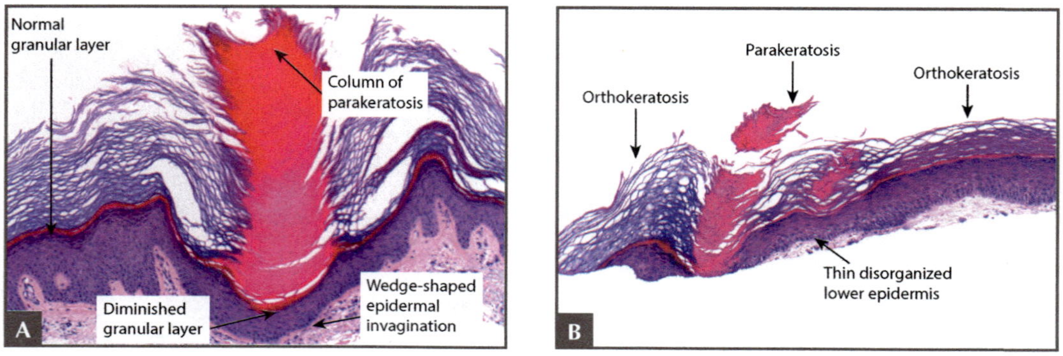

Figure 4.31 Porokeratosis. **A** The layered parakeratosis is the cornoid lamella. **B** DSAP. Note the actinic changes in the lower epidermis.

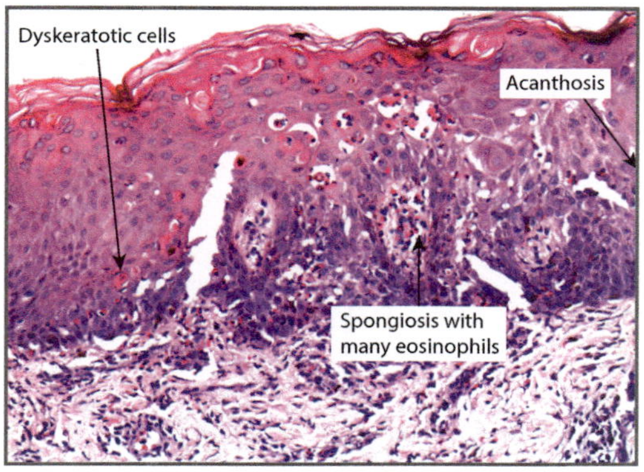

Figure 4.32 Incontinentia pigmenti, vesicular. Note the presence of dyskeratotic and squamoid cells in the spongiotic epidermis and the numerous eosinophils.

PERFORATING DISORDERS

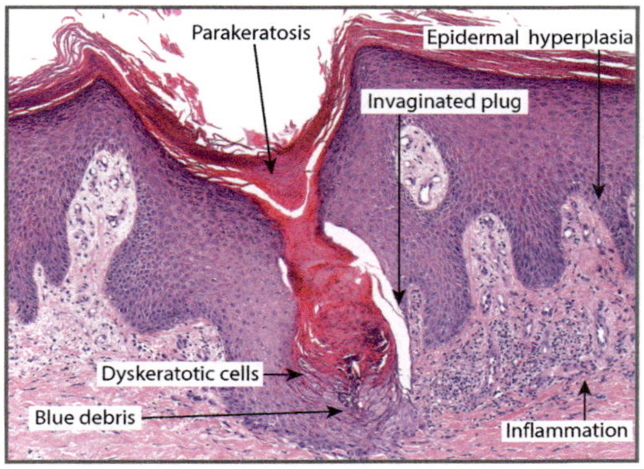

Figure 4.33 Kyrle's disease. Note the "busy" invaginated plug.

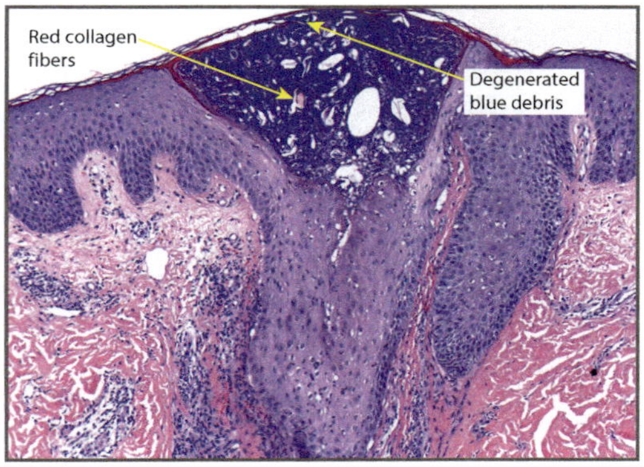

Figure 4.34 Perforating folliculitis. Note the blue material within the dilated infundibulum with a few red collagen fibers.

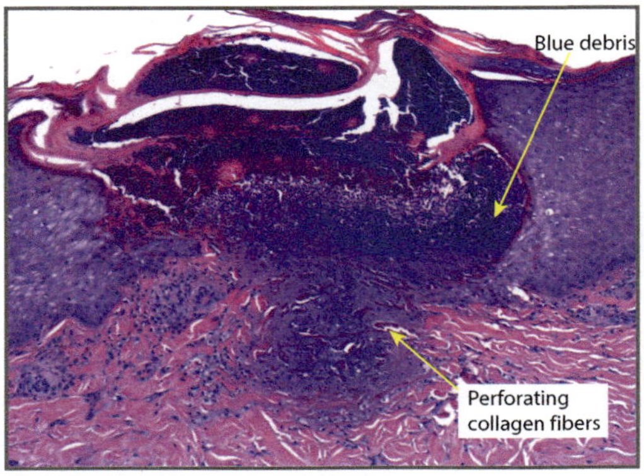

Figure 4.35 Perforating collagenosis. Note the short canal filled with blue debris and the red collagen fibers extruding from the dermis.

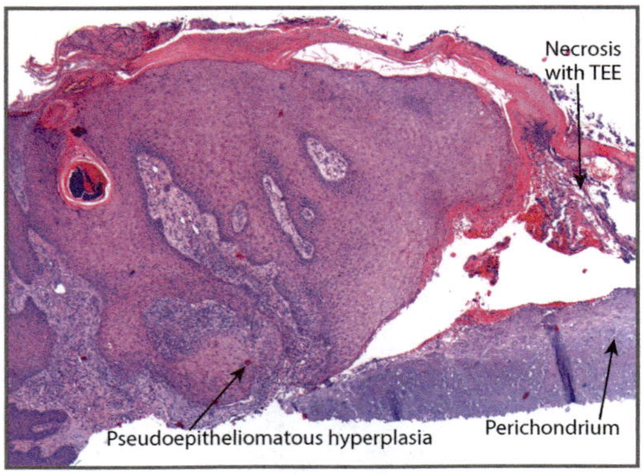

Figure 4.36 Chondrodermatitis nodularis helicis. There is an epidermal ulceration with necrosis of the dermis overlying the perichondrium.

INFECTIONS

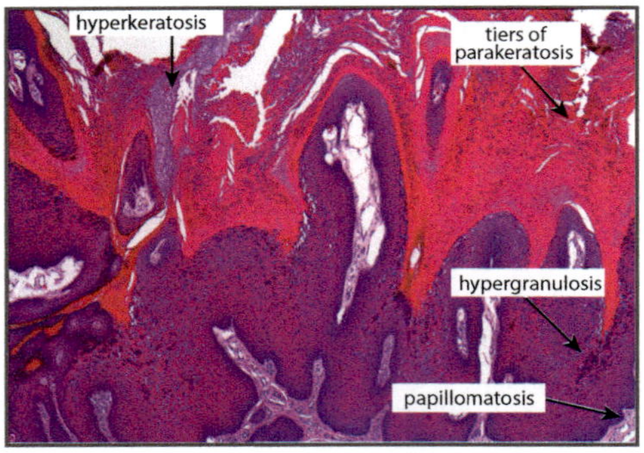

Figure 4.37 Verruca vulgaris. The lateral rete ridges point toward the center of the lesion.

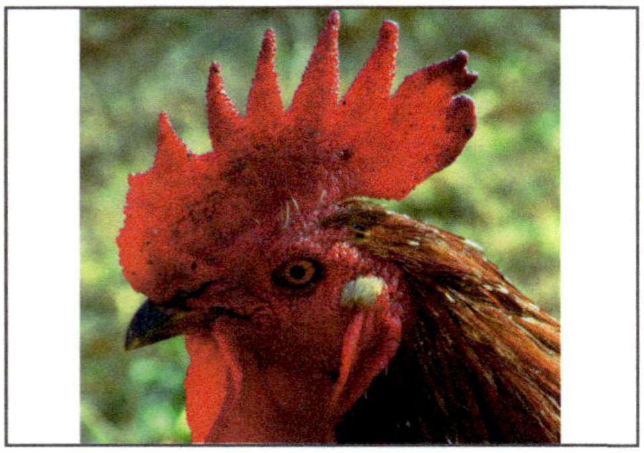

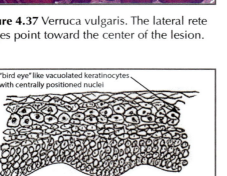

Photomnemonic 4.5 The papillomatous epidermis with thick hyperkeratosis and parakeratosis in verruca vulgaris resembles a rooster comb.

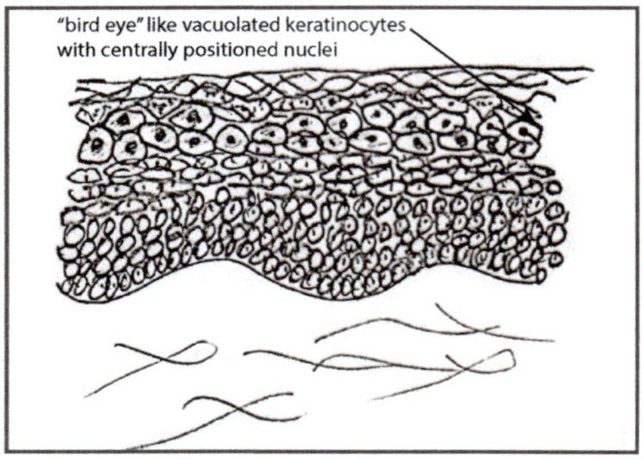

Figure 4.38 Verruca plana. Note the normal basket-weave stratum corneum and the "bird eye"-like cells.

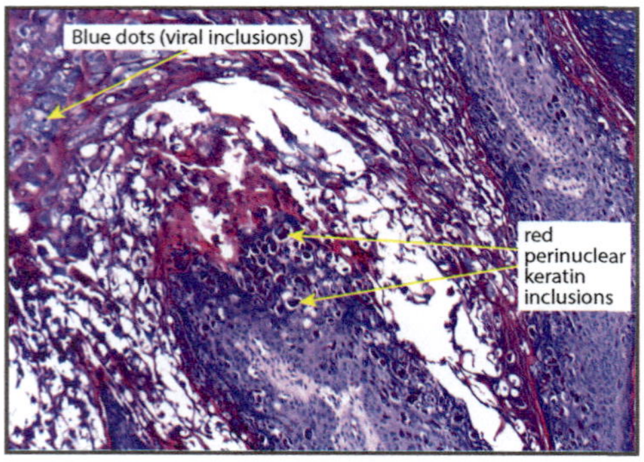

Figure 4.39 Plantar wart (myrmecia).

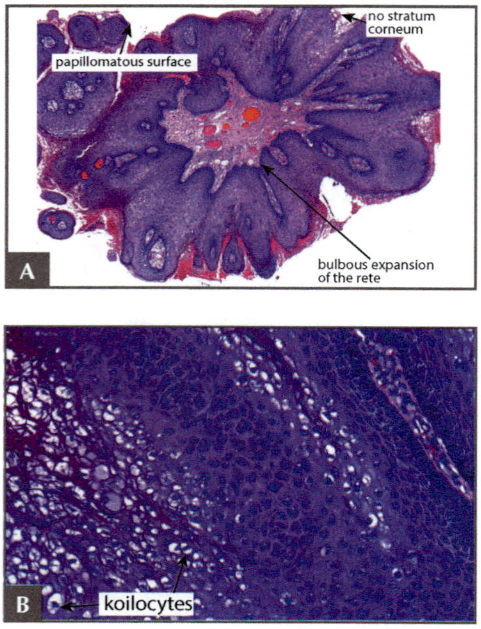

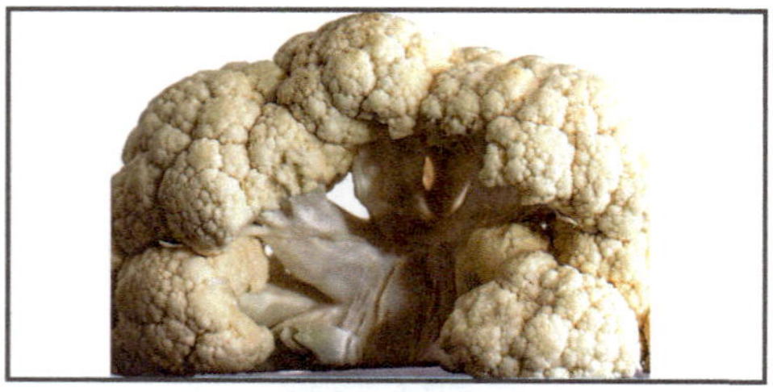

Photomnemonic 4.6 Bulbous endo-exophytic acanthosis resembles the branches in a cauliflower.

Figure 4.40 Condyloma acuminatum. **A** Note the bulbous endo-exophytic acanthosis with inward orientation of the rete. The epidermis looks pale due to the vacuolization.
B Koilocytes in HPV lesions. Note the shrunken raisin-like nuclei.

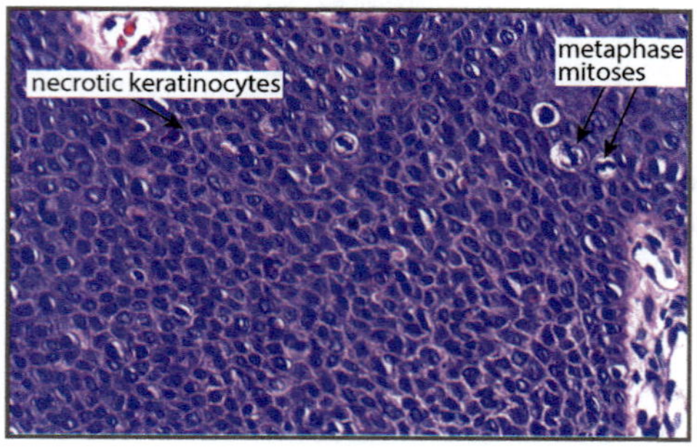

Figure 4.41 Bowenoid papulosis.
The epidermis appears "windblown" due to the crowded atypical keratinocytes, the necrotic keratinocytes, and the increased mitotic count.

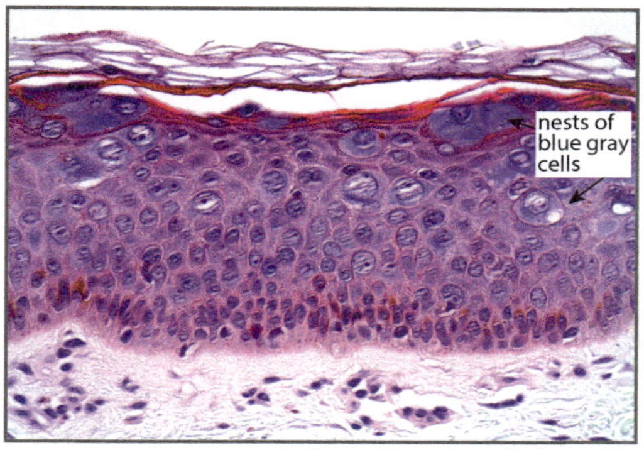

Figure 4.42 Epidermodysplasia verruciformis (EDV). Note the blue–gray cells with perinuclear halo in the spinous and granular layer similar to the bird eye cells in verruca plana.

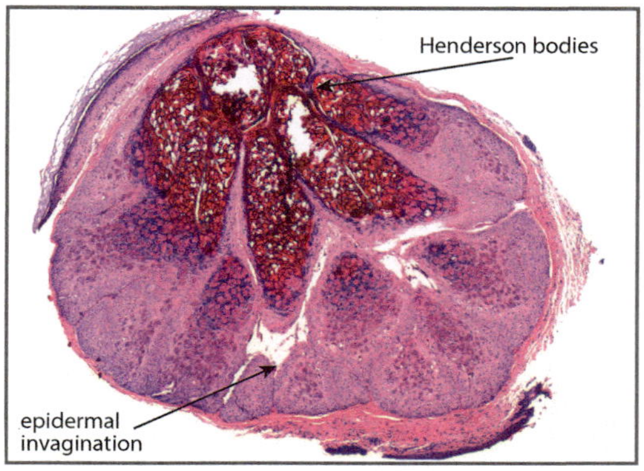

Figure 4.43 Molluscum. Note the viral red intracytoplasmic inclusions (Henderson bodies).

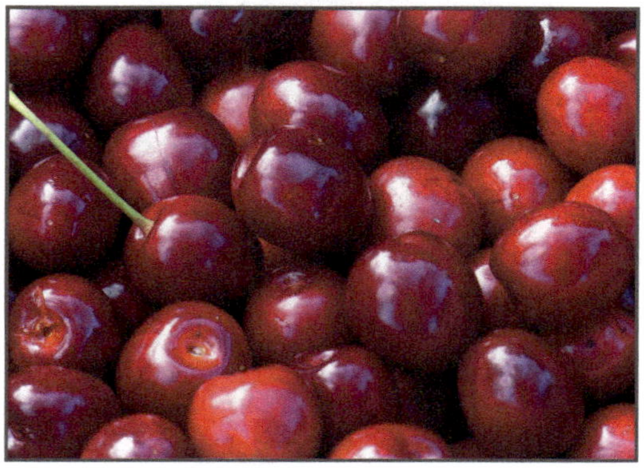

Photomnemonic 4.7 The Henderson bodies in molluscum resemble red cherries.

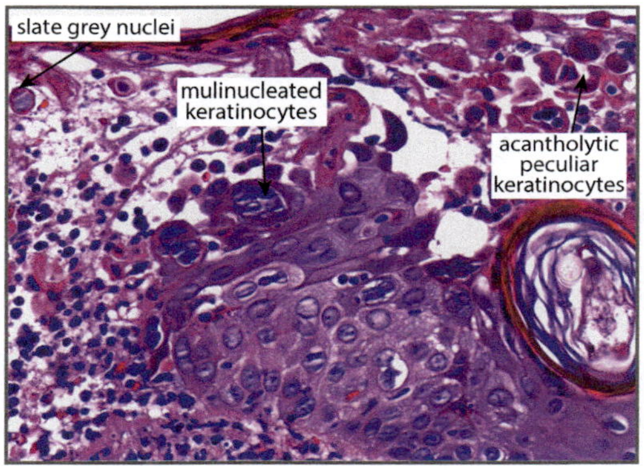

Figure 4.44 HSV lesion. Note the different nuclear abnormalities in the affected cells.

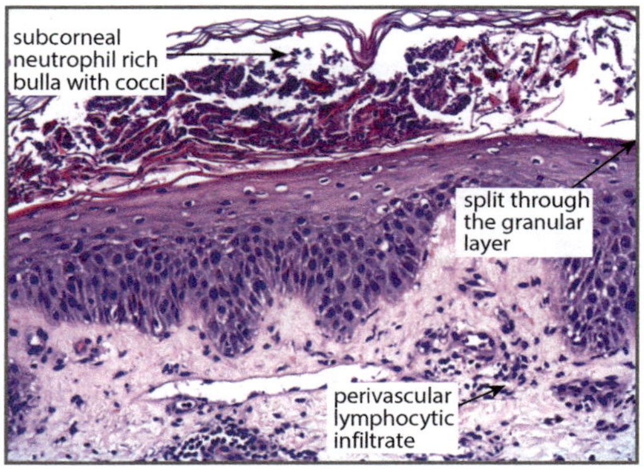

Figure 4.45 Bullous impetigo. Note the absence of acantholysis compared to pemphigus foliaceus.

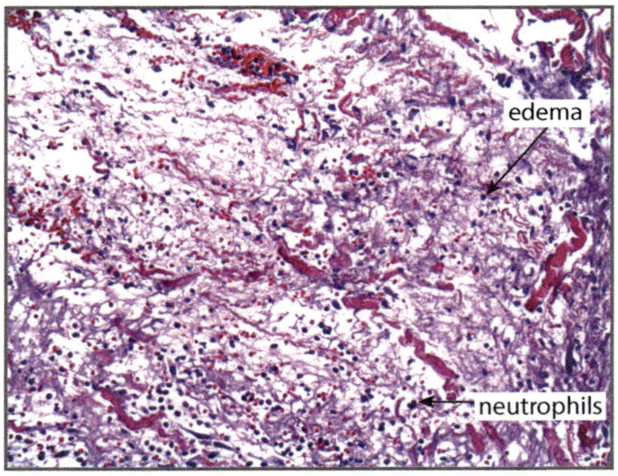

Figure 4.46 Cellulitis. Neutrophils and edema dissect the collagen.

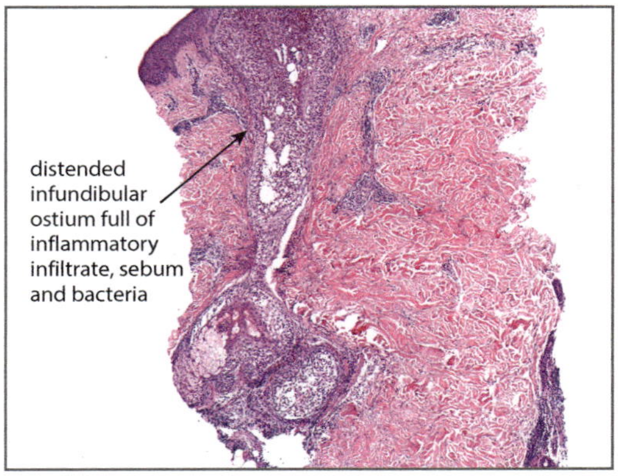

Figure 4.47 Folliculitis. The inflammation affects the infundibular portion of the follicle (the uppermost part of the follicle).

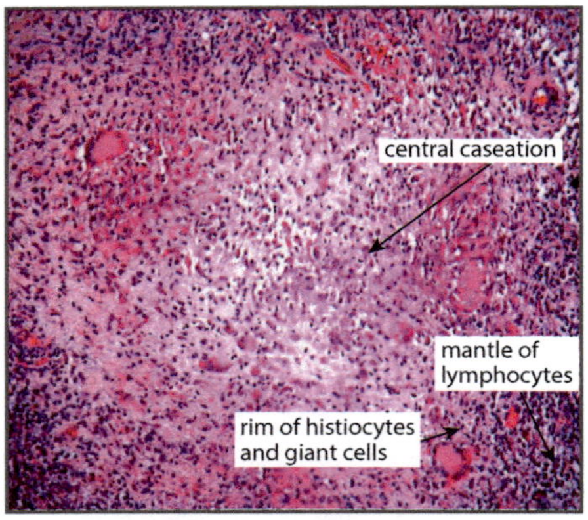

Figure 4.48 Tuberculosis cutis. Classic presentation of the caseating tuberculoid granulomas.

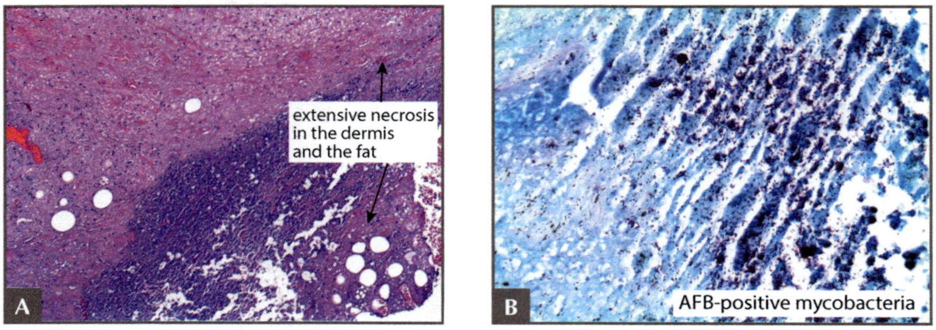

Figure 4.49 Buruli ulcer. **A** Atypical mycobacterial infection caused by *M. ulcerans*. Note the extensive necrosis. **B** Infectious panniculitis with numerous extracellular clusters of AFB-positive mycobacteria.

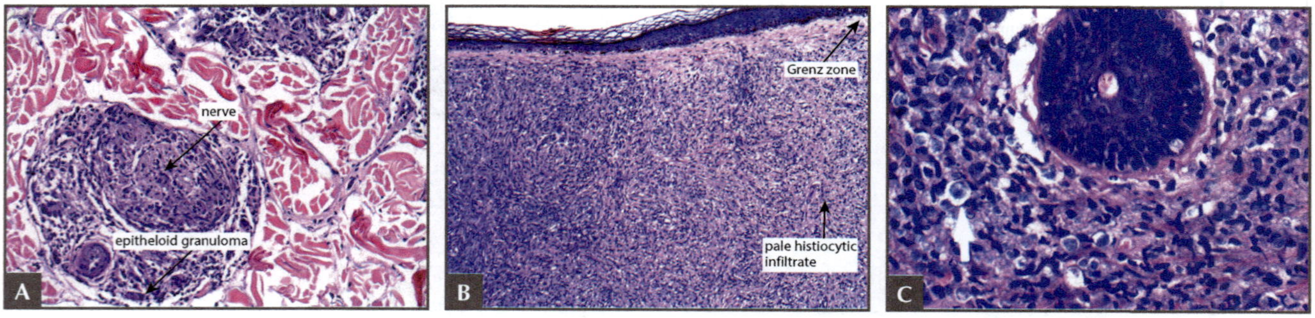

Figure 4.50 Leprosy. **A** Tuberculoid leprosy. The granulomas wrap up neural structures, vessels, follicle, and sweat glands. **B** Lepromatous leprosy. Note the Grenz zone separating the atrophic epidermis from the dense pale histiocytic infiltrate in the dermis. **C** Lepromatous leprosy. The arrowhead points to globi (intra- and extracellular encapsulated masses of bacilli).

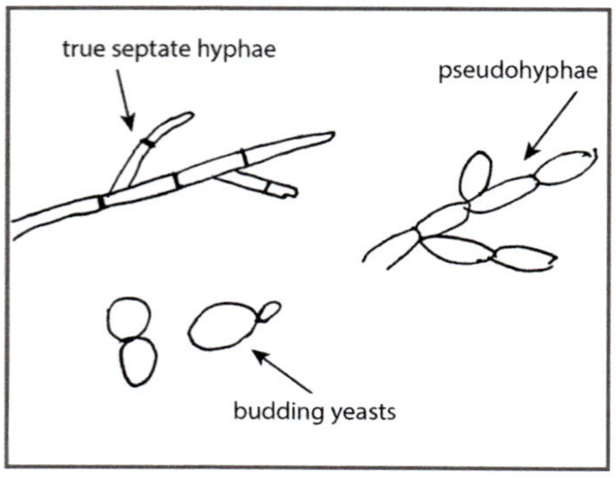

Figure 4.51 Schematic presentation of the most common fungal forms.

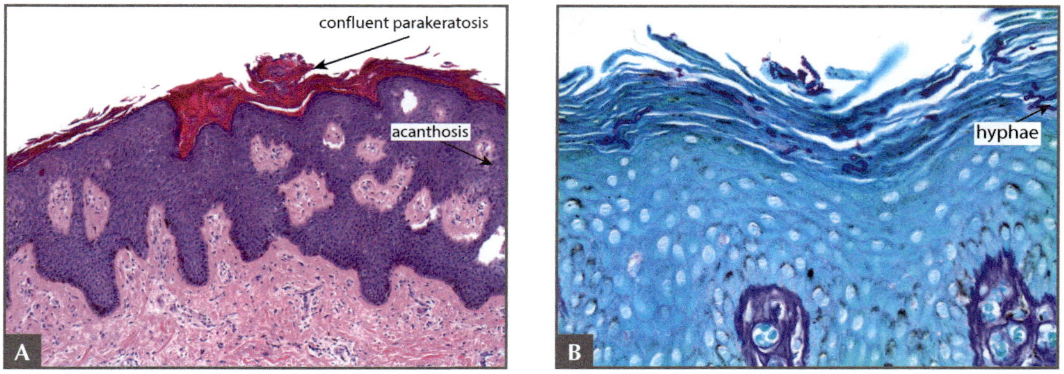

Figure 4.52 Dermatophytosis. **A** Tinea corporis. There is acanthosis covered by confluent parakeratosis. **B** The PAS stain of the same case highlights hyphae in the stratum corneum.

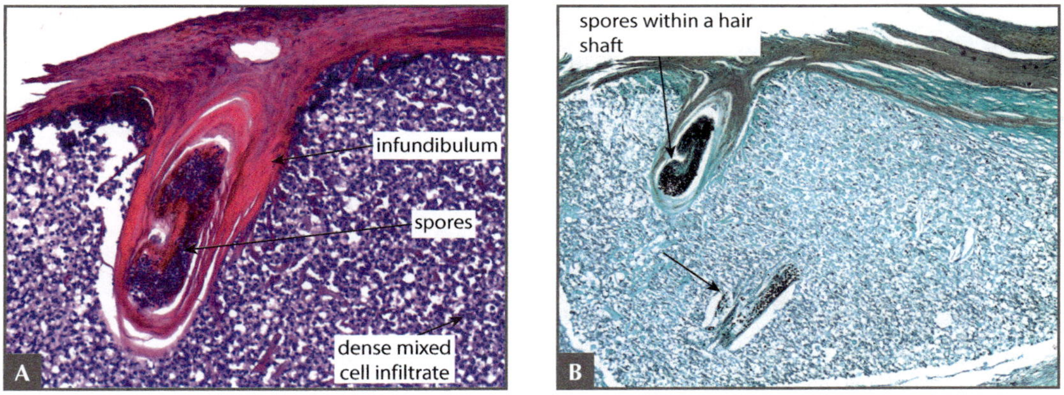

Figure 4.53 Majocchi's granuloma. **A** Note the hair shaft within the infundibular ostium is filled with spores. There is dense inflammatory infiltrate in the dermis. **B** GMS stain highlights the spores.

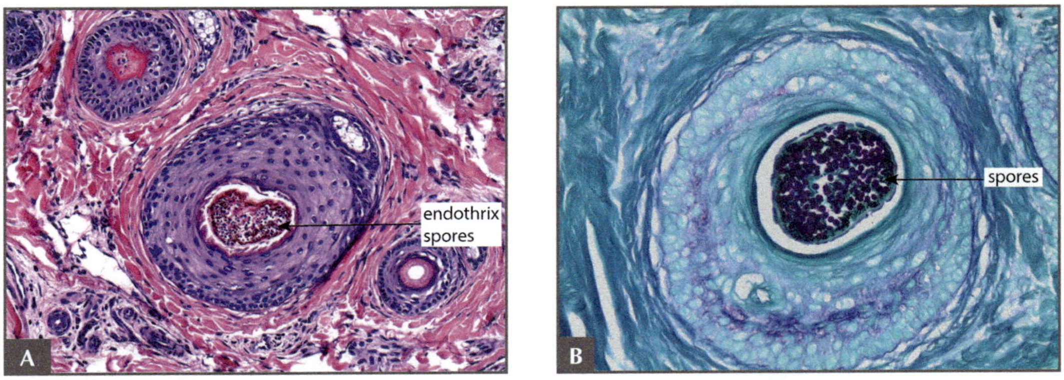

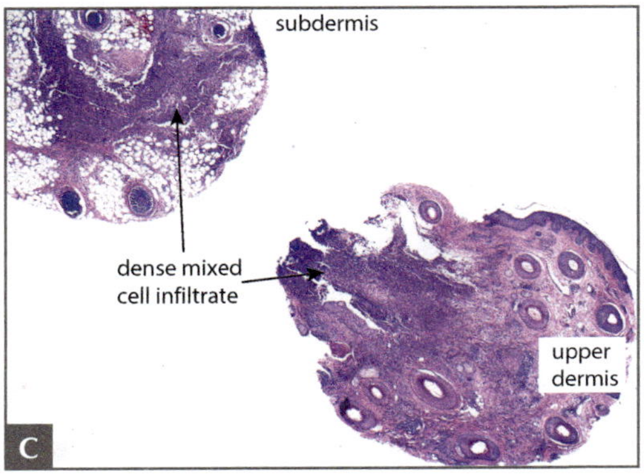

Figure 4.54 Tinea capitis (horizontal sections). **A** Note the spores within the hair shaft. **B** PAS-positive spores. **C** Kerion (inflammatory tinea capitis). There is dense mixed-cell infiltrate (abscess) extending from the upper dermis to the subdermis.

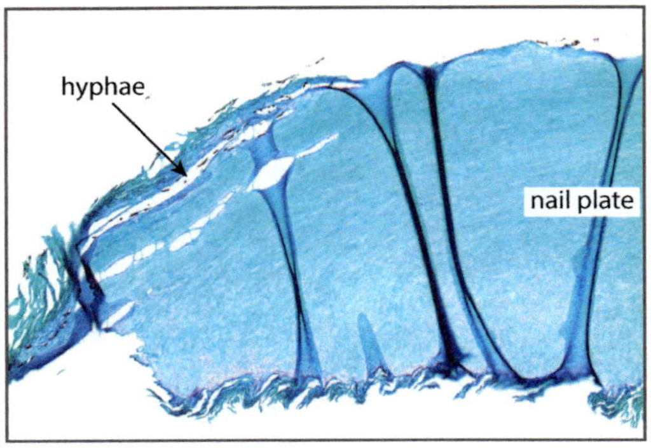

Figure 4.55 White superficial onychomycosis, PAS stain. The hyphae are located in the superficial layers of the nail plate.

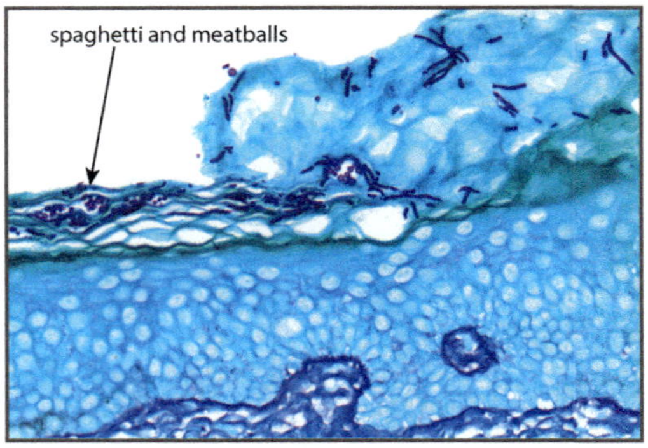

Figure 4.56 Tinea versicolor, PAS stain.

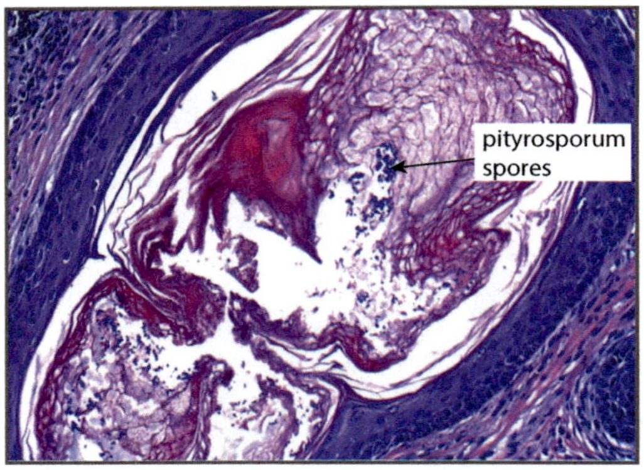

Figure 4.57 Pityrosporum folliculitis. There is a dilated infundibulum with small round blue spores.

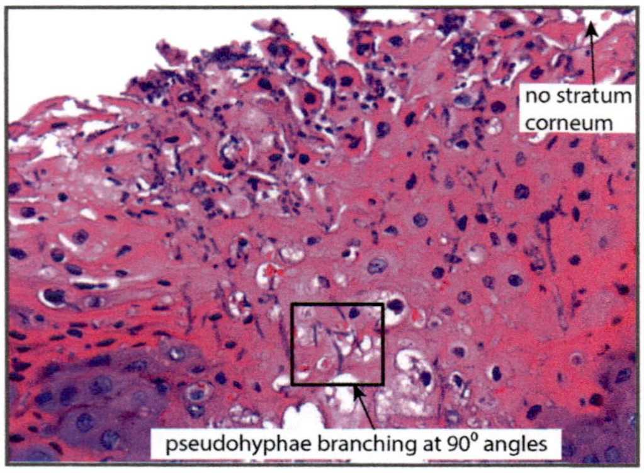

Figure 4.58 Oral candidiasis. Note the numerous pseudohyphae.

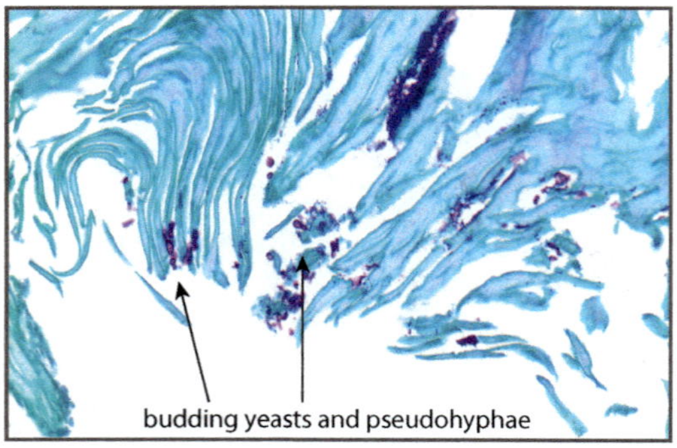

Figure 4.59 Candida onychomycosis. There is no nail plate invasion. There are budding yeasts and pseudohyphae located on the undersurface of the nail plate.

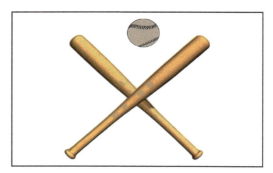

Photomnemonic 4.8 In Mucomycosis, the plump hyphae branch at 90° like crossed baseball bats; the collapsed ring-like hyphae resemble the baseball ball.

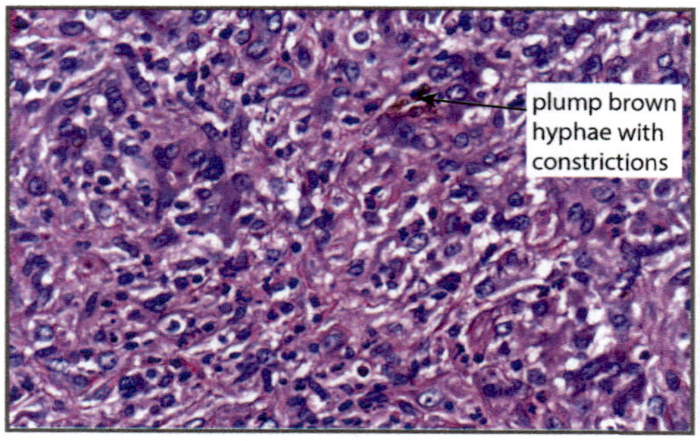

Figure 4.60 Phaeohyphomycosis. Note the plump brown hyphae within the dense mixed-cell infiltrate.

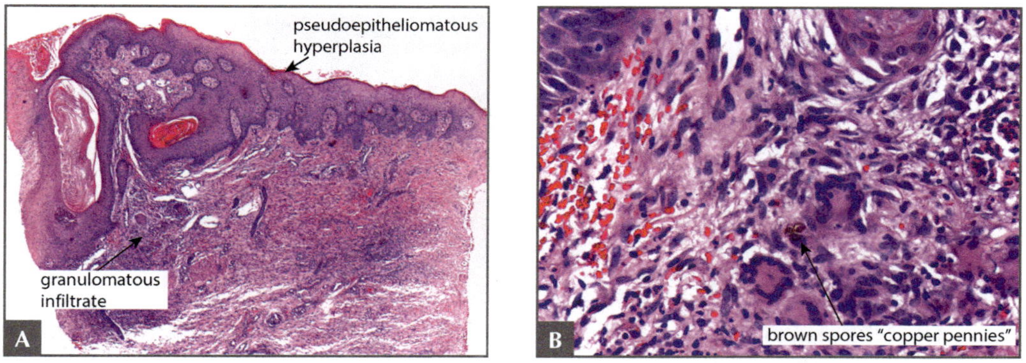

Figure 4.61 Chromoblastomycosis. **A** Note the pseudoepitheliomatous hyperplasia. **B** Note the "copper pennies" in the granulomatous infiltrate.

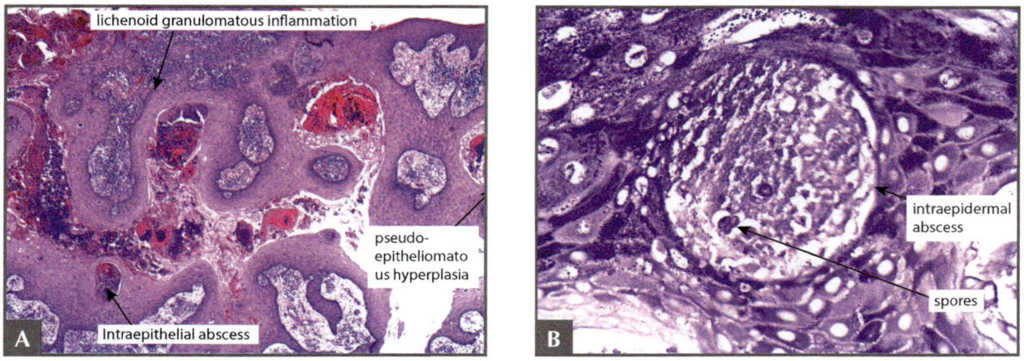

Figure 4.62 North American blastomycosis. **A** This tangentially bisected specimen demonstrates the pronounced pseudoepitheliomatous hyperplasia which together with the intraepidermal abscesses simulates the silhouette of keratoacanthoma. **B** Thick-walled spores highlighted by the PAS stain.

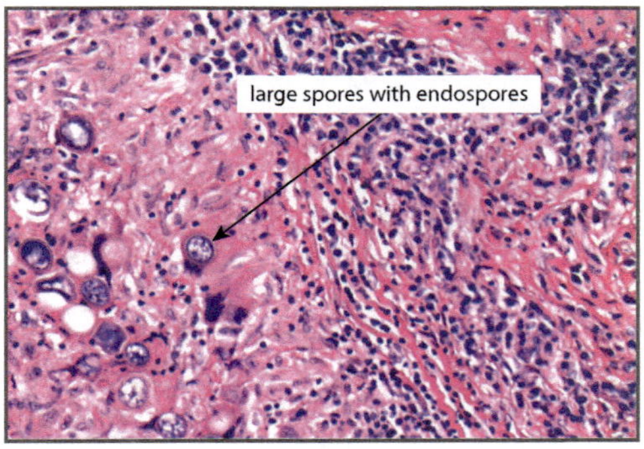

Figure 4.63 Coccidioidomycosis. Note the granulomatous inflammation with the numerous large spores containing endospores.

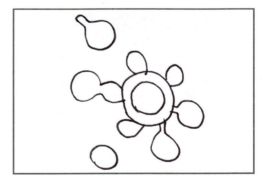

Figure 4.64 Paracoccidioidomycosis. The spores show a narrow single bud and sometimes are arranged as a marine wheel.

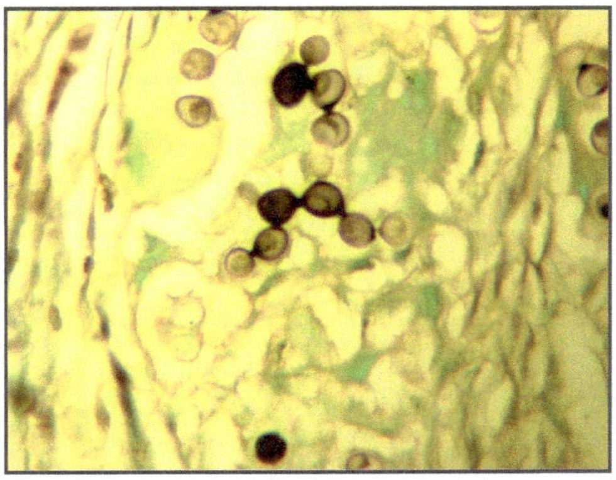

Figure 4.65 Lobomycosis, GMS stain. Lemon-shaped spores in the dermis, scarce inflammation. (Image courtesy of Antonio Schettini, MD.)

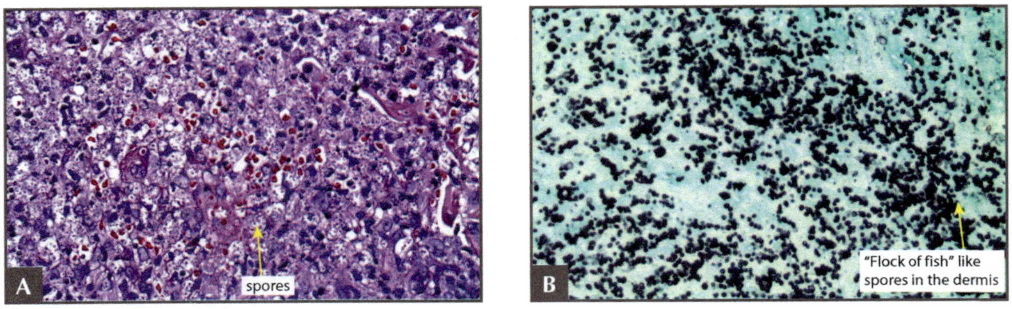

Figure 4.66 Histoplasmosis. **A** Note the small spores within the cytoplasm of histiocytes. **B** GMS stain highlights the spores.

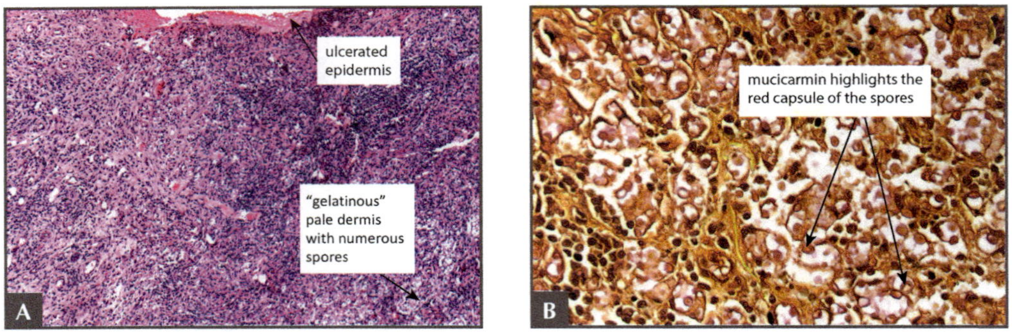

Figure 4.67 Cryptococcosis. **A** In a specimen from an immunocompromised patient note the gelatinous pale stroma with mild inflammation, no granulomatous pattern. **B** Mucicarmine highlights the red capsule of the spores.

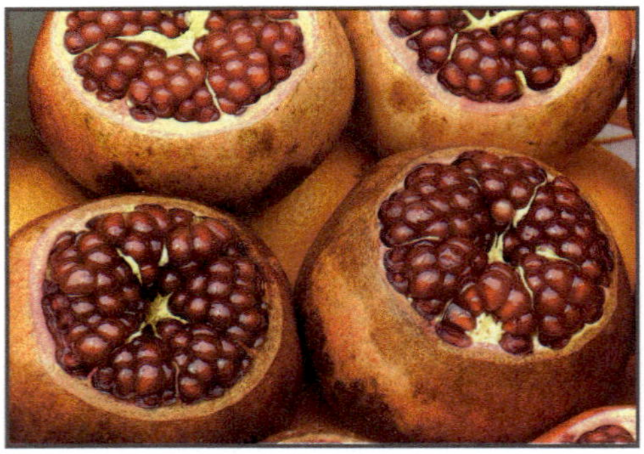

Photomnemonic 4.9 The sporangia in rhinosporidiosis resemble a transversely cut pomegranate.

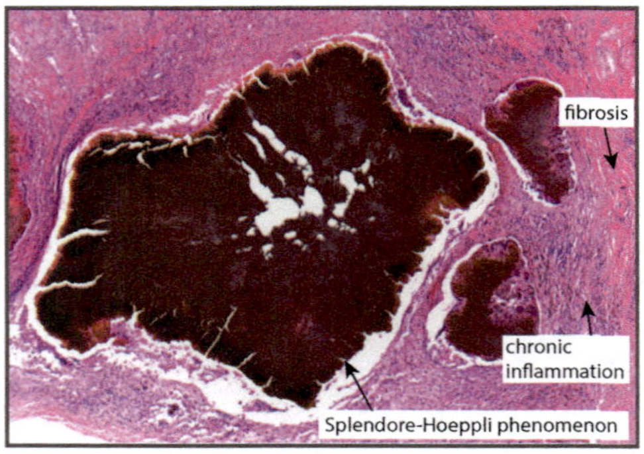

Figure 4.68 Eumycetoma. Note the large black sulfur grains in the fibrotic dermis with the Splendore-Hoeppli phenomenon.

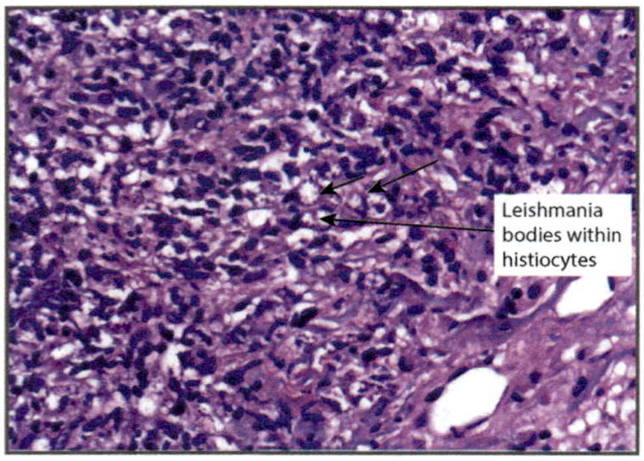

Figure 4.69 Leishmaniasis. The infiltrate in the dermis is pale due to the predominant histiocytes. The *Leishmania* bodies are seen as small intracellular dots.

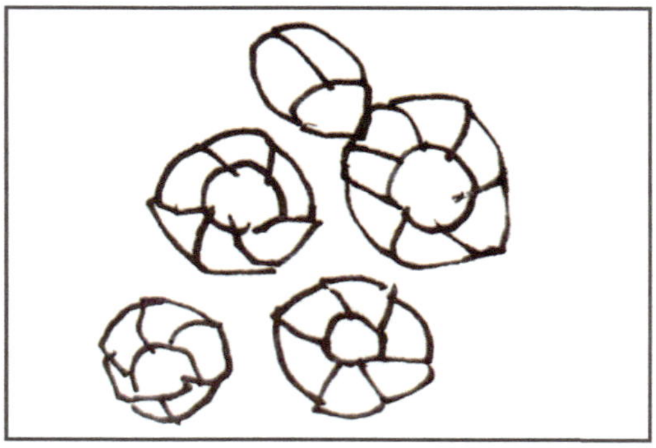

Figure 4.70 The sporangia in protothecosis resemble morula-like structures.

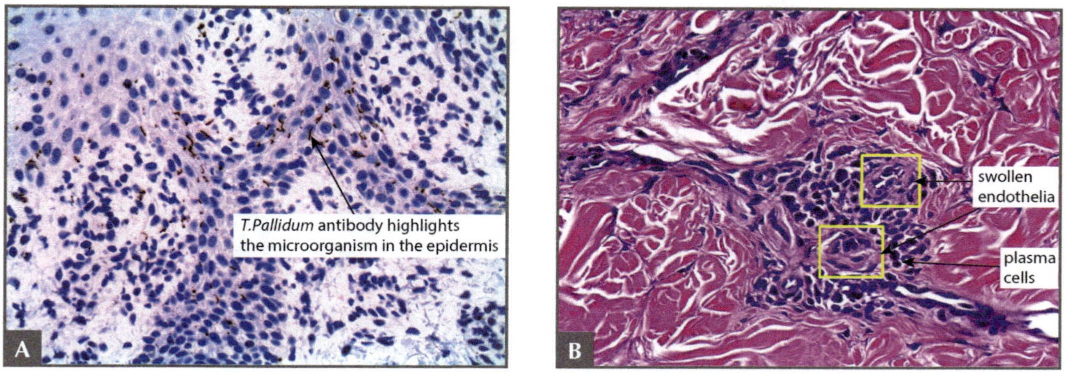

Figure 4.71 Syphilis. **A** The immunohistochemistry for *T. pallidum* is positive in the acanthotic epidermis. **B** Syphilitic endarteritis in secondary syphilis.

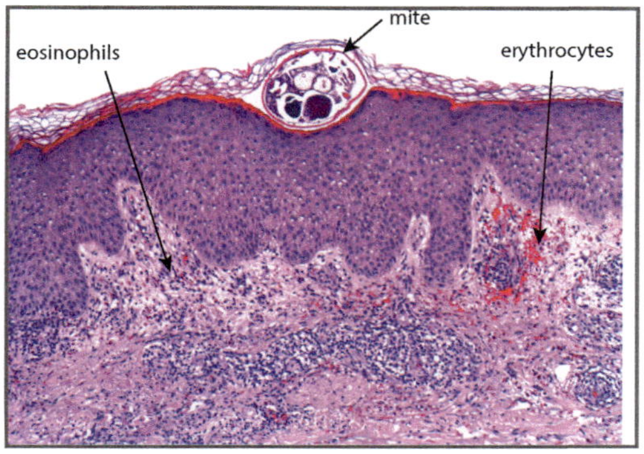

Figure 4.72 Scabies. The exoskeleton of the mite is present in the stratum corneum. There are typical arthropod-like features in the dermis.

HAIR AND NAIL DISORDERS

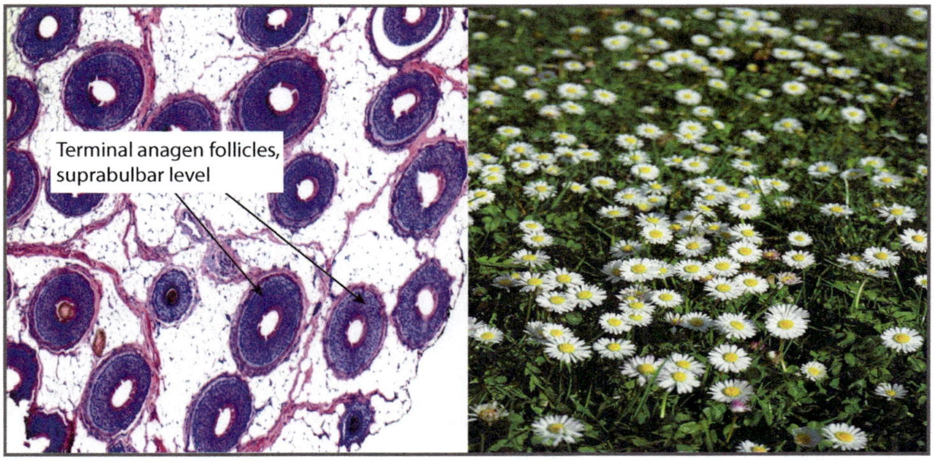

Figure 4.73 and Photomnemonic 4.10 Non-scarring alopecia. The random distribution of the follicular bulbs in the fat resembles a lawn of daisies on horizontal sections (bulbar level). Image modified from Miteva M., *Am J Dermatopathol* 2013; 35: 529.

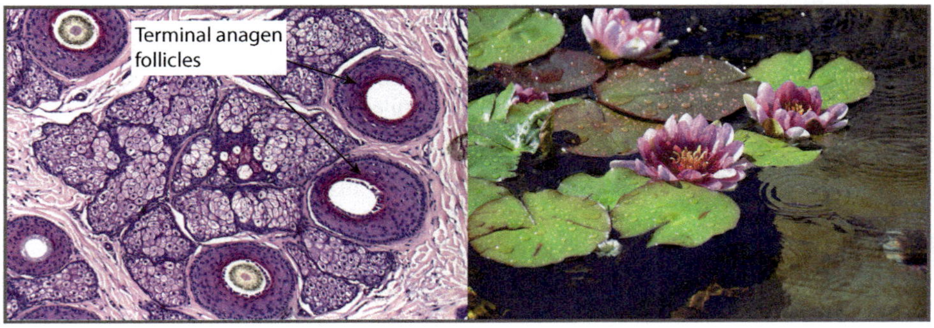

Figure 4.74 and Photomnemonic 4.11 Non-scarring alopecia. The isthmus level on horizontal sections resembles a pond with water lilies due to the similarity of the follicular units with their sebaceous glands to the islands of water lilies with their big leaves.

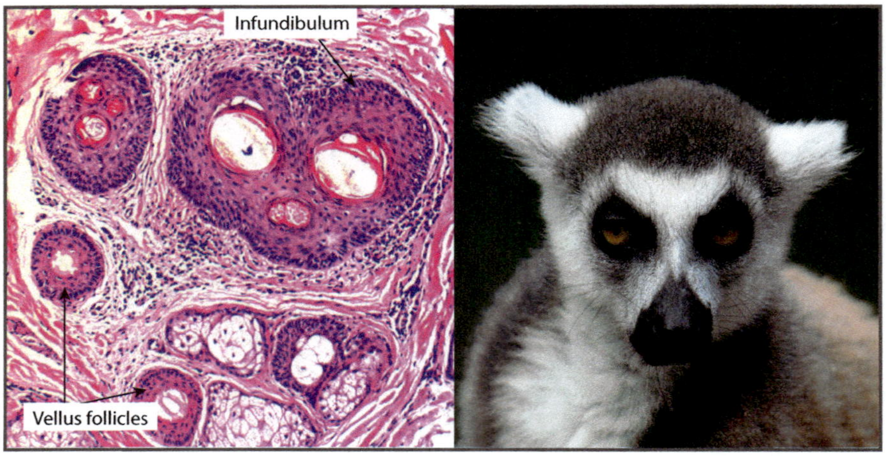

Figure 4.75 and Photomnemonic 4.12 Non-scarring alopecia. The infundibulum is characterized by grouping the emerging 2–3 hairs into one infundibular opening which resembles a monkey/skeleton face.

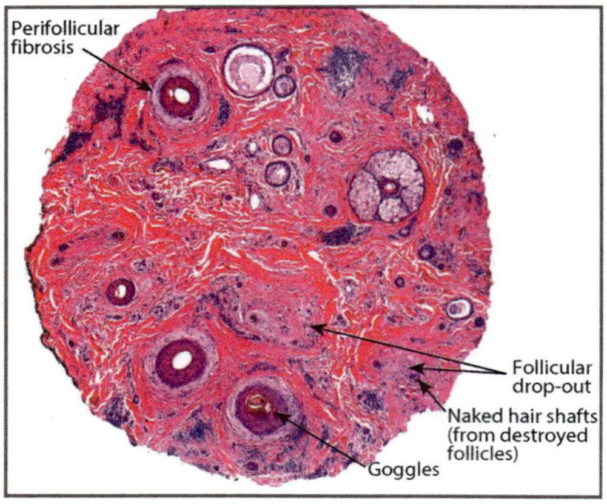

Figure 4.76 Central centrifugal cicatricial alopecia. Note the altered follicular architecture and the only focally preserved sebaceous glands.

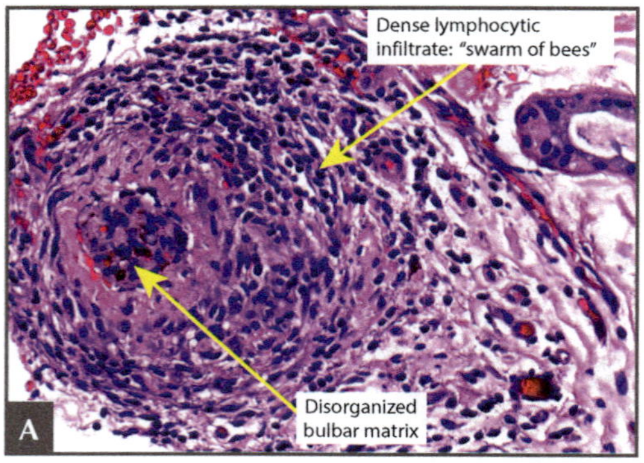

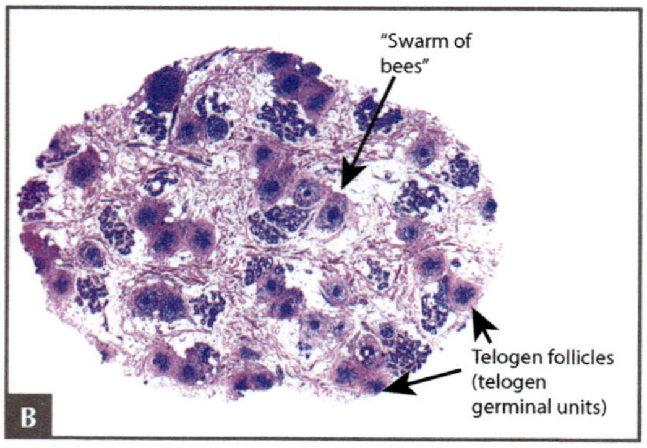

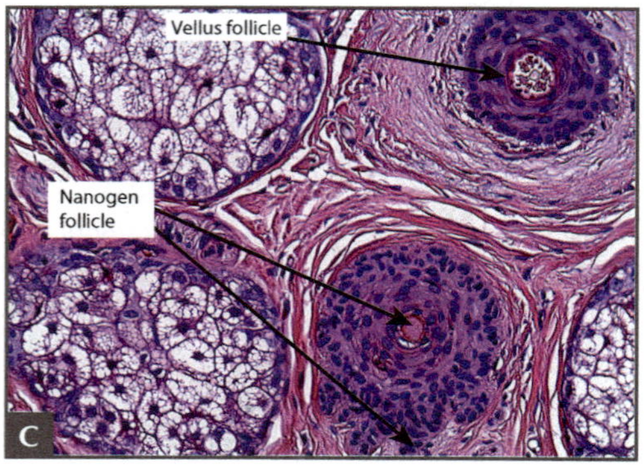

Figure 4.77 Alopecia areata (AA). **A** Acute stage AA. There is dense peribulbar lymphocytic infiltrate. **B** Subacute AA. At the bulbar level, note the predominant number of telogen follicles (mostly telogen germinal units in this case) which resemble clovers; some bulbs are affected by "swarm of bees"-like inflammation. The overall picture can be associated with a swarm of bees in a field of clovers. **C** Chronic stage AA. Note the vellus follicle with "pencil-like" thin hair shaft, and the nanogen follicle with keratotic material in the hair canal (but no real hair shaft) and serrated epithelial borders.

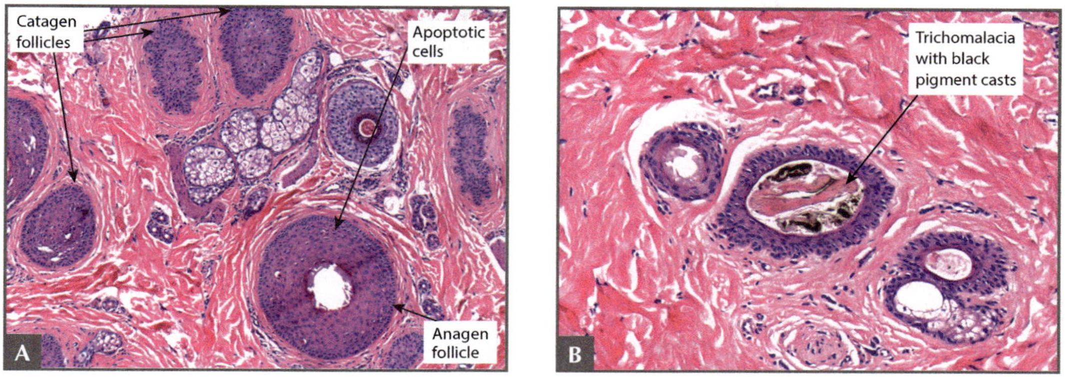

Figure 4.78 Trichotillomania. **A** Note the grouping of catagen follicles (with apoptotic cells). The present terminal anagen follicles also show apoptotic cells as a sign of catagen involution. **B** The same case showing trichomalacia and pigment casts.

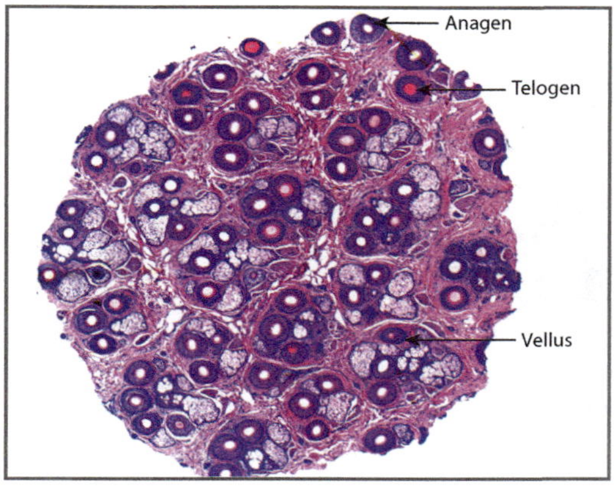

Figure 4.79 Chronic telogen effluvium. At the level of the isthmus in this "busy" slide there is preserved follicular architecture with no follicular miniaturization. The counts and ratios are similar to normal scalp.

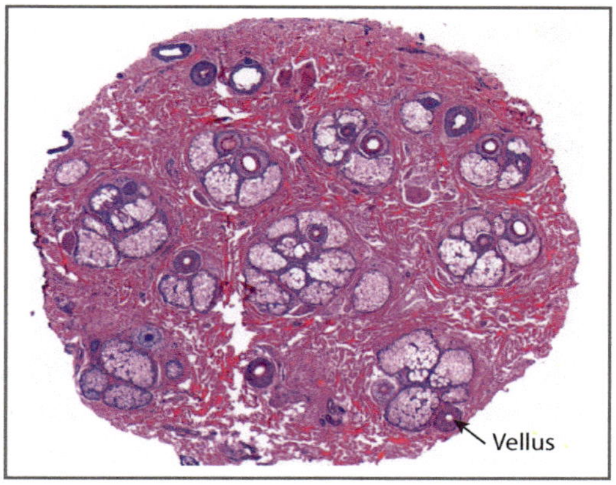

Figure 4.80 Androgenetic alopecia. At the level of the isthmus there is a predominant number of vellus follicles. In this particular case the terminal:vellus ratio is 0.2:1.

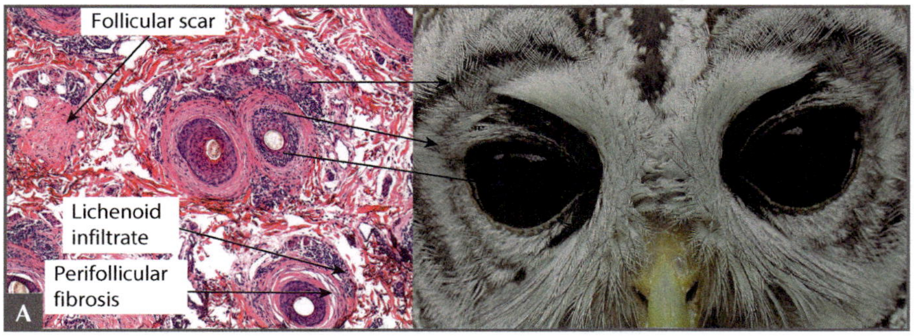

Figure 4.81A and Photomnemonic 4.13A Lichen planopilaris: the affected follicles show perifollicular lichenoid inflammation (the owl's eyebrows), perifollicular fibrosis (the concentric circles of feathers around the eyes), and hair shafts with their sheaths (the iris and the pupil).

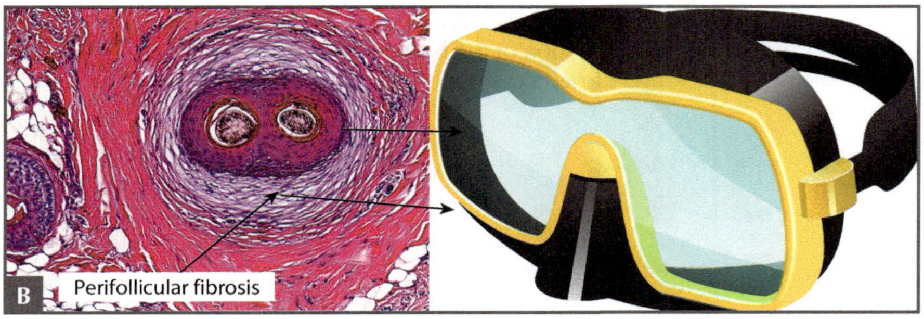

Figure 4.81B and Photomnemonic 4.13B A similar sign is the goggles sign in lichen planopilaris is the goggles sign in scarring alopecia: the perifollicular fibrosis corresponds to the frame of the glasses and the fused outer root sheaths to the glasses.

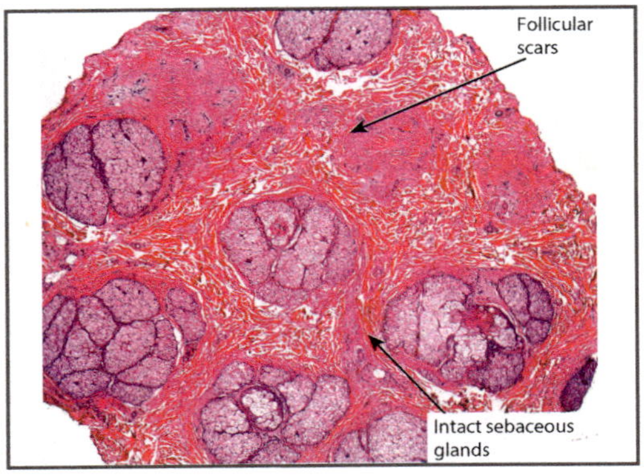

Figure 4.82 Traction alopecia. Note the absence of follicles in this specimen.

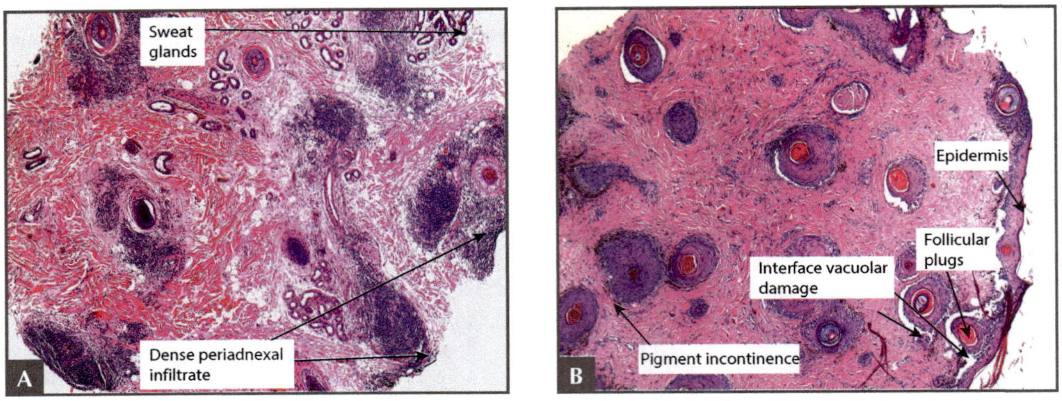

Figure 4.83 Discoid lupus erythematosus (DLE). **A** At the level of the bulbs there is dense periadnexal and perivascular infiltrate. **B** DLE at the level of the infundibulum.

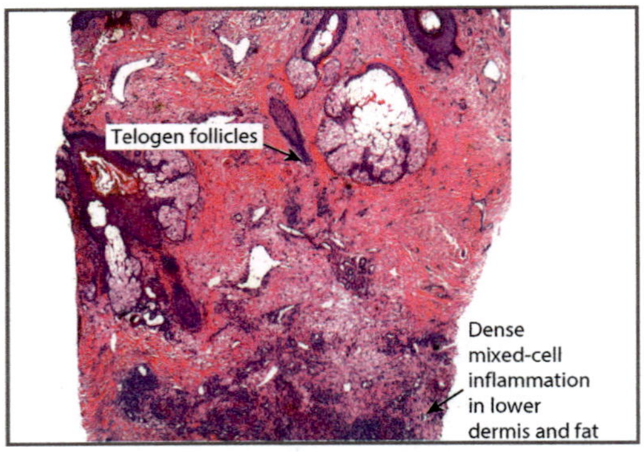

Figure 4.84 Dissecting cellulitis of the scalp. This is a vertical section from an early diagnosed case which shows non-scarring pattern. Note the dense inflammation in the deep part.

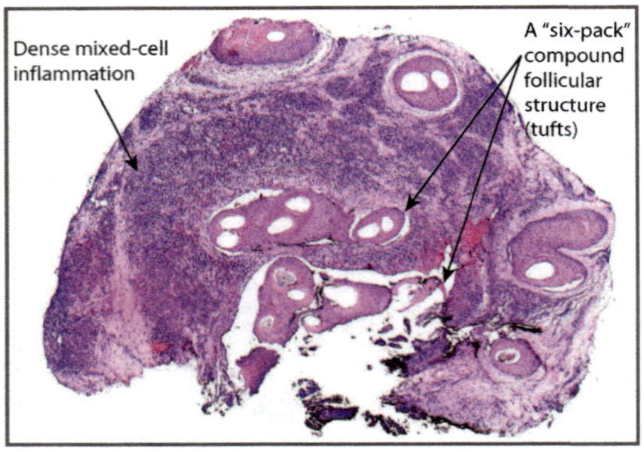

Figure 4.85 Folliculitis decalvans. Note the compound follicular structures, the dense inflammation and the absence of sebaceous glands at the level of the isthmus.

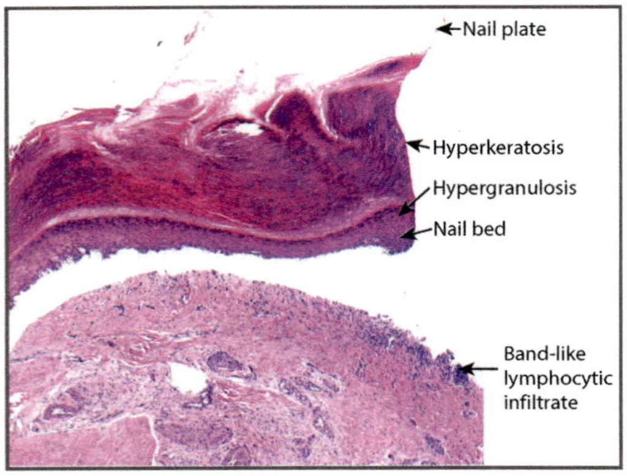

Figure 4.86 Nail bed lichen planus. There is a cleft between the nail bed and the dermis which is most likely artifactual in this case, but it can be observed also as a result of liquefactive degeneration of the basal layer in lichen planus (Max Joseph cleft).

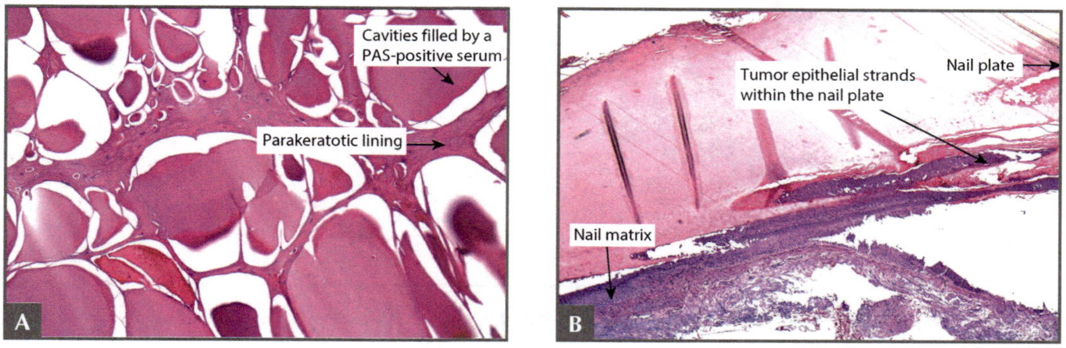

Figure 4.87 Onychomatricoma. **A** Transverse view from a nail clipping from onychomatricoma showing the cavities in the dystrophic nail plate. **B** Excisional specimen from onychomatricoma. Note the parallel digitate epithelial proliferations of tumor cells within the nail plate.

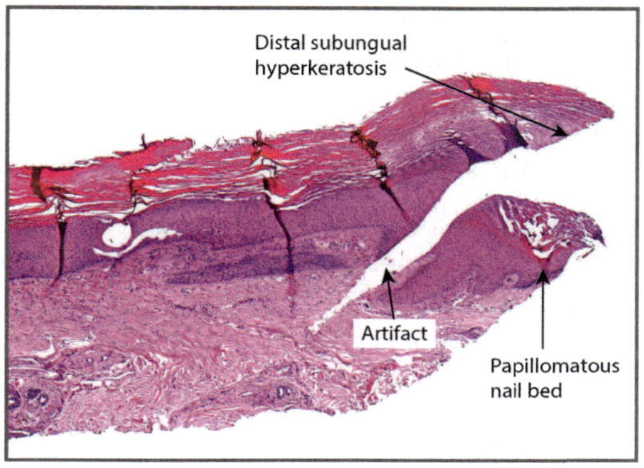

Figure 4.88 Onychopapilloma. In this excisional specimen there is papillomatous acanthosis of the nail bed and distal subungual hyperkeratosis.

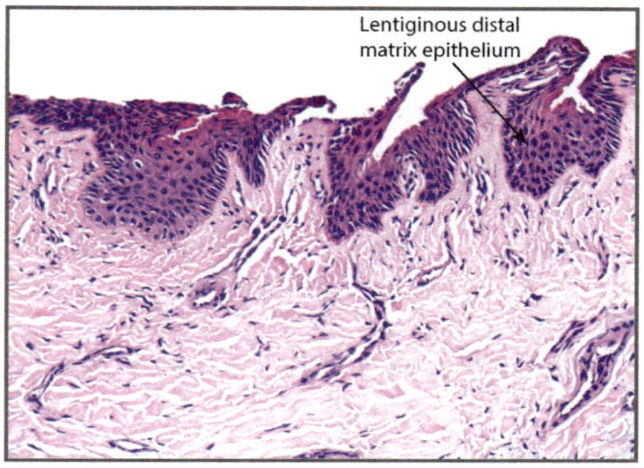

Figure 4.89 Shave biopsy of the distal matrix shows slight lentiginous hyperplasia.

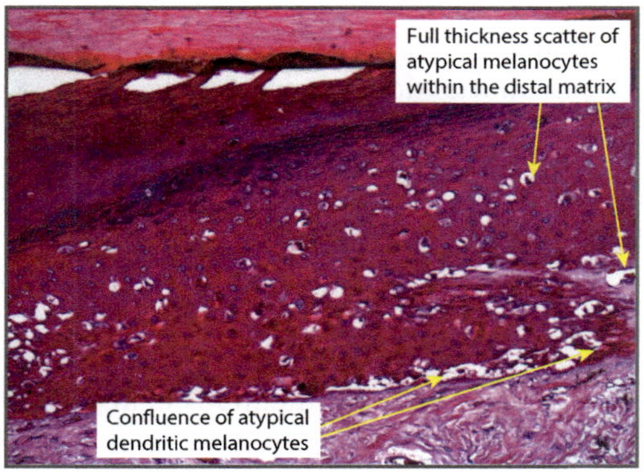

Figure 4.90 Subungual melanoma in situ. Note the scatter of atypical melanocytes and their confluence.

5 | Skin tumors

KERATINOCYTIC TUMORS (Tumors of the epidermis)

Andrew Miner and Mariya Miteva

Definition: Commonly referred to as non-melanocytic skin neoplasms, these are a large group of benign hyperplastic and malignant neoplasms arising from the epidermis.

General concepts

- **Most benign tumors** have a well-circumscribed silhouette characterized by epidermal hyperplasia (acanthosis, papillomatosis) and inconspicuous keratinocytes with preserved intercellular bridges, low nuclear/cytoplasmic ratio, and no atypia.
  - *Clonal pattern:* intraepidermal "nests of clonal keratinocytes" (intraepidermal epithelioma or Borst-Jadassohn phenomenon) in seborrheic keratosis, large cell acanthoma, basal cell carcinoma and squamous cell carcinoma. It has recently been shown that the clonal keratinocytes strongly express epidermal growth factor receptor (EGF-R)
  - *Squamous eddies:* whorled epithelial formations of glassy eosinophilic keratinocytes (inflamed seborrheic keratosis, inverted follicular keratosis)
- **Most malignant tumors** are characterized by epidermal hyperplasia or/and epidermal atrophy and atypical and pleomorphic keratinocytes with increased nuclear/cytoplasmic ratio, necrotic keratinocytes, and an increased number of atypical (asymmetric or multipolar) mitoses; in invasive carcinomas the atypical keratinocytes infiltrate the dermis, subdermis and their adjacent structures with potential for metastasis.

On high power

BENIGN TUMORS (ACANTHOMAS, KERATOSES)

Seborrheic keratosis (SK)

- Benign basaloid and squamoid proliferation
- Overlying lamellar (loose) keratin more common than compact hyperkeratosis
- Varying degrees of papillomatosis and acanthosis
- Horn pseudocysts filled with loose keratin
- Squamous eddies (mostly in inflamed seborrheic keratosis)

NB Clinically and histologically seborrheic keratoses have many shapes, sizes, and forms.

Variants:

- Acanthotic (dome-shaped surface with a flat bottom, basal layer hyperpigmentation) **(Figure 5.1A)**
- Flat (macular/incipient) seborrheic keratosis: subtle acanthosis and hyperkeratosis
- Reticulated (lace-like anastomosing strands of basaloid cell)
- Inflamed (hyperkeratosis, exo/endophytic growth with focal areas of squamous changes that may simulate squamous cell carcinoma: squamous eddies, necrotic keratinocytes and dermal inflammatory infiltrate) **(Figure 5.1B)**
- Clonal (nests of basaloid keratinocytes within the epidermis) **(Figure 5.1C)**

- Inverted follicular keratosis (endophytic growth associated with a hair follicle, squamous eddies) **(Figure 5.1D)**

Lichenoid keratosis (lichen planus like keratosis)

See Chapter 3, Interface dermatitis

Porokeratosis

See Chapter 4, Selected genodermatoses

Clear (pale) cell acanthoma

- Sharply demarked area in the epidermis of clear and enlarged cells (positive for PAS due to accumulation of glycogen and impaired melanin transfer from melanocytes) **(Figure 5.2)**
- Intact basal layer
- Diminished granular layer with overlying confluent parakeratosis and dispersed neutrophils

Differential diagnosis: Clear cell acanthoma is more of a horizontal process while trichilemmoma is endophytic. Both share parakeratosis and variable amounts of clear cell changes due to increased glycogen. Clear cell acanthoma lacks the peripheral palisade and pink cuticle of trichilemmoma.

Warty dyskeratoma

- Endophytic growth along a cystically dilated follicular structure
- Suprabasal acantholysis with villi protruding into the cystic cavity **(Figure 5.3)**
- Dyskeratotic cells: corps ronds and grains (see Chapter 1)

Acantholytic acanthoma

- A circumscribed and symmetrical acanthotic lesion
- Hyperkeratosis and hypergranulosis
- Acantholysis throughout the entire epidermis sparing the basal layer

NB Acantholytic acanthoma lacks the atypia of an acantholytic actinic keratosis.

Large cell acanthoma

- Often clinically mistaken for melanocytic neoplasm
- Similar to solar lentigo/flat seborrheic keratosis on pathology but with large keratinocytes (twice as big as regular keratinocytes)
- Lacks the degree of atypia for actinic keratosis or squamous cell carcinoma in situ

Epidermolytic acanthoma

- Acanthosis
- Ragged vacuole-like changes within the superficial epidermal layers (epidermolysis due to mutations in keratins 1 and 10)
- Unless widespread, these areas of epidermolysis are of no clinical relevance but are a histological curiosity

NB Similar diffuse epidermal changes characterize bullous congenital ichthyosiform erythroderma (epidermolytic hyperkeratosis).

Psoriasiform acanthoma

Isolated acanthotic lesion showing classic features for psoriasis
(Table 5.1)

ATYPICAL KERATINOCYTIC PROLIFERATIONS/INTRAEPIDERMAL CARCINOMAS

Actinic keratosis

- A form of intraepithelial neoplasia on sun-damaged skin

NB Look for solar elastosis.

Table 5.1 Summary of the most common features in benign acanthomas

	Warty dyskeratoma	Acantholytic acanthoma	Large cell acanthoma	Epidermolytic acanthoma	Psoriasiform acanthoma
Main histologic finding	Cystic cavity filled with keratotic debris Dyskeratosis Suprabsal acan-tholysis	Acanthosis with hyperkeratosis – the acantholysis involves *the entire epidermis*	Flat lesion, no acanthosis *Large keratinocytes* (twice the size of normal keratino-cytes) Hyperpigmented basal layer	Epidermolytic hyperkeratosis: clear spaces around nuclei in *the granular and upper spinous layers*	Classic *psoriasis features:* • suprapapillary thinning • regular elongated rete ridges • parakeratosis • hypogranulosis
Similar inflammatory counterpart	Darrier's disease	Pemphigus vulgaris Hailey-Hailey disease	Solar lentigo/flat seborrheic keratosis	Epidermolytic hyperkeratosis	Psoriasis

- The hyperchromatic, atypical, often enlarged nuclei are limited to the basal cell layer or lower layers of the epidermis; the superficial epidermal layers flatten out and mature
- The granular layer may or may not be intact (controversial)
- Overlying "pink and blue" stratum corneum: blue orthokeratosis over the follicular infundibula (compare to parakeratosis involving the follicular infundibula in Bowen's disease) and pink parakeratosis over the interfollicular epidermis **(Figure 5.4A)**

NB Alternating atrophy and hyperplasia of the epidermis is common.

Variants:

- Hypertrophic (hyperkeratosis and acanthosis) **(Figure 5.4B)**
- Atrophic (epidermal atrophy)
- Lichenoid (dense band-like infiltrate) **(Figure 5.4C)**
- Acantholytic (shows acantholysis)

Squamous cell carcinoma in situ (Bowen's disease)

- Psoriasiform/plaque-like acanthosis
- Full thickness atypia of the epidermis with loss of maturation (transepidermal atypia) **(Figure 5.5A)**
- Crowding of atypical keratinocytes
- Necrotic keratinocytes
- The atypia can extend down the adnexal structures but it does not invade the dermis
- Atypical vacuolated (koilocytic-like) and pagetoid (pale) cells (see Chapter 1 for the immunohistochemical expression of pagetoid cells in Bowen's disease vs melanoma vs Paget's disease)
- Atypical mitotic figures **(Figure 5.5B)**

NB While most commonly the granular layer is lost, there are many cases of clear full-thickness atypia with preserved granular layer.

Erythroplasia of Queyrat (Bowen's disease on the penile or vulvar mucosa)

- Epidermal acanthosis with parakeratosis
- Partial or full-thickness epidermal atypia **(Figure 5.6)**
- Possible dyskeratosis and possible lymphohistiocytic dermal infiltrate with plasma cells

Bowenoid papulosis

See Chapter 4, Infections

MALIGNANT TUMORS

Basal cell carcinoma (BCC)

This is the most common human malignancy.

- The tumor arises from the follicular germs (germinative cells) (see Adnexal tumors)
- Lobules, strands, nodules, and cords of basaloid cells with scant cytoplasm
- Apoptosis
- Characteristic is the peripheral palisade of elongated basaloid cells
- Clefts between the tumor aggregates and the stroma – the tumor cells lack hemidesmosomes to attach to the dermis
- The stroma may show mucinous degeneration and amyloid (comes from the degenerated keratin released from the apoptotic tumor cells in the dermis)

NB Recurrent BCC may have no epidermal connection.

Most common variants:

- Superficial (buds of tumor cells extend from the epidermis in a horizontal pattern) **(Figure 5.7A)**
- Nodular (large tumor lobules in the dermis) **(Figure 5.7B, C)**
- Infundibulocystic (oblong and round nests surround keratin-filled cystic structures)
- Fibroepithelioma of Pinkus (see Adnexal tumors)
- Keratotic (nodular BCC with central squamous differentiation)
- Micronodular* (small round tumor nests showing infiltrative growth in fibrotic stroma; no retraction clefts) **(Figure 5.7D)**
- Morpheaform/sclerosing* (strands, tongues, and columns of basaloid cells within a sclerotic stroma; no attachment to the epidermis; no retraction clefts; the differential diagnosis includes microcystic adnexal carcinoma and desmoplastic trichoepithelioma (see Adnexal tumors)

NB *The micronodular and morpheaform BCCs have an infiltrative, poorly delineated widespread growth and therefore show aggressive behavior.

- Basosquamous/metatypical (infiltrating jagged tongues of basaloid tumor cells admixed with tumor tongues whose cells show intercellular bridges and cytoplasmic keratinization for squamous differentiation)

BCC immunohistochemistry: BerEp4+, p63+, EMA and CEA–

Squamous cell carcinoma (SCC)

The tumor arises from the keratinocytes of the epidermis, de novo, or within preexisting AK or squamous cell carcinoma in situ.

- The tumor cells have eosinophilic (pink) glassy cytoplasm, large vesicular nuclei, prominent nucleoli

NB Look for intercellular bridges and horn pearls (small whorled foci of keratinization with/without necrotic keratinocytes) as a clue to the squamous differentiation.

Worse prognosis:

- Tumor thickness: tumors thinner than 2 mm rarely metastasize whereas tumors thicker than 5 mm have a 20% chance to metastasize
- High-risk locations: scalp, lip, nose, eyelid, ears
- Lymphovascular or perineural invasion (perineural lymphocytes are a clue to perineural invasion)
- Poorly differentiated tumors
- Acantholytic tumors

Keratoacanthoma-like SCC

This has been a controversial entity for decades, with some considering it a benign and others a malignant proliferation. There are reports of perineural invasion and metastatic keratoacanthoma in the literature.

- Well-differentiated multilobular exo/endophytic cyst-like invagination of the epidermis
- Keratin-filled central crater with peripheral "lip-like" epidermal borders **(Figure 5.8A)**
- Pushing lower border in the dermis: tongues of tumor cells
- Intraepidermal neutrophilic abscesses
- The tumor cells are enlarged and atypical keratinocytes with eosinophilic glassy cytoplasm **(Figure 5.8B)**

Invasive SCC

1. *Well-differentiated SCC*
    - Clearly of keratinocyte origin (intercellular bridges, horn pearls) **(Figure 5.8C)**
    - Mild to moderate atypia
2. *Moderately differentiated SCC*
    - While keratinocyte origin is at least focally clear, there are atypical or bizarre cells in at least one portion of the tumor **(Figure 5.8D)**
3. *Poorly differentiated/spindled SCC*
    - This term is often reserved for tumors requiring immunohistochemistry to establish the diagnosis
    - Spindled cells or otherwise difficult to ascertain atypical cells of origin invade the dermis and its structures as irregular masses, strands, and tongues **(Figure 5.8E)**
    - No/minimal keratinization
    - Prominent inflammatory infiltrate

SCC immunohistochemistry: Broad-spectrum cytokeratins (MNF116)+, EMA+, CAM5.2-, and BerEp4–

NB SCC is typically graded by the most poorly differentiated area: if a fairly typical well differentiated tumor has a small focus of moderate differentiation, it will be called "moderately differentiated" or "well to moderately differentiated."

Verrucous carcinoma

An uncommon variant of SCC

- Well-differentiated, low-grade SCC with low propensity for invasion and metastasis
- Characteristic silhouette: papillomatous acanthosis with bulldozing invasive downgrowth of the rete in the dermis
- Deceptively bland cytology: minimal atypia of the cells and very low mitotic rate

Four main types of verrucous carcinoma exist, differing by location:

- Epithelioma cuniculatum (plantar foot)
- Oral florid papillomatosis
- Buschke-Lowenstein tumor (on genital mucosa in immunocompromised, associated with HPV 6 and 11)
- Pretibial papillomatosis cutis carcinoides (in long-standing ulcers)

CYSTS

Andrew Miner and Mariya Miteva

Definition: Cutaneous cysts are typically cavities with an epithelial lining and contents which may or may not contain adnexal structures. Hybrid forms of cysts exist.

General concepts

The diagnosis is usually based on the type of cyst wall lining.

- **With epithelial lining:**
  - *Stratified squamous epithelium:* epidermoid cyst, trichilemmal cyst, vellus hair cyst, milia
  - *Stratified squamous epithelium with cyst wall components*: steatocystoma, dermoid cyst
  - *Mixed squamous and non-squamous ciliated epithelium*: bronchogenic cyst
  - *Pseudostratified columnar epithelium*: median raphe cyst
- **With no epithelial lining:** mucocele, digital mucous cyst, ganglion cyst

On high power

WITH EPITHELIAL LINING

Epidermoid cyst (infundibular cyst)

Most common type of cutaneous cyst

Originates from the infundibular portion of the hair follicle, which shows the same pattern of keratinization as the surrounding epidermis

Lining: Ordered, normal layers of the epidermis, including a granular layer

(Figure 5.9)

Adnexal structures: None

Content: Lamellar ("loose") keratin

Often there is rupture of the cyst wall with foreign body giant cell reaction. These giant cells may be engulfing the keratin (see Chapter 3, Granulomatous dermatitis).

Pilar cyst (trichilemmal/isthmus-catagen cyst)

More common on the scalp but can occur anywhere on the body

Originates from the isthmus portion of the hair follicle where the inner root sheath keratinizes abruptly (without a granular layer)

(Figure 5.10)

Lining: Reminiscent of epidermis but with "abrupt" keratinization and no granular layer; no intercellular bridges between the keratinocytes

Adnexal structures: None

Contents: Thick, compact homogenous keratin; occasional calcification

Vellus hair cyst

Most common in young people; present as multiple skin-colored or brown; sometimes many lesions may arise suddenly (eruptive vellus hair cysts)

Originates from the infundibular portion of the vellus follicles

Lining: Ordered, normal layers of epidermis, preserved but thin granular layer

(Figure 5.11)

Adnexal structures: Vellus hair shafts

Contents: Keratin and several vellus hair shafts, rarely telogen-like structures

NB Small epidermoid cyst(s) containing vellus hairs in the upper and mid dermis: think vellus hair cysts.

Milium/milia

These are primary (on the face) or secondary (in bullous disorders)

Originate from the infundibular portion of the vellus follicles (but contain no vellus hairs in contrast to vellus hair cysts) or from the eccrine ducts (secondary milia)

Lining: Ordered, normal layers of epidermis

Adnexal structures: None

Contents: Keratin

NB A very small epidermoid cyst in the upper dermis: think milia.

(Figure 5.12)

Steatocystoma

Cystic invagination with sebaceous glands in the lining and loose, oily cyst contents; often contains vellus hair follicles in the cyst wall. Solitary lesions are known as steatocystoma simplex; multiple lesions are known as steatocystoma multiplex (associated with pachyonychia congenita type 2 and keratin 17 mutations)

Lining: Thin stratified squamous epithelium with characteristic pink, rugged "shark tooth"- like cuticle

(Figure 5.13, Photomnemonic 5.1)

Lining of the cyst originates from the cuticle lining of the sebaceous ducts (see Chapter 1, Figure 1.41)

Adnexal structures: Sebaceous glands within the wall (not always present, may require multiple step sections)

Contents: Sebum

Dermoid cyst

Present at birth; clinically most common on the lateral eyebrow of a young child

Lining: Ordered, normal layers of epidermis with preserved granular layer

Adnexal structures: Mature hair follicles, sebaceous glands, and even eccrine/apocrine glands can be seen

Contents: Lamellar keratin and sometimes fragmented hair shafts and sebum

Differential diagnosis: Dermoid cysts differ from epidermoid cysts in that they have large cystic cavities with adnexal structures in their walls and from steatocystoma by the absence of pink cuticle lining.

Bronchogenic cyst

Usually located on the neck and thoracic wall

Originates from an embryonic defect leading to abnormal ventral budding of the tracheobronchial tree and lies in the subdermis

Lining: Ciliated or non-ciliated columnar or cuboidal epithelium; areas of stratified squamous epithelium

(Figure 5.14)

Adnexal structures: None or rarely seromucinous glands; cyst wall may contain smooth muscle or cartilage
Contents: Water and proteinaceous mucin (may appear empty)

Median raphe cyst

Located on the ventral penis or perineum up to the anus

Originate from an embryonic defect during the development of the male genitals

Silhouette of the cystic cavity is irregular and angulated and there is no connection to the epidermis
Lining: Pseudostratified columnar epithelium; stratified squamous epithelium may be seen
Adnexal structures: Usually none
Contents: Fluid secretions in pseudostratified columnar variants but loose keratin in stratified squamous variants

WITH NO EPITHELIAL LINING

NB The following cysts have no epithelial lining and therefore are not true cysts (pseudocysts).

Digital mucous cyst

Located on the dorsal finger close to the distal interphalangeal joint (DIJ) to which it is attached by a pedicle

Originates from myxoid degeneration of the synovial lining of the adjacent DIJ's capsule

- Wall composed of compressed collagen fibers and acid mucopolysaccharides (mucin) **(Figure 5.15)**
- Cystic space filled with mucin

Mucocele

Mucous pseudocyst of the oral cavity
Originates from traumatic injury to the excretory salivary ducts, which results in a pool of mucin in the dermis

- Cyst-like cavity with mucin in the dermis **(Figure 5.16A)**
- Pseudocyst wall contains granulation tissue with inflammation **(Figure 5.16B)**

Ganglion cyst

Located close to a joint or a tendon (on hand, wrist or foot)
Originates from myxoid degeneration of a joint capsule or a tendon sheath

- Wall is thick and composed of dense layered fibrous tissue **(Figure 5.17)**
- Cystic space contains mucin

NB A ganglion is a pseudocyst; contrast a synovial cyst, which is a true cyst with an epithelial lining.

SOFT TISSUE TUMORS

Andrew Miner and Mariya Miteva

Definition: Soft tissue pathology is a large subspecialty of pathology distinct from but often overlapping with skin pathology. It studies the heterogeneous group of tumors with differentiation towards the mesenchymal tissue (fibrohistiocytic, histiocytic, vascular, and tumors from the adipose tissue, muscle, cartilage, and bone).

General concepts

CLASSIFICATION

The World Health Organization (WHO) classifies soft tissue tumors into:

1. Benign (most do not recur)
2. Intermediate, locally aggressive (require a wide excision in healthy tissue)
3. Intermediate, rarely metastasizing (to lymph nodes and lung)
4. Malignant, with significant risk for distant metastases (20–100%)

Only the most common soft tissue tumors are included here.

For the current classification of benign, intermediate, and malignant soft tissue tumors, see http://www.iarc.fr/en/publications/pdfs-online/pat-gen/bb5/bb5-classifsofttissue.pdf [Accessed: 5 July 2016]

CELL MORPHOLOGY

See Chapter 1 for details about fibroblasts, myofibroblasts, histiocytes, giant cells, smooth muscle cells, vascular structures, and adipose tissue.

On low power

- Most malignant soft tissue tumors (sarcomas, from the Greek word *sarx* meaning flesh) are poorly circumscribed while most benign tumors are well circumscribed.
- Mitotic figures may be seen in benign soft tissue tumors but atypical (multipolar) mitotic figures are suggestive of a more sinister process.

- Some malignancies, such as dermatofibrosarcoma protuberans, may have less atypia than benign fibrohistiocytic lesions, such as benign fibrous histiocytoma.

GROWTH PATTERNS

- **Whorled:** Wavy concentric arrangement of the fascicles **(Photomnemonic 5.2)**
- **Storiform:** An irregularly whorled pattern **(Photomnemonic 5.3)**
- **Plexiform:** From plexus; web-like or network-like arrangement **(Photomnemonic 5.4)**
- **Rosette-like:** The arrangement of the cells in a rose-like pattern or in a halo around a central acellular area **(Photomnemonic 5.5)**
- **Honeycomb:** This pattern usually refers to infiltration of the tumor into the fat tissue **(Photomnemonic 5.6)**
- **Fascicular:** Arranged in the form of a stack of logs **(Photomnemonic 5.7)**

IMMUNOHISTOCHEMICAL MARKERS

See Chapter 1

FIBROHISTIOCYTIC TUMORS

Dermal and/or subcutaneous mesenchymal tumors which show fibroblastic, myofibroblastic, and histiocytic (macrophage-like) differentiation

Skin tag (acrochordon, fibroepithelial polyp)

A very common skin lesion

- A polypoid papillomatous silhouette with normal/acanthotic epidermis
- A core of loose connective tissue **(Figure 5.18)**
- In older/giant lesions fibroadipose tissue can be found (fibrolipoma)

Fibrous papule (angiofibroma)

- Isolated facial lesion or part of tuberous sclerosis and MENI syndrome
- Perifollicular fibrosis (mostly around vellus telogen follicles which are common on the face) **(Figure 5.19)**
- Fine, dilated capillaries with perivascular "onion-like" fibrosis
- Stellate (angulated) fibroblasts in the collagenous stroma (these are F.XIIIa-positive fibroblasts)

Hypertrophic scar and keloid

Both represent an excessive scar growth as a response to trauma.
(Figure 5.20, Table 5.2)

Table 5.2 Summary of the pathologic differences between hypertrophic scars and keloids

	Hypertrophic scar	Keloid
Growth pattern	In early lesions: parallel In developed: whorled	Whorled with tongue-like pushing edge in the dermis
Cellularity	Cellular: fibroblasts and myofibroblasts	Less cellular: scattered fibroblasts and myofibroblasts
Collagen	Thinner collagen fascicles (mostly in developed lesions)	Thick hyalinized "glassy" collagen
Vessels	Vertical slender vessels	Few

Dermatofibroma (DF)

Also called benign fibrous histiocytoma (BFH)

- Epidermal acanthosis with hyperpigmented basal layer (simulating lentigo) **(Figure 5.21A)**
- Poorly defined tumor without a capsule
- The spindled fibroblasts are organized in a storiform and fascicular pattern
- The cells surround small individual hyalinized collagen bundles at the periphery (collagen trapping/collagen balls) **(Figure 5.21B)**
- If the tumor extends in the fat tissue, it extends down the fibrous septa (compare to the infiltrative honeycomb pattern of DFSP)

Cellular DF

- Dense storiform/fascicular pattern **(Figure 5.21C)**
- Extends into the superficial fat tissue but in a bulging pattern (compare to the honeycomb pattern in DFSP)
- Look for collagen trapping at the periphery as a clue to the diagnosis

NB CD34 positive at periphery only (diffuse CD34 positivity should lead to re-evaluation).

Epithelioid DF

- Epithelioid cells with eosinophilic cytoplasm and vesicular nuclei
- Immunohistochemistry is needed to distinguish from cellular neurothekeoma, perineurioma, hypopigmented blue nevus, and interstitial Spitz nevus

Hemosiderotic DF

- Also called "aneurysmal", which can be confused with the angiomatoid fibrous histiocytoma (a distinct low-grade malignancy that shares the EWSR1/ATF1 and FUS/ATF1 translocations with clear cell sarcoma)

- Dense cellular proliferation
- Cleft-like or cystic-like pseudovascular spaces (no endothelial lining) and hemosiderin **(Figure 5.21D)**

Lipidized DF

- Common on leg (also called "ankle-type DF")
- Numerous foamy cells present among the spindle cells **(Figure 5.21E)**

NB Always look at the periphery of the tumor for the characteristic collagen trapping of DF.

NB The DF variants which show cellular pleomorphism (not all cells look alike) and atypia (some cells are larger with prominent nuclei) are associated with an increased risk of local recurrence.

Immunohistochemistry: rarely required or helpful:

- Cellular DF can be CD34-positive at the periphery, but this should fade at the center of the lesion
- Factor XIIIa is positive but it is a non-specific marker and helpful only rarely

Dermatomyofibroma

A common location is the scapula/shoulder.

- Densely cellular "plaque-like (horizontal)" proliferation of spindled cells in the dermis parallel to the epidermis
- Fascicular pattern **(Figure 5.22)**
- The hair follicles sometimes remain intact "entrapped" within the fascicles

NB No collagen trapping and no epidermal acanthosis compared to DF.

Acquired digital fibrokeratoma (ADFK)

Dome-shaped papule on acral skin

- Hyperkeratosis and acanthosis
- Verticalized interwoven collagen bundles **(Figure 5.23)**
- Verticalized fine vessels

NB ADFK with nerve bundles in the dermis: think accessory digit.

Giant cell tumor of the tendon sheath (GCTTS)

Benign commonly recurrent tumor of tendons; common on hand joints; CSF1 gene on chromosome 1 translocations are common

- Multilobular plexiform growth
  - Spindle and more plump cells, including foamy cells
  - Osteoclast-like giant cells **(Figure 5.24)**
- Hemosiderin, hemosiderophages
- Normal mitotic figures common
- Collagenous stroma

Nodular fasciitis

A rapidly growing soft tissue tumor on extremities of young women after trauma; recurrence is rare

- A poorly demarcated proliferation of myofibroblasts in a random pattern (resembles a tissue culture of fibroblasts) and in a more organized storiform pattern focally **(Figure 5.25)**
- The cells are spindled to plump
- The stroma is variably myxoid
- Collagen is sparse
- Look at the margins for inflammatory cells

Proliferative fasciitis

A variant of nodular fasciitis which shows numerous myofibroblasts resembling ganglion cells (multipolar cells with dendrites) **(Figure 5.26)**

Storiform collagenoma (sclerotic fibroma)

Associated with Cowden's disease but also seen as isolated lesion

- Hypocellular eosinophilic proliferation of collagen organized in a whorled and storiform pattern
- Cleft-like spaces between the short eosinophilic strands **(Figure 5.27)**

Myofibroma

Multiple lesions in children (at birth or develop in the first 2 years); single lesions in adults

- Pale silhouette (due to the pronounced stromal hyalinization)
- Plexiform arrangement of lobules **(Figure 5.28A)**
- Peripheral short fascicles of spindled and plump elongated cells (myofibroblasts which are SMA-alpha(+) and desmin(-))
- Delicate collagen bundles
- Angulated vascular spaces mostly among the cells in the lobules (hemangiopericytoma type) **(Figure 5.28B)**

NB Necrosis, hyalinization, calcification, and hemorrhage are more common in the adult type.

Atypical fibroxanthoma (AFX)

Tumor of the elderly involving the head and neck; typically on very sun-damaged skin

It has no aggressive behavior, therefore metastatic cases are better classified as pleomorphic dermal sarcoma (see below).

NB AFX is characterized by striking *pleomorphism* (variability in the shape and size of the cells/and or their nuclei) + *polymorphism* (variability in the type of cells and their growth patterns).

- It is a tumor of myofibroblastic and fibrohistiocytic differentiation
- Thin or ulcerated epidermis with a collarette (elongated rete on both sides of the tumor) **(Figure 5.29A)**
- Well-circumscribed, highly cellular dermal proliferation (with NO subcutaneous involvement)

> • NB Look for solar elastosis

- The adnexal structures are pushed aside but usually spared
- Atypical, bizarre spindle cells, plump cells, epithelioid or clear cells **(Figure 5.29B)**
- Giant cells can be seen
- Numerous mitoses, including atypical

Immunohistochemistry:
- Cytokeratin and melanocytic markers(–) (to exclude poorly differentiated squamous cell carcinoma and melanoma)
- Desmin(–) (to exclude leiomyosarcoma)

Confirmative stains: CD10 and procollagen 1(+)

Dermatofibrosarcoma protuberans

Affects a wide range of ages and physical locations (without palms or soles)

90% of the tumors are characterized by t(17;22)(q22;q13), resulting in the fusion of alpha chain type 1 of collagen gene and platelet-derived growth factor beta gene

It has a high recurrence rate and can rarely metastasize.
- A storiform pattern
- Bland spindle cells, often very uniform
- The cells infiltrate the adipose tissue and the fat lobules appear entrapped within the tumor in a *honeycomb* pattern **(Figure 5.30)**. (This is found even in the atrophic variant)
- Only rare mitotic figures unless *fibrosarcomatous* change is present (long fascicles of atypical cells resembling a "herringbone" pattern)

> NB Only with fibrosarcomatous change does DFSP typically develop pleomorphism and atypia and is associated with a higher risk for metastasis and recurrence.

Pleomorphic dermal sarcoma (PDS, malignant fibrous histiocytoma)

Head and neck tumor on sun-damaged skin which is similar to AFX on pathology but with deep extension and metastatic potential

Distinguishing features:
- Deep extension into the subcutaneous fat (not seen in AFX) **(Figure 5.31A)**
- Perineural or intravascular extension seen in a significant percentage
- Necrosis supports the diagnosis (no necrosis in AFX)

Epithelioid sarcoma

A slow-growing nodule in young adults, with predilection for fingers, hands, and forearms

> NB It originates from primitive mesenchymal cells with capacity for epithelial differentiation.

- Dermal and subcutaneous nodules of tumor cells surround central necrosis
- Atypical epithelioid (prominent eosinophilic cytoplasm) and spindle cells
- Fusion of adjacent necrotic nodules results in a *geographic necrosis pattern* **(Figure 5.32)**
- Hyalinized/fibrous stroma with hemorrhage and mucin

> NB Confluent 'rheumatoid nodule-like" aggregates intermingled with atypical epithelioid cells confluencing in a geographic pattern: think epithelioid sarcoma.

Immunohistochemistry: High and low molecular cytokeratins(+), EMA(+), CD34(+/–), desmin(–)

HISTIOCYTIC TUMORS

Histiocytes are monocytes derived from the bone marrow which in the tissues acquire the ability to phagocytize.

For an overview of all members of the "histiocytic family" and their immunohistochemical profile, see Chapter 2, Table 2.3.

Xanthogranuloma

Clinically, a yellow papule or nodule with the majority of cases above the neck; occurs in children (juvenile xanthogranuloma) and in adults
- Epidermal collarette
- Dense dermal "pale" infiltrate of mononuclear cells with vesicular nuclei; some cells are foamy
- Giant cells the Touton type in developed/older lesions (Touton giant cells have a "foamy" peripheral rim as they form from the foamy histiocytes) **(Figure 5.33A)**
- Minimal atypia and only rare to no mitotic figures
- Inflammatory cells, particularly eosinophils **(Figure 5.33B)**
- Older lesions resemble DF

Immunohistochemistry: F.XIIIa, CD68, CD163(+) and S100 and CD1a(–)

Reticulohistiocytic granuloma (reticulohistiocytoma)

A solitary and a multicentric form exist

- Grenz zone
- Dermal dense nodular pink infiltrates of histiocytes with light "ground-glass" and dark "dusty-rose colored" eosinophilic cytoplasm **(Figure 5.34)**
- Mixed inflammatory infiltrate with eosinophils (early); giant cells and fibrosis (later)

NB F.XIIIa is positive in solitary reticulohistiocytoma and is negative in multicentric reticulohistiocytosis.

Differential diagnosis:

- Xanthogranuloma (more foamy cells, no ground-glass cells)
- Granular cell tumor (the cells have distinct cell membranes and granular cytoplasm)

Xanthoma

Cutaneous eruptions with variety of clinical presentation and associations, often including elevated lipids

- All varieties have in common collections of foamy macrophages (bubbly cytoplasm loaded with lipid material displace the nuclei at the periphery)
- Extracellular lipid material ("pools of pale material" surrounded by macrophages) can be observed in hyperlipidemia
- Cholesterol esters are birefringent under polarized light (usually present in tuberous and tendinous xanthomas)
- Cholesterol clefts are fusiform spaces caused by the dissolving out of cholesterol crystals in paraffin embedded tissue

(Table 5.3)

Rosai-Dorfman disease

Systemic and cutaneous forms exist, with the cutaneous form showing more indolent, self-regressing course. Clinically is manifested by papules and nodules coalescing into plaques

NB On pathology the buzzword is "emperipolesis" (intact lymphocytes or plasma cells engulfed wholly by macrophages) **(Figure 5.36A)**.

- The dermis and subcutaneous fat are completely filled by dense sheets or large nodules of lymphocytes, plasma cells, and histiocytes **(Figure 5.36B)**
- On low power may appear as a lymph node in the dermis
- Late stages may show fibrosis and/or storiform pattern

Immunohistochemistry: S100(+), CD68(+), CD1a(–)

Necrobiotic xanthogranuloma (NXG)

A disorder of questionable inflammatory or neoplastic origin

- Dense dermal infiltrate of histiocytes (usually foamy), granulomas, Touton giant cells, and foreign body giant cells

Table 5.3 Helpful diagnostic features in differentiating xanthoma varieties

Name	Clinical features	Histologic clues	Lab findings
Planar xanthoma	Palms or intertriginous thin yellow plaques	Often subtle superficial dermal foamy cells	Range from normal to type IIa (intertriginous) and III (palmar) hyperlipidemia
Tuberous xanthoma	Extensor surfaces	Foamy cells; inflammatory cells; foreign body granulomas; cholesterol clefts	Common in type III, seen in other hyperlipidemias
Tendinous xanthoma	Hand, foot, and Achilles tendons	Foamy cells in the subcutaneous tissue and underlying fascia, tendons	Type III hyperlipidemia and others
Xanthelasma **(Figure 5.35A)**	Periorbital skin	Dermal foamy cells in eyelid skin (the presence of thin epidermis, vellus follicles, and skeletal muscle at the base is a clue to location)	About 50% of patients have hyperlipidemia
Verruciform xanthoma **(Figure 5.35B)**	Oral > genital > other locations	Rounded "premature" parakeratosis and foamy cells in dermal papillae	Usually no hyperlipidemia
Eruptive xanthoma **(Figure 5.35C)**	Buttocks and proximal extremities	Foamy cells, extracellular pools of lipid and inflammatory cells, including neutrophils	Elevated chylomicrons

Table 5.4 Summary of the features distinguishing NXG, necrobiosis lipoidica, and xanthogranuloma

	Necrobiosis lipoidica	Xanthogranuloma	NXG
Necrosis	Necrobiosis of collagen	No	Necrosis
Sclerosis	Prominent	No	No
Infiltrate pattern	Palisading, in tiers	Nodular	Nodular or diffuse dense
Cells	Histiocytes	Histiocytes Touton giant cells	Foamy histiocytes Touton giant cells Foreign body giant cells
Other features	Lymphoid follicles Plasma cells	Eosinophils	Lymphoid follicles Plasma cells Neutrophilic debris Cholesterol clefts

- Cholesterol clefts are surrounded by palisading foamy cells
- Neutrophilic debris
- Plasma cells and lymphoid follicles may be present

(Table 5.4)

Langerhans cell histiocytosis (LCH)

The Langerhans cell is an antigen-presenting cell, processing antigens and presenting them to other cells of the immune system (see Chapter 1).

There exists some debate as to whether to classify Langerhans cell histiocytoses (LCH) as a malignancy. Recent discovery of V600E mutations in the BRAF gene support a neoplastic process. In any event, collections of Langerhans cells can range from solitary skin lesions to extensive multisystem involvement and potentially lethal disease.

> NB All forms of LCH contain infiltrates of Langerhans cells in the dermis.

There are two types of infiltrate: 1) lichenoid (a band-like infiltrate in the dermis, associated with epidermal acanthosis) **(Figure 5.37A)**, and 2) nodular (infiltrates of Langerhans cells and eosinophils in reticular dermis)

- Numerous round to epithelioid cells with kidney-shaped nuclei with longitudinal grooving (resembles a coffee bean)
- The cytoplasm is gray–blue and somewhat granular
- Eosinophils are common
- Histiocytes are common in older, more developed lesions

> NB Epidermotropism is common – it can simulate Pautrier's microabscesses.

Immunohistochemistry is helpful: Langerin (CD207 identifies transmembrane protein associated with the Birbeck granules)), CD1a, S100 (+) **(Figure 5.37B)**

VASCULAR TUMORS

These tumors are primary composed of vascular endothelial cells (see Chapter 1).

It is useful to describe vascular tumors in terms of their benign, intermediate (tufted angioma, Kaposi's sarcoma, kaposiform hemangioendothelioma, retiform angioendothelioma and papillary intralymphatic angioendothelioma), and malignant potential (angiosarcoma).

Several patterns can be detected:

- Thin slit-like (collapsed) and cystically dilated (cavernous) vascular channels (cavernous pattern) **(Photomnemonic 5.8)**
- Cellular proliferation of spindled cells (in spindle-cell hemangioma or Kaposi's sarcoma)
- Cellular epithelioid proliferation (of vascular endothelial cells in angiolymphoid hyperplasia with eosinophilia or epithelioid angiosarcoma)
- Thrombosed lumina (arteriovenous hemangioma, deep venous hemangioma) **(Figure 5.38)**
- "Hobnail" cells (prominent endothelial cells that protrude into the lumina (targetoid hemosiderotic hemangioma, angiolymphoid hyperplasia with eosinophilia)

Angiokeratoma

- Thin-walled dilated capillaries with red blood cells in the papillary dermis (cavernous channels)
- The vessels are "enveloped" by the epidermis **(Figure 5.39)**
- The epidermis shows hyperkeratosis

Types of angiokeratoma:

- *Solitary angiokeratoma*: Sporadic lesion, occasionally with thrombi and can be confused with melanocytic lesion
- *Angiokeratoma circumscriptum*: Congenital cluster of angiokeratomas, usually on extremity
- *Angiokeratoma of Fordyce*: Vulvar or scrotal angiokeratomas
- *Angiokeratoma corporis diffusum*: Diffuse angiokeratomas seen in Fabry's disease

NB Superficial thin lymphatic vessels enveloped by the epidermis similarly to angiokeratoma but containing pink proteinaceous material (instead of red blood cells) are best characterized as a superficial *lymphangioma* or *lymphangioma circumscriptum* **(Figure 5.40)**.

NB Angiokeratoma-like surface with a deep lobular proliferation of small vessels characterizes verrucous hemangioma which is a combined vascular malformation of capillaries, lymphatics, and veins **(Figure 5.41)**.

Cherry angioma

- Epidermal collarette
- Atrophy of the epidermis
- Proliferation of interconnecting vascular channels (venous capillaries and postcapillary venules) in the upper dermis (the name comes from the clinical "cherry"-like appearance) **(Figure 5.42)**

Arteriovenous hemangioma

- Proliferation of both arteries and veins
- Thrombosed lumina are common

Venous lake

- A common location is the lip
- By definition this is a solitary dilated vessel and not a collection of multiple vessels

Glomus tumor and glomulovenous malformation (glomangioma)

These proliferations are derived from the perivascular glomus cells in the dermis.

The more cellular proliferations are termed glomus tumors (cells > vessels), while mostly vascular proliferations (vessels > cells) are termed glomangiomas.

NB Glomus tumors may arise within blood vessels and nerves.

The malignant counterpart is glomangiosarcoma (40% risk of metastasis)

- Varying proportions of glomus cells organized in sheets (abundant eosinophilic cytoplasm and uniform punched out nuclei) **(Figure 5.43A)**
- Small blood vessels with several layers of glomus cells (in glomus tumors) or numerous dilated with angulated shape vessels surrounded by fewer layers of glomus cells (in glomangioma) **(Figure 5.43B)**
- The stroma can be myxoid

Immunohistochemistry for smooth muscle cells: SMA, H-caldesmon(+)

Differential diagnosis: It may resemble eccrine spiradenoma on lower power (look for ductal differentiation and several populations of cells) and intradermal nevus with pseudovascular spaces (look for pigment and melanocytes with intranuclear inclusions).

Lobular capillary hemangioma (pyogenic granuloma)

- Commonly an ulcerated surface with an epidermal collarette

NB Note the *lobular silhouette* resembling the architecture of the human placenta.

- The lobules contain capillaries lined by bland endothelial cells, and granulation tissue and are separated by fibrous septa **(Figure 5.44)**
- The capillaries are larger and tightly packed in the upper lobules
- In the lower lobules the capillaries are small, indistinct, and less tightly packed
- A feeding vessel can be seen in the vicinity

Variants: Intravenous, subcutaneous

NB A "dirty"-looking pyogenic granuloma with neutrophils, nuclear dust, and bacteria clusters: think bacillary angiomatosis (infectious proliferation almost exclusively in immunosuppressed individuals caused by *Bartonella quintana* and *Bartonella henselae*).

Spindle-cell hemangioma (formerly known as spindle-cell hemangioendothelioma)

Vascular proliferation on the extremities in young people

- Large dilated thrombosed vessels next to collections of closely packed spindled cells with slit-like spaces
- Intracytoplasmic vacuoles (miniature lumina)
- Papillae of endothelial cells may form intravascular structures, "Roman bridges", in small vessels apart from the tumor bulk

Infantile hemangioma

A benign vascular proliferation either congenital or developing during infancy which resolves spontaneously in the majority of cases

- Multiple lobules separated by fibrous tissue (lobular architecture similar to the human placenta)
- Prominent (plump) endothelial cells but no atypia
- Frequent mitoses
- A feeding vessel may be observed in the vicinity

NB Differential diagnosis: Rapidly involuting congenital hemangioma (RICH) and non-involuting congenital hemangioma (NICH) are present fully formed at birth. Histologically, RICH and NICH are similar to infantile hemangioma but lack the mitotic figures. In immunohistochemistry, infantile hemangioma is positive for GLUT1, while RICH and NICH are negative.

Microvenular hemangioma

- Thin, collapsed slit-like venules
- Collagenous stroma

NB The collapsed vessels can involve the arrector pili muscle **(Figure 5.45)**.

Angiolymphoid hyperplasia with eosinophilia (epithelioid hemangioma)

Superficial proliferation classically around the ear but also reported on other sites

- *Lobular architecture* **(Figure 5.46A)**
- Small to medium-sized thin-walled blood vessels
- Hobnail endothelial cells with intracytoplasmic vacuoles (this phenomenon represents an attempt for endothelial formation) **(Figure 5.46B)**
- *Nodular lymphoid aggregates* commonly including eosinophils

Tufted angioma

Slowly progressive red to violaceous plaque typically affecting children

- Closely set convolutes of poorly canalized capillaries in the dermis surrounded by pericytes (ovoid angiomatoid lobules resembling "cannon balls") **(Figure 5.47A)**
- Enlarged endothelial cells **(Figure 5.47B)**
- Mitotic figures common
- Lymphatic channels may be found at the periphery of the lobules as semi-lunar clefts; these are D2-40(+) **(Figure 5.47C)**

Kaposi's sarcoma

Clinical types:

- Mediterranean elderly males (classic)
- HIV-related (epidemic)
- African (endemic)
- Immunosuppression-related (from 1 month up to 10 years after organ transplantation)

NB Minimal cytologic atypia; severe atypia should make one consider angiosarcoma.

1. **Patch stage:**
   - Jagged outlined vessels dissect the collagen bundles
   - Tiny clefts along the adnexal structures (which can be mistaken for microvenular hemangioma)
   - Patchy infiltrates of lymphocytes and plasma cells in early lesions
2. **Plaque stage:**
   - Slit-like vascular spaces with hemorrhage; hemosiderin common **(Figure 5.48A)**
   - PAS(+) cytoplasmic hyaline bodies (partially digested erythrocytes)
   - Spindled cells
3. **Tumor stage:**
   - Dense nodular proliferation of spindled cells **(Figure 5.48B)**
   - Small vascular clefts between the tumors fascicles
   - Newly formed vascular structures protruding into existing ectatic vascular space (promontory sign) **(Figure 5.48C)**

Differential diagnosis: Hemosiderotic DF (no real vascular spaces but cystic clefts with hemorrhage defined to them); angiosarcoma (nuclear pleomorphism, mitoses)

NB **Immunohistochemistry:** HHV8 **(Figure 5.48D)**.

Intermediate malignant vascular tumors

(Table 5.5)

Table 5.5 Intermediate malignant vascular tumors

	Kaposiform hemangioendothelioma	Retiform hemangioendothelioma	Papillary intralymphatic angioendothelioma (Dabska tumor)
Affected population	Children	Young adults	Children
Prognosis	Progressive congenital or acquired proliferation with rare metastases	Rare metastases but common recurrence primarily of young adults	Favorable prognosis; however, can be locally invasive and have the potential to metastasize
Pathologic features	"Cannon balls" (sometimes glomeruloid) of blood vessels in the dermis Numerous fibrin thrombi	"Rete testis-like" proliferation of: • Branching blood vessels with hobnail endothelial cells • Lymphocytes both within lumina and in the dermis • Less cavernous compared to Dabska tumor **(Figure 5.49)**	Cavernous spaces with surrounding prominent inflammation Lined by hobnail or columnar endothelium Papillary projections with fibrous avascular cores

Angiosarcoma

Clinical types:

1. Head and neck violaceous plaque on sun damaged skin
2. Post radiation (typically 10+ years)
3. Chronic lymphedema (e.g. Stewart-Treves syndrome after mastectomy and lymphadenectomy)

NB Often severely atypical endothelial cells; numerous mitotic figures and atypical mitotic figures are common.

- Prominent dilated vessels in the upper dermis
- Look for jagged, angulated vascular spaces (sometimes only at the margins of the specimens)
- The atypical cells have hyperchromatic nuclei and protrude and pile in the lumina (multilayering)
- A promontory sign can be found also in angiosarcoma
- In the deep part of the specimen: cohesive sheets of spindled or epithelioid cells **(Figure 5.50)**

Immunohistochemistry:

- Poorly differentiated angiosarcoma may require immunohistochemistry to aid the diagnosis
- CD34 and CD31 are helpful vascular markers (CD31 can also highlight histiocytes and CD34 can highlight numerous fibrohistiocytic cells, and these properties can be a pitfall)
- ERG, a nuclear marker, is a sensitive and specific vascular marker; ERG will stain some genitourinary cancers, but this is rarely in the differential diagnosis when evaluating possible angiosarcoma
- FLI-1 is a nuclear transcription factor (the first nuclear stain for endothelial cells) which is positive in all differentiated vascular neoplasms

SMOOTH MUSCLE TUMORS

The smooth muscle in the skin gives rise to the smooth muscle tumors: the arrector pili muscle of the hair follicles (piloleiomyoma), the walls of the blood vessels (angioleiomyoma), the dartos muscle (genital leiomyoma).

For an overview of the smooth muscle cells and their immunohistochemical profile, see Chapter 2.

Piloleiomyoma

Often present clinically as multiple red-brown papules

NB Multiple cutaneous and uterine lesions should entertain the possibility of Reed syndrome (a defect in fumarate hydratase that predisposes to renal cell carcinoma).

- The tumor is not encapsulated and is located in the reticular dermis
- Short intersecting fascicles among variable amount of collagen **(Figure 5.51)**
- Cigar-shaped vesicular nuclei with highly eosinophilic cytoplasm

Differential diagnosis: A cellular scar – both can stain for SMA(+); but desmin(-) in a scar

Angioleiomyoma

Often painful lesions on lower extremities although reported in many sites

- Well-circumscribed, very compact eosinophilic tumor with a fibrous capsule (a pink ball in the lower dermis and subdermis) **(Figure 5.52A)**
- Spindle cells with cigar-shaped vesicular nuclei arranged in tight interlacing fascicles **(Figure 5.52B)**
- Three pathologic types exist based on the type of vessels involved:
  - Solid type (slit-like channels)
  - Cavernous (dilated vascular channels but without distinct walls)
  - Venous (thick walls)

Atypical intradermal smooth muscle neoplasm (formerly cutaneous leiomyosarcoma)

It derives either from the arrector pili muscle (dermal location; good prognosis) or from the vessel walls (subdermal location; very aggressive and may metastasize)

- Increased atypia and nuclear hyperchromasia (compare to banal piloleiomyoma) **(Figure 5.53)**
- Big, bizarre, giant smooth muscle cells
- Numerous mitotic figures and/or atypical mitotic figures can occur (more than 2 mitotic figures/10 high power fields)

Immunohistochemistry: SMA+, desmin (+in 75%), cytokeratin (+ in 30%)

TUMORS OF FAT

Benign tumors of fat range from run-of-the-mill fat collections (simply called lipomas) to the more vascular angiolipoma. Malignant tumors of fat are called liposarcomas and range from atypical lipomatous tumor (also called well-differentiated liposarcoma) to pleomorphic liposarcoma, dedifferentiated liposarcoma, and myxoid liposarcoma.

For an overview of adipose tissue, see Chapter 1.

Lipoma

Common lesion in wide range of skin sites

- Banal mature adipose tissue without atypia
- Small, thin vasculature

Table 5.6 Summary of the most common types of liposarcoma

	Well-differentiated liposarcoma	Pleomorphic liposarcoma	Myxoid/round cell liposarcoma
General notes	Also called atypical lipomatous tumor Most commonly retroperitoneal; extremely rare in the skin MDM2 is amplified in addition to other markers such as CDK4 in FISH studies	Multiple genetic abnormalities but CDK4 and MDM2 are not reliably amplified Although rare, most common cutaneous site is the extremities	Most common in the deep soft tissue of the thigh More common in people under age 30 Fusion gene of FUS with DDIT3 common
Pathologic features	Often banal in appearance with only focal atypia Suspicion must be high in lesions from the spermatic cord or retroperitoneum	Bizarre nuclear features common Rare lipoblasts often present	Myxoid cells and background Sometimes round cells prominent Delicate network of branching blood vessels referred to as "chicken-wire" vasculature Severe atypia and mitotic figures typically absent

- Mast cells
- A variant of simple lipoma is the mobile encapsulated lipoma **(Figure 5.54)**

Angiolipoma

Often tender on extremities or trunk

- Encapsulated mature fat with more than about 20–25% of the lesion composed of mature-looking blood vessels
- Blood vessels commonly contain fibrin thrombi **(Figure 5.55)**
- Possible mucin in the stroma (myxoid stroma)

NB A cellular variant may be confounded with Kaposi's sarcoma or other vascular malignancies; however, while fibrin thrombi are present in angiolipoma, they are rare in vascular malignancies.

Spindle-cell/pleomorphic lipoma

Most common in men on the neck and upper chest

- Most specimens have mixed mature adipocytes and spindle cells **(Figure 5.56)**
- Rope-like collagen bundles are present
- Myxoid background common
- Some cases consist almost entirely of spindle cells

Liposarcoma

(Table 5.6)

TUMORS OF BONE

Osteoma cutis

Commonly occurs in sites of prior trauma such as acne scars or previous skin cancer surgeries

- Bone formation within the dermis **(Figure 5.57)**
- Osteocytes in the lacunae are essential for diagnosis

Primary cutaneous osteosarcoma

Exceedingly rare; limited to case reports

- Osteoid formation with a wide variety of phenotypes of the non-osteoid tumor cells
- Sometimes resembles undifferentiated pleomorphic sarcoma or has chondroid or giant-cell rich areas

MELANOCYTIC TUMORS

Definition: Benign or malignant, usually pigmented proliferations composed of melanocytes, nevus cells, or melanoma cells.

For melanocytic lesions of the nail unit, see Chapter 4, Hair and nail disorders.

General concepts

- **Melanocytes** are *solitary* round small cells with *dendrites* in the *basal layer*. They have regular oval nuclei and scant cytoplasm. (See Chapter 1 for morphology of melanocytes and immunohistochemical stains for melanocytic lesions.)

- **Nevus cells** are *round* with regular oval nuclei or *spindled-shaped*; they *group in clusters* and rarely show mitoses.
  - Type **A** (**A like an apple**) are epithelioid cells (round to cuboidal): larger pale nucleus and more cytoplasm; present in the junctional zone and upper dermis and form nests **(Figure 5.58A)**
  - Type **B** (**B like blue**) small blue cells like lymphocytes due to dark nuclei and scant cytoplasm; present in the mid dermis and aggregate in cords **(Figure 5.58B)**
  - Type **C** (**C like a clove**) are elongated with spindled nuclei resembling fibroblasts; they may form neural-like structures; present in the lower dermis **(Figure 5.58C)**
- **Melanoma cells** are *rounded or spindled* with irregular *large hyperchromatic nuclei (larger than the nuclei of keratinocyte)* and red nucleoli, organized in *clusters or sheets*; mitoses are common

- NB Large pale melanocytes with dusty, fine granular cytoplasm are a clue to 1) nevus of special sites (including scalp nevi), 2) atypical nevus, or 3) melanoma.

- **Nests:** Clusters of three or more nevus/melanoma cells; (cords are linearly arranged cells)
- **Maturation:** Decrease in size of nests, nuclei, and pigment with progressive descent in the dermis

NB Most nevi mature except for blue nevi.

- **Symmetry:** If an imaginary central line divides the lesion into two, those two halves should look similar in shape, thickness and number and position of nests and cells
- **Circumscription:** The lateral epidermal shoulder of the lesion ends with a well-defined nest
- **Pagetoid spread:** Presence of melanocytes in the suprabasal layers

On low power

- **Benign lesions** are usually well-circumscribed, monotonous throughout, and symmetric, with features of maturation and absent cytologic atypia.
- **Malignant lesions** are poorly circumscribed, large, and asymmetric, with absent maturation and with features of cytologic atypia.
- Distinction by the silhouette of the base:
  1. *Flat:* dysplastic nevus, halo nevus
  2. *Wedge-shaped:* Spitz nevus, deep penetrating nevus
  3. *Uneven:* congenital nevus
  4. *Convex:* cellular blue nevus
  5. *Jagged:* melanoma

On high power

Lentigo simplex (simple lentigo)

- Elongated hyperpigmented rete ridges **(Figure 5.59, Photomnemonic 5.9)**
- Increased number of single normal-looking melanocytes at the tips of the rete ridges
- Pigment through the epidermis and in the stratum corneum
- Melanophages may be found in the upper dermis

NB The following syndromes include multiple lentigines:
- Carney complex: epithelioid blue nevi, lentiginoses, myxomas of the heart and skin, endocrine tumors, psammomatous schwannoma
- NAME: lentigines, atrial myxomas, blue nevi
- LAMB: lentigines, atrial myxomas, myxoid neurofibromas, blue nevi
- LEOPARD: lentigines, ECG conduction abnormalities, ocular hypertelorism, pulmonary stenosis, abnormal genitalia, retarded growth, and deafness
- Peutz–Jeghers: perioral lentiginoses, benign colon polyps
- Laugier–Hunziker syndrome: labial and oral lentigines, longitudinal nail pigmentation

Melanotic macule (labial, genital, and volar)

- Fewer elongated and more plump rete ridges with pigmented basal layer **(Figure 5.60, Photomnemonic 5.10)**
- Increased number of melanocytes in the basal layer
- Melanophages in the upper dermis

Lentiginous junctional nevus

- Elongated rete ridges with increased number of melanocytes
- Small nests at the dermoepidermal junction **(Figure 5.61)**

Compound nevus (junctional + dermal component)

- Elongated rete ridges with increased number of melanocytes
- Small nests and cords at the dermoepidermal junction and in the papillary dermis
- The cells in the upper dermis are larger and contain more melanin than the deeper ones **(Figure 5.62A)**

Compound nevus of special sites

NB Special sites include breast, scalp, auricular region, umbilicus, genital, flexural, and acral sites.

NB Nevi of special sites mimic dysplastic nevi and even melanoma due to asymmetry, large confluent nests, and focal intraepidermal ascent of nevus cells.

- *Architecture:*
  - Poor circumscription
  - The nests vary in size, shape, and position
  - The nests may be quite big and show confluence at the dermoepidermal junction **(Figure 5.62B)**
- *Cytology:*
  - Nevus cells may be large, with abundant cytoplasm which contains fine dusty melanin **(Figure 5.62C)**
  - Prominent eosinophilic nucleoli
  - The cells may be dyscohesive

Acral nevus

NB On dermoscopy the pigment is in the furrows (sulcus superficialis) between the dermatoglyphic ridges (crista superficialis), whereas in melanoma it is in the ridges.

- Similar pathologic features to nevi of special sites
- The nests are located around the crista limitans (which is the junctional projection of sulcus superficialis)
- Additional features include: columns of upward spread of melanocytes throughout the epidermis including the stratum corneum **(Figure 5.63)**

Intradermal nevus

- Nevus cells are confined to the dermis, arranged in nests and cords **(Figure 5.64A)**
- Clefts and spaces among nests and cords (from processing) which simulate lymphatic vessels
- The nevus cells show intranuclear pseudoinclusions: the cytoplasm extends in the nuclei **(Figure 5.64B)**
- Multinucleate nevus cells

Ancient nevus (on the face in older people):

- Over time, intradermal nevi, just like some people, may "become fat and neurotic" by developing degenerative changes: fat tissue in the nevus, thrombi, neurotization (nerve fibers or Meissner's corpuscle-like structures, see Figure 5.58C) **(Figure 5.64C)**

Balloon cell nevus

- Mature nevus cells are admixed with large pale cells with central small nucleus and vacuolated cytoplasm

NB For comparison: adipocytes have flat nuclei at the periphery **(Figure 5.64D)**.

- The cells are pale because melanin is absent due to melanosome degeneration

Congenital nevus (CN)

- CN has a silhouette of a papillomatous surface and a wedge-shaped bottom (mammillated brown papule clinically)
- The surface may simulate seborrheic keratosis **(Figure 5.65A)**
- The dermal papillae are filled with small melanocytes arranged in bands
- In the compound type: nests are present at the dermoepidermal junction and in the upper dermis
- The melanocytes are arranged in single file among collagen bundles (splaying of melanocytes) and extend along the adnexal structures (follicles, sweat glands), nerves, and vessels **(Figure 5.65B)**
- Maturation

NB Giant congenital nevi and nevi after birth can show pagetoid melanocytes.

NB A proliferative nodule: an intratumoral cellular aggregation of large epithelioid cells with prominent nucleoli that merges with the bland nevus cells in the upper dermis.

Deep penetrating nevus

- Pyramidal shape ("an upside down pyramid") **(Figure 5.66)**
- Nests of nevus cells at the dermoepidermal junction
- Loosely arranged/or in fascicles epithelioid or spindled nevus cells extend deep around blood vessels, nerves, and the cutaneous adnexa
- Pigmented melanocytes
- Maturation

Halo nevus

- A compound nevus whose dermal component disappears due to CD8+lymphocyte- mediated apoptosis
- A symmetric lesion with a flat base of brisk lymphocytic infiltrate **(Figure 5.67)**
- The nevus cells are uniform from side to side and mature with depth
- Possible melanophages, giant cells, and mast cells

Recurrent nevus

A recurrent nevus has three zones from the bottom to the top:

1. Residual dermal nevus cells or scattered nests
2. A zone of dermal fibrosis (some nests can be entrapped in the fibrosis)
3. Solitary melanocytes, single pagetoid cells, and small nests at the dermoepidermal junction restricted to the area of the scar

(Figure 5.68)

Differential diagnosis: In recurrent melanoma the epidermal melanocytic proliferation is typically at the margin of the scar and extends beyond its lateral borders.

Blue nevus

Common blue nevus

- Pigmented spindled and slender dendritic (bipolar) nevus cells among thickened collagen bundles in upper/mid dermis **(Figure 5.69A)**
- Dendritic nevus cells have fine granular cytoplasm versus melanophages which have coarse chunks of melanin
- Melanophages

> NB If melanophages predominate, the lesion may mimic a tattoo: look for dendritic cells.
>
> If sclerosis predominates, the lesion may mimic a dermatofibroma: HMB-45 stains strongly throughout the entire lesion in blue nevi.

Cellular blue nevus

- Bulky, heavily pigmented tumor occupying the reticular dermis with a convex silhouette at the bottom **(Figure 5.69B)**
- The tumor extends along the adnexal structures and nerves and ends up bulging into the fat with a bulbous bottom **(Photomnemonic 5.11)**
- The tumor is multilobular and highly cellular:
  - Pigmented spindled cells lie back-to-back more at the periphery **(Figure 5.69C)**
  - Cuboidal cells with pale cytoplasm (epithelioid cells) lie in nests, sheets, and fascicles **(Figure 5.69D)**
- Many melanophages among sclerotic collagen bundles
- Entrapped collagen balls at the periphery (like in dermatofibroma)

> NB Deeply pigmented epithelioid cellular blue nevi are part of Carney complex.

> NB Deeply pigmented blue nevi may be difficult to distinguish from animal-type melanoma (look for mitoses, atypia, and necrosis).

Spitz nevus

A small, symmetric mostly compound nevus made of large epithelioid and spindle cells

- **Epidermal component** (usually does not go beyond the dermal part):
  - The epidermis is "hyper": hyperkeratosis, hypergranulosis, and hyperplastic pointed rete ridges

  > NB Compare to consumption of the epidermis in melanoma **(Figure 5.70A)**.

  - Ovoid large nests, vertically oriented at the dermoepidermal junction; the nests are surrounded by artifactual clefts
  - The nevus cells are large ovoid or spindled and may have prominent nucleoli **(Figure 5.70B, C)**
  - Bizarre giant nevus cells are possible
  - Pagetoid melanocytes in the lower half of the epidermis are common in young children (but consider melanoma in adults!)
  - Kamino bodies: extracellular pink globules at the dermoepidermal junction (contain basement membrane proteins)

  > NB Kamino bodies, together with good symmetry, and uniformity of the nests and sheets help to distinguish from melanoma.

- **Dermal component:**
  - Maturation
  - Up to two mitoses in the entire lesion and no mitoses in depth
  - "Outlier cells" at the bottom of the lesion: single epithelioid nevus cells in the reticular dermis **(Figure 5.70D)**

  > NB Compare to the solid fascicles and invasive tongues in melanoma.

Pigmented spindle cell nevus of Reed

Similar to Spitz nevus with the following differences:

- Only spindled, pigmented melanocytes are organized in *vertical nests* at the dermoepidermal junction **(Figure 5.70E)**
- Confluence of the nests
- Pigmented ortho- and parakeratosis
- A band of melanophages in the papillary dermis

Atypical (dysplastic, Clark's) nevus (AN)

A compound nevus with *architectural* and *cytologic* atypia of three grades (mild, moderate, and severe)

- Lentiginous hyperplasia extending beyond the dermal component (shoulder phenomenon)
- Single melanocytes and nests along the basal layer, mostly arranged at the tips and the sides of the rete ridges **(Figure 5.71A)**
- The nests may show confluence and bridging
- The cells show random (but not uniform!) atypia and can be: 1) large epithelioid with dusty cytoplasm, hyperchromatic nuclei, and prominent nucleoli, or 2) slender due to shrinkage artifact **(Figure 5.71B)**
- Stromal response: lamellar and concentric fibroplasia around the rete ridges

(Table 5.7)

MALIGNANT MELANOMA (MM)

General concepts

See also Table 5.7

Architectural features favoring melanoma

- Broad lesion
- Asymmetry

Table 5.7 Distinguishing atypical nevus from melanoma requires a complex analysis

	Atypical nevus	Melanoma
Architecture		
Breadth	Usually less than 6 mm	Usually more than 6 mm (ranges from 1 mm to many cm)
Symmetry	Overall symmetric	Asymmetric
Circumscription	Lentiginous component goes beyond the dermal but finishes with a nest	Poor circumscription: usually single cells at the periphery
Single cells vs nests	Nests predominate	Single cells and confluence of single cells predominate
Involvement of suprapapillary plates	Absent	Present
Pagetoid scatter in the epidermis	"Pseudopagetoid scatter": only a focal scatter of individual cells	Present
Configuration of the epidermis	Regular lentiginous hyperplasia	Irregular hyperplasia with epidermal consumption
Host response	Absent/patchy lymphocytic infiltrate	Brisk band-like infiltrate
Diffuse fibrosis	Absent/present	Present
Regression	Absent	Present often
Cytologic features		
Atypia	Random	Uniform
Nuclear size	Increased but focally	Increased, uniform
Nuclear hyperchromatism	Present but focally	Present, uniform
Maturation	May be absent	Absent
Dermal mitoses	Absent	Present (absent in melanoma in istu)

- Poor circumscription
- Predominance of single cells over nests
- Confluence of melanocytes (they are so close to each other that keratinocytes "seem to disappear" among them)
- Uneven epidermal contour (consumption of the epidermis)
- Scatter of melanocytes above the basal layer

NB Trauma can cause scatter of melanocytes but usually focal and limited to a few cells; acral nevi show suprabasal scatter.

Cytologic features favoring melanoma

NB There is no specific cell morphology to define MM.

- *Small melanocytes with angulated/stellate nuclei* in lentigo maligna
- *Large round/oval or epithelioid melanocytes with pale or "dusty" cytoplasm* due to brown fine granular pigment (including pagetoid cells in the epidermis)

NB Scalp nevi in children may show such cells.

- *Spindled melanocytes* (the nuclei in melanoma are more hyperchromatic compared to dysplastic nevi and Spitz nevi and are arranged haphazardly)
- *Dendritic melanocytes* in lentigo maligna, acral lentiginous melanoma, subungual melanoma

NB Suprabasal scatter of dendritic melanocytes with different length of their dendrites is a clue to MM.

Immunohistochemistry

See Chapter 1

Prognostic factors in melanoma

- **Breslow's thickness:** Measures the tumor thickness on 10× magnification from stratum granulosum to the deepest invasive tumor cell
  - Thin melanomas are defined by Breslow <1 mm
  - Melanomas with Breslow ≥1 mm usually require sentinel lymph node biopsy
- **Clark's level:** Measures the level of invasion
  - Clark I: melanoma in situ
  - Clark II: tumor in the papillary dermis
  - Clark III: tumor fills and expands the papillary dermis
  - Clark IV: tumor infiltrates the reticular dermis
  - Clark V: invasion in the fat
- **Ulceration:** Important sub-stratifying factor: switches from "a" to "b" for tumor stages T1, 2, and 3 (see TNM classification; www.uicc.org)

NB When ulceration is present, Breslow is measured from the bottom of the ulceration.

- **Mitoses:** Most important prognostic factor in thin melanomas where 1 mitosis/mm² changes staging from T1a to T1b
- **Regression:** A fibrous stroma replaces the dermal portion at the center of the tumor and is associated with lymphocytic infiltrate, dilated vessels, and melanophages **(Figure 5.72)**
  - **Tumoral melanosis** defines absence of melanoma cells but dense collections of melanophages
- **Brisk lymphocytic infiltrate:** Lymphocytes infiltrate among tumor cells
- **Microscopic satellites:** Any bigger than 0.05 mm nest of metastatic tumor cells discontinuous from the primary tumor (but not separated only by fibrosis or inflammation)
- **Lymphovascular invasion:** Melanoma cells within the lumen of blood vessels or lymphatics or both **(Figure 5.73)**

On low power

- **Non-tumorogenic radial growth phase melanoma**
  - Restricted to the epidermis: melanoma in situ, lentigo maligna
  - Microinvasive: superficial spreading melanoma (a few cells in the papillary dermis without capacity to survive, proliferate, and form tumor masses)
- **Tumorogenic vertical growth phase melanoma**
  - At least one cluster (nest) of cells in the dermis is larger than the largest junctional nest and/or there is a mitosis in the dermis
  - The dermal component has capacity for survival and proliferation with expansive growth
  - It can develop in any type of non-tumorogenic melanoma or arise de novo as in nodular melanoma

On high power

Melanoma in situ and lentigo maligna

NB Lentigo maligna is melanoma in situ on sun-damaged skin. Lentigo maligna melanoma is vertical growth developing in lentigo maligna.

- Lentiginous and focally nested proliferation of atypical melanocytes along the dermoepidermal junction and extending along the hair follicles (down to the level of the sebaceous gland) **(Figure 5.74)**
- *Contiguous* junctional proliferation of atypical melanocytes with ovoid, stellate, spindled nuclei appearing as flattened ("pressed against the cell wall"); may have dendrites
- *Atrophic epidermis*
- Suprabasal (pagetoid) spread of melanocytes
- Regression and lymphocytic infiltrate may be found
- Solar elastosis in lentigo maligna

Superficial spreading melanoma

1. **Radial growth phase:**
   - *Lentiginous* and nested proliferation of atypical melanocytes along the dermoepidermal junction with pagetoid spread **(Figure 5.75A)**
   - *Uniform* cytologic atypia (large cells with abundant dusty cytoplasm)
   - Nests can be of different size and coalesce
   - Dermal melanophages and brisk lymphocytes
   - Regression can be found
2. **Vertical growth phase** includes the superficial portion with the following additional dermal components:
   - Nests and sheets of atypical melanocytes **(Figure 5.75B)**
   - No maturation
   - Mitoses
   - Pushing border

Nodular melanoma

- A dome-shaped or polypoid tumor

NB The tumor may be symmetric.

- The overlying epidermis is usually thinned
- There may be in situ component but it does not extend three rete ridges beyond the dermal component on either side
- Cohesive nodule of nests in the dermis, without maturation and with pushing border **(Figure 5.76A)**
- The cells are: 1) epithelioid with large pleomorphic nuclei and dusty cytoplasm, or 2) spindled cells **(Figure 5.76B)**
- Mitoses

Acral lentiginous melanoma (ALM)

- Poor lateral circumscription
- Irregular elongated rete ridges

- Buckshot scatter of pagetoid melanocytes in the epidermis (rather than in columns) **(Figure 5.77A)**
- Atypical junctional melanocytes: hyperchromatic nuclei, prominent nucleoli, and dendritic processes

- NB The junctional melanocytes, the junctional nests, and the keratinocytes are dyscohesive and form cavities (lacunae); junctional cavitation is a clue to ALM **(Figure 5.77B, C)**

- In the vertical growth phase: sheets of atypical cells; often the cells are of spindled morphology and are entrapped in a fibrotic stroma (desmoplastic reaction)

Subungual melanoma

See Chapter 4, Hair and nail disorders

Nevoid melanoma

NB On low power nevoid melanoma simulates a banal nevus due to its verrucous/nodular architecture with symmetric outlines and sharp circumscription **(Figure 5.78A)**.

On high power:
- Variable junctional component
- Sheets of type-A nevus cells with mild nuclear pleomorphism in the dermis **(Figure 5.78B)**

- NB Mitoses are usually multiple and are a clue to the diagnosis

- No maturation

Desmoplastic melanoma

- Overlying melanoma in situ component
- Spindled non-pigmented melanocytes in haphazard fascicles dissect the dermis
- Patchy lymphoid cells (germinal center-like aggregation)
- Common neurotropism (malignant spindled cells wrap up nerve fibers; do not mistake with the benign phenomenon of "neurotization" in dermal nevi)

NB S100 must be performed to distinguish desmoplastic melanoma from fibrohistiocytic neoplasms; MART-1 is usually negative.

ADNEXAL TUMORS

Definition: Adnexal tumors are generally divided into follicular, eccrine/apocrine and sebaceous neoplasms based on their differentiation. They originate from pluripotent stem cells (in the epidermis and the appendageal structures) which undergo neoplastic transformation and therefore may result in more than one lineage of appendageal differentiation.

General concepts

Epithelioma: A benign epithelial tumor

Carcinoma: A malignant epithelial tumor

Adenoma: A benign tumor formed from glandular structures in epithelial tissues

Cystadenoma: A cystic adenoma

Adenocarcinoma: A malignant tumor from epithelial tissue that has glandular origin or glandular characteristics

Hamartoma: A tumor-like malformation arising from the abnormal mixture of normally present for this location tissue components

Nevus: A type of hamartoma with excessive tissue from epidermal, mesenchymal, adnexal, nervous, or vascular elements

SWEAT GLAND (ECCRINE AND APOCRINE) NEOPLASMS

General concepts

The anatomy of the sweat glands and the useful immunohistochemical markers are described in Chapter 1.

The most common sweat gland neoplasms are classified according to three features:

1. The segment of the gland from which the tumor arises (differentiation towards secretory portion, dermal duct, acrosyringium), *and*
2. The type of gland (eccrine or apocrine), *and*
3. Benign vs malignant

(Table 5.8)

On low power

Helpful photomnemonics for some glandular neoplasms can be found in their descriptions below.

Other clues:
- "Seborrheic keratosis" with vascular cores: think poroma

Table 5.8 Classification of the most common sweat gland neoplasms

	Eccrine differentiation	Apocrine differentiation
Acrosyringium (acro-end, syringium tube, pore)	Syringoma	–
	Eccrine syringofibroadenoma	(The apocrine glands open in the pilosebaceous units)
	Poroma	–
	Porocarcinoma	–
Dermal duct (upper straight and lower spiral part)	Dermal duct tumor (poroma)	–
	Spiradenoma	Cylindroma
	Nodular hidradenoma	–
	Chondroid syringoma (mixed tumor)	Chondroid syringoma (mixed tumor)
	Eccrine hidrocystoma	Apocrine hidrocystoma
Secretory portion (sweat coils)	Spiradenoma	–
	Cylindroma	Cylindroma
	Nodular hidradenoma	–
	Papillary eccrine adenoma	Tubular apocrine adenoma
	Chondroid syringoma (mixed tumor)	Chondroid syringoma (mixed tumor)
	–	Hidradenoma papilliferum
	Mucinous eccrine adenocarcinoma	–
	Aggressive digital papillary adenocarcinoma	–
	–	Paget's disease
Mixed	Syringocystadenoma papilliferum	
	Microcystic adnexal carcinoma	

- Pale, cystic and "hemorrhagic" poroma in the dermis, with pink, clear, and squamoid cells organized in rosettes around dilated vessels: think nodular hidradenoma
- Hidradenoma papilliferum-like dermal tumor extending to the surface: think syringocystadenoma papilliferum
- Basaloid (blue) epithelioid cords, "syringoma-like structures in fibrotic stroma from the top to the bottom of the specimen: think microcystic adnexal carcinoma (MAC)

Stromal reaction:

- Fibrotic (sclerotic) stroma: syringoma, tubular apocrine/papillary eccrine adenoma, MAC
- Bluish-gray-purple compact stroma: chondroid syringoma
- Loose fibrous stroma: syringofibroadenoma

On high power

BENIGN TUMORS

Syringoma

- The tumor is situated in the upper dermis and is non-circumscribed
- Small round (or cord like) ducts lined by two layers of cells with a lumen, which may contain pink debris (sweat) and is outlined by a pink cuticle **(Figure 5.79)**
- Some ductal structures have elongated comma-like tails (tadpoles) **(Photomnemonic 5.12)**
- In the clear cell variant the cells are pale due to accumulation of glycogen
- Fibrotic stroma
- Milia-like structures are possible

Poroma

- Well-circumscribed intraepidermal proliferation extends in interconnected anastomosing masses into the dermis **(Figure 5.80A)**
- The stroma between the epithelial masses shows dilated vessels
- The cells are very monomorphic, smaller than keratinocytes, cuboidal in shape, and connected by bridges (poroid cells) **(Figure 5.80B)**

NB Ductal lumina lined by a pink cuticle (PAS-positive) can be a clue to the diagnosis.

Variants:

- **Hidroacanthoma simplex:** Entirely intraepithelial variant of poroma
- **Dermal duct tumor:** Entirely dermal variant of poroma **(Figure 5.80C)**

Eccrine syringofibroadenoma (ESF)

- Slender epithelial cords of acrosyringeal cells (forming lumina) with broad connection to the epidermal surface invade the dermis in a net-like/web-like pattern **(Figure 5.81, Photomnemonic 5.13)**
- The stroma among the cords is loose and fibrovascular (hence **fibro**adenoma)

Differential diagnosis: Pinkus tumor – ESF has ductal structures and no follicular structures such as basaloid buds (follicular germs)

Nodular hidradenoma

NB A heterogeneous tumor (solid and cystic areas, and different types of cells).

- Well-circumscribed, lobular, non-encapsulated dermal tumor (less than a third of the tumors connect to the surface)
- Cystic and hemorrhagic areas due to tumoral degeneration **(Figure 5.82A)**
- Several types of cells can be detected **(Figure 5.82B)**:
  - Clear cells
  - *Polyhedral/polygonal/fusiform pink cells, particularly around dilated vessels*
  - Pink cuboidal (poroid) cells
  - Squamoid (epithelioid) cells usually clustered in small morula-like structures
  - Mucinous cells
- The cells are organized in rosettes around dilated vessels (which may be surrounded by glassy hyalinized collagen) **(Figure 5.82C)**

Eccrine and apocrine hidrocystoma

NB The epidermis is thin and flat (clue to eyelid location).

- One (in eccrine hydrocystoma) or several (in apocrine hydrocystoma) cystic spaces in the dermis
- The cyst lining is made of a single layer of cuboidal cells

1. **Eccrine hidrocystoma** is a retention cyst from the ductal epithelium
2. **Apocrine hidrocystoma** is a cystadenoma – a cystic tumor from the secretory coils: look for papillary projections with decapitation secretion **(Figure 5.83)**

Papillary eccrine adenoma/Tubular apocrine adenoma

These are two counterparts of the same tumor.

1. **Eccrine:** A cribriform pattern of cystic ductal structures with intraluminal papillary projections
   - The ducts are lined by two layers of cells
   - NB This duct lining is a sign of benignity.
   - Cellular debris and granular material in the lumina is possible
   - Sclerotic stroma
2. **Apocrine:** Similar features but the structures are more tubular than cystic and show decapitation secretion **(Figure 5.84)**

Hidradenoma papilliferum

Adenoma of apocrine differentiation (from genital apocrine glands)

- No connection to the surface
- Well-circumscribed and encapsulated dermal nodule of tubular and cystic structures organized in a maze-like pattern **(Figure 5.85, Photomnemonic 5.14)**
- Two layers of cells line the lumina: inner columnar (secretory) cell and outer cuboidal (myopeithelial cells)
- Papillary projections and decapitation

NB Mitoses are not a sign for malignancy.

Syringocystadenoma papilliferum

NB This is the most common tumor arising in the postpubertal nevus sebaceus.

- *Exophytic* papillomatous (verrucous) surface with epidermal hyperplasia **(Figure 5.86A, Photomnemonic 5.15)**
- Cystic and tubular glands form *papillary* projections which connect to the surface and fill the dermis in a lace-like pattern
- The glands are lined by two layers of cells (inner columnar, outer cuboidal) and show decapitation **(Figure 5.86B)**

NB Note the cores of plasma cells among the papillary projections.

Eccrine spiradenoma

- One or several well-demarcated, encapsulated blue lobules in the dermis (one or more blue balls in the dermis) **(Figure 5.87A)**
- A "tightly packed", very cellular tumor made of two type of cells showing:
  - Small dark nuclei (at the periphery): undifferentiated cells
  - Large pale nuclei in the center, arranged in rosettes around ductal lumina: secretory cells
- Pink hyaline droplets among the tightly packed cells (PAS-positive protein aggregates)
- NB Lymphocytes are dispersed within the tumor **(Figure 5.87B)**.

- The stroma can show dilated vessels, cystic and hemorrhagic changes (due to tumoral degeneration in older lesions)

Cylindroma

This tumor is the "apocrine" cousin of eccrine spiradenoma.

NB Some lesions are best characterized as cylindrospiroadenomas.

- "Jigsaw puzzle" of numerous closely set islands of basaloid cells of similar dual morphology **(Figure 5.88)**
  - Dark nuclei palisading at the periphery
  - Pale vesicular nuclei in the center
- Each island is enveloped in pink (hyaline) sheath
- Ductal differentiation (round white circles lined by pink cuticle within the islands)
- Hyaline droplets
- Linked to the CYLD gene mutation (Brooke Spiegler syndrome: cylindroma, spiradenoma, trichoepithelioma)

Chondroid syringoma (mixed tumor of skin)

A circumscribed nodular pseudoencapsulated tumor of mixed (epithelial and mesenchymal) differentiation

Epithelial component:
- Differentiation is towards the eccrine/apocrine ductal and secretory segment of the glands
- Two types of ductal structures:
  - Tubular branching structures: lined by two layers of cells (luminal cuboidal and peripheral flattened) as in tubular apocrine adenoma **(Figure 5.89A)**; aggregates of epithelial cells without ductal lumina
  - Small non-branching tubular lumina: numerous small round ducts lined by a single layer of cells (flat cells) like in syringoma **(Figure 5.89B)**

Stroma:
- Myxoid matrix (contains acid mucopolysaccharides) with focal calcifications, sebaceous/matrical differentiation
- Hyaline epithelial cells, appearing plasmocytoid, are surrounded by halo-like chondrocytes (this gives the stroma the "chondroid" appearance) **(Figure 5.89C)**

NB The stroma is produced by the outer layer of the cells lining the tubulo-glandular structures.

MALIGNANT TUMORS

Porocarcinoma

Malignant asymmetric poroid tumor with areas of necrosis, mitoses, marked atypia, pagetoid spread

NB Distinguishing porocarcinoma from metastatic adenocarcinoma may be difficult. The presence of ductal structures with a PAS-positive pink cuticle excludes metastasis.

Microcystic adnexal carcinoma (MAC)

MAC is a low-grade sweat gland carcinoma of the head and neck of unclear adnexal origin: possible folliculo-apocrine differentiation

NB It shows deeply infiltrating growth: from the top to the bottom of the specimen, invading the subdermis.

- Scattered keratocysts on the top (micro**cystic** adnexal carcinoma) **(Figure 5.90A)**
- Cords and strands of basaloid epithelioid cells showing ductal lumina invade the dermis and the subdermis (microcystic **adnexal** carcinoma) **(Figure 5.90B)**
- Sclerotic (paucicellular) stroma

NB Perineural invasion is almost always present (80%).

(Table 5.9)

Primary cutaneous mucinous eccrine adenocarcinoma (MEC)

It can develop as a primary or as a secondary metastatic carcinoma (from breast and gastrointestinal tract) to the skin

Table 5.9 Main differential diagnoses for MAC

Features	Microcystic adnexal carcinoma	Morpheaform basal cell carcinoma	Desmoplastic trichopeithelioma
Horn cysts	Yes	No	Yes
Ductal differentiation	Yes	No	No
Infiltrative growth	Yes	Yes	No
Sclerotic stroma	Yes	Yes	Yes
"Papillary mesenchymal bodies"	No	No	Yes
Perineural invasion	Yes	No	No
Clefts separating the tumor islands from the stroma	No	Yes	No

- Well-circumscribed but not encapsulated neoplasm with a honeycomb silhouette **(Figure 5.91A)**
- Solid round, cribriform or irregular nests or cords of dark and pale cells (like in the normal secretory coils) with minimal or mild atypia **(Figure 5.91B, Photomnemonic 5.16)**
  - Some nests show tubular lumina
  - The nests are suspended in a pool of mucin
  - The nests with the mucinous stroma are compartmentalized by thin fibrovascular septa

Immunohistochemistry (in a primary lesion): CEA+; EMA+; CK7+; CK5/6 and p63+ indicating the presence of myoepithelial cells and CK20- (positive in MEC metastatic from the gastrointestinal tract)

Aggressive digital papillary adenocarcinoma (ADPA)

NB Thick stratum corneum is a clue to acral location (fingers, toes, palms, and soles).

- The features are similar to papillary eccrine adenoma but more anaplastic: infiltrative pattern with necrosis, cellular atypia, and mitoses **(Figure 5.92A)**
- Solid islands of cuboidal, columnar cells
- Tubuloalveolar or tubular structures of same cells
- *Papillary projections* lined by atypical cells protrude into dilated lumen **(Figure 5.92B)**
- *Atypia and marked mitotic activity*

Extramammary Paget's disease (EMPD)

Primary EMPD (I EMPD) is a rare cutaneous adenocarcinoma of the apocrine glands in the groin/perianal area

Secondary EMPD (II EMPD) is a metastatic disease to the skin from an underlying malignancy (genitourinary or gastrointestinal carcinoma) (25–50% of the EMPD cases)

NB Mammary Paget's disease is always associated with an intraductal breast carcinoma.

- Epidermis can be hyperplastic
- Large round pale cells with ample cytoplasm, vesicular nuclei, and prominent nucleoli invade the epidermis individually and in clusters (nests) **(Figure 5.93)**
- No intercellular bridges

NB Compare EMPD to Bowen's disease. **(Table 5.10)**

- The cells stain with mucicarmin and PASD because they contain mucin
- All layers are involved except for the basal cells, which are flattened
- The cells do not invade the dermis directly but extend down the follicles and sweat glands

(Table 5.10)

FOLLICULAR NEOPLASMS

General concepts

The anatomy of the pilosebaceous structures is described in Chapter 1.

- **Follicular germs:** Small crowded palisading aggregates of basaloid (blue) cells with oval nuclei and scant cytoplasm; in postnatal life they are located at the level of the isthmus and look like buds
- The germinative cells are BEREP4+
- **Follicular mesenchyme** envelops the follicle: The dermal papilla (plump fibroblasts with overlapping crowded nuclei) and the connective tissue sheath, which is made of thin fibrillary type I collagen

Table 5.10 Immunohistochemical pattern in EMPD vs melanoma vs Bowen's disease

	Melanoma	I EMPD	II EMPD	Bowen's disease
Melanocytic markers (MART-1, S100, HMB-45)	+	–	–	–
CK7, CAM5.2	–	+	+	–
EMA	–	+	+	+/–
BEREP4	–	+	–	–
CEA	**–**	**+**	**+**	**–**
GCDFP15		+	–	
CK20, CDX2		–	+ (large intestinal/rectal carcinoma)	–
Uroplakin		–	+ (uroepithelial carcinoma)	
PSA		–	+ (prostate carcinoma)	
p16		–	+ (cervical carcinoma)	

- **Matrical cells (hair bulb):** Oval basophilic vesicular nuclei; mitoses are normal
- **Supramatrical cells:** Larger elongated cells with more eosinophilic cytoplasm

The matrical cells differentiate into the hair shaft and into the inner root sheath

- **Hair shaft:** Compact anuclear keratinized cells of salmon–yellow color
- **The inner root sheath** contains bright red trichohyaline granules (prior to its keratinization at the isthmus)
- **The outer root sheath (trichilemma)** contains pale and clear epithelial cells (due to glycogen), columnar in shape, palisading at the periphery above the basement membrane, and round in the center; the cells are much paler at the level of the bulb and eosinophilic at the level of the isthmus
- **Trichilemmal keratinization:** Abrupt differentiation towards the outer root sheath without trichohyaline granules
- **Sebaceous mantle:** Cords of undifferentiated basaloid cells that emanate from the infundibulum and droop down aside the follicle like a mantle/skirt. It gives rise in puberty to the fully developed sebaceous lobules and glands which in senescence involute to become undifferentiated mantles again

(Table 5.11)

Table 5.11 Most common follicular neoplasms classified by the segment of the follicular epithelium towards which they differentiate

Differentiation	Follicular neoplasm(s)
Differentiation towards the follicular germs (germinative cells)	Basal cell carcinoma
Biphasic (epithelial + mesenchymal) differentiation (germinative cells and mesenchymal papilla)	Fibroepithelioma of Pinkus Trichoblastoma Trichoepithelioma Lymphadenoma
Differentiation towards the matrix	Pilomatricoma
Differentiation towards outer root sheath (at the bulb) Differentiation towards outer root sheath (at the isthmus)	Trichilemomma Tumor of the follicular infundibulum
Differentiation towards the infundibulum	Trichoadenoma
Panfollicular differentiation (from all parts of the follicle)	Trichofolliculoma Pilar sheath acanthoma
Differentiation towards the follicular mantle	Fibrofolliculoma Trichodiscoma

On low power

Helpful photomnemonics for some follicular neoplasms can be found in their descriptions below.

On high power

Basal cell carcinoma (BCC)

See Keratinocytic tumors

Fibroepithelioma of Pinkus

The **epithelial** component differentiates towards the germinative cells and the stroma differentiates towards the follicular mesenchyme (hence fibro**epithelioma**).

- Fenestrated pattern: strands of epithelial cells branch and interconnect **(Figure 5.94)**
- Buds (germinative cells) along the epithelial strands **(Photomnemonic 5.17)**
- The stroma framed by this fenestrated tumor is fibrotic

NB Larger tumors form clefts from the stroma (similar to basal cell carcinoma).

Trichoblastoma/Trichoepithelioma

The epithelial component differentiates towards the germinative cells (trichoblasts) and the stroma differentiates towards the follicular mesenchyme.

- No epidermal connection (in around two-thirds of cases)
- Islands of palisading basaloid cells (germinative cells), embedded in the stroma without clefts (retraction artifacts are characteristic for basal cell carcinoma) **(Figure 5.95A)**
- The islands vary in shape and morphology: 1) Solid small/large; 2) racemiform (from raceme – a pedicle on which flowers are held); 3) cribriform (sieve-like); 4) retiform (fenestrated, net-like); 5) columnar (cords and strands)
- The stroma is fibrotic: wiry delicate collagen (from the connective tissue sheath) with plump or spindle fibroblasts which attempt to form papillary mesenchyme (papillary mesenchymal bodies) **(Figure 5.95B)**

Trichoepithelioma (TEP)

A more superficial variant of trichoblastoma showing:

- More cribriform pattern
- Horn cysts **(Figure 5.95C)**

NB Calcifications, amyloid, and foreign body granulomas are common in TEP.

Desmosplastic TEP

- Narrow strands of basaloid cells **(Figure 5.95D)**
- Fibrotic stroma (desmoplastic refers to a fibrotic stromal reaction pattern in tumors)

- Horn cysts
- Foreign body granulomas

NB Differential diagnosis: MAC (see MAC).

Lymphadenoma

Another variant of trichoblastoma showing:

- Rhomboid islands of 1) palisading basaloid cells at the periphery, and 2) large pale cells with vesicular cytoplasm in the center **(Figure 5.95E, F; Photomnemonic 5.17)**
- The follicular structures are infiltrated with lymphocytes

Syndromes with trichoblastomas/trichoepitheliomas

- *Brooke Fordyce syndrome:* Multiple trichoblastomas
- *Brooke Spiegler syndrome:* Spiradenomas, cylindromas, and trichoepitheliomas (cribriform trichoblastomas)
- *Rombo syndrome:* Atrophoderma vermiculata, milia, hypotrichosis, basal cell carcinomas, trichoepitheliomas, peripheral cyanosis
- *Bazex syndrome:* Atrophoderma vermiculata, hypotrichosis, hypohidrosis, trichoepitheliomas, basal cell carcinomas
- *Gardner's syndrome:* Epidermoid cysts, desmoid tumors, multiple trichoepitheliomas, fibromas, lipomas, leiomyomas, osteomas
- *Rassmusen syndrome:* Trichoepitheliomas, milia, cylindromas

Pilomatrixoma (pilomatricoma) (PMX)

Circumscribed nodular/cystic tri-colored masses and tongues in the dermis (blue, salmon color, and pale pink) composed of cells of mixed differentiation

1. Matrical and supramatrical: basaloid blue cells **(Figure 5.96)**
2. Hair shaft: anucleated eosinophilic "shadow/ghost" cells and yellow orange cornified cells
3. Inner root sheath: transitional cells with bright red trichohyaline granules

NB Evolving lesions may show increased mitoses; old lesions show less basaloid and more shadow cells.

- Calcification, even bone formation (ossification) is possible (in old lesions)
- Foreign body granulomas are possible
- The stroma is fibrotic

Differential diagnosis: Pilomatrix carcinoma shows more infiltrative growth with atypia, necrosis and mitoses

Trichilemmoma

- Exo (*grows outwards*)/endophytic (*grows inwards*) epidermal based "pale" tumor with a collarette
- The surface may be verrucous
- The tumor has a rounded (multi)lobular contour outlined by a thin pink basement membrane **(Figure 5.97A)**
- The cells are pale and bland, with clear cytoplasm (due to glycogen) arranged in a palisade on the basement membrane; they show differentiation toward the outer root sheath at the level of the bulb **(Figure 5.97B)**
- Droplets of basement membrane material (hyaline droplets) and squamous eddies are possible

Desmoplastic trichilemmoma

Jagged epithelial strands extend from the trichilemmal lobules in fibrotic stroma **(Figure 5.97C).**

NB This simulates invasive tumor growth: look for features of a typical trichilemmoma.

Tumor of the follicular infundibulum

- A horizontal plate-like tumor of fenestrated pattern
- Multiple connections to the epidermis **(Figure 5.98)**
- The cells are pink and pale: they differentiate towards the outer root sheath at isthmus level
- Small vellus follicles enter the plate from below and "lose their identity" by becoming part of the tumor mass
- The stroma is fibrotic

Differential diagnosis: From fibroepithelioma of Pinkus: the cells are pink and pale (differentiation is towards the outer root sheath) and do not form buds (of basaloid germinative cells)

Trichoadenoma

Differentiation towards the follicular infundibulum results in **infundibulo-cystic structures**; numerous closely set round cystic structures with features of epidermal cysts in the upper dermis **(Figure 5.99, Photomnemonic 5.19)**

NB The cysts lie back to back (crowded specimen).

- When the inner lining is pink and crenulated, this is a clue to sebaceous duct differentiation (the sebaceous duct opens in the infundibulum)
- Foreign body granulomatous reaction to ruptured cysts is possible
- Fibrotic stroma

Trichofolliculoma (TF)

This is a hamartoma with differentiation towards all parts of the hair follicle (panfollicular differentiation).

NB TF is a highly organized and highly differentiated tumor which shows follicular structures in different stages of the hair cycle (anagen, telogen) and of different types (terminal, vellus) **(Figure 5.100, Photomnemonic 5.20).**

- The center is a dilated cystic cavity lined by squamous epithelium (infundibular differentiation)
- Radiating from the center are small but well-differentiated mature follicles (which all have features of a hair follicle starting with the papilla at the bottom, matrix cells, hair shaft, root sheaths)
- The follicles can be anagen, telogen, and vellus
- Interfollicular bridges connect the radiating follicles
- The surrounding stroma is fibrotic and "encapsulates" the tumor with a cleft from the dermis

Sebaceous TF

The radiating follicles have attached, well-differentiated sebaceous lobules and show sebaceous ducts.

Pilar sheath acanthoma

This is a tumor of *panfollicular* differentiation (*pan* means all, everything).

- A markedly dilated cystic cavity filled with keratin opens to the surface (a pore-like opening)
- Elongated rete and small projections of epithelial cells (with infundibular characteristics: eosinophilic keratinocytes) emanate from the cystic cavity into the dermis (dilated pore of Winer) **(Figure 5.101)**
- When lobulated masses of infundibular keratinocytes emanate from the cystic cavity into the dermis, this is called pilar sheath acanthoma

Fibrofolliculoma/Trichodiscoma

Fibrofolliculoma is a *fibroepithelial* tumor with differentiation towards the sebaceous mantle.

- A central cystically distorted infundibulum with emanating delicate thin *epithelial* cords of basaloid cells (mantle differentiation) extending in the stroma in a fenestrated pattern
- The epithelial cords are interconnected
- The stroma is *fibrotic*

> NB The tumor's silhouette resembles trichofolliculoma but there are no mature follicular structures, just thin mantle structures.

Trichodiscoma is the "*stromal counterpart*" of fibrofolliculoma.

- Fibrillar (ribbon-like) collagen bundles
- Mucin giving loose appearance to the stroma
- Mature sebaceous lobules, assimilated to "hands of bananas", lie alone (not attached to follicles) in the stroma
- Small clusters of blood vessels

SEBACEOUS NEOPLASMS

General concepts

- **Germinative cells** (peripheral basaloid cells) stain positive with androgen receptor (AR)
- **Mature sebocytes** (centrally located, contain compartmentalized multiple intracytoplasmic vacuoles): Stain positive with EMA, adipophilin, and CK7
- **Sebaceous duct:** Keratinizing stratified squamous epithelium with granular layer and inner crenulated pink cuticle

On low power

- A conglomerate of mature sebaceous glands in the dermis: think sebaceous hyperplasia
- **Multilobular pale-pink tumor** with mature sebaceous lobules connecting directly to the surface: think sebaceous adenoma
- **Multinodular blue tumor** with less prominent sebaceous lobules in the dermis: think sebaceoma

On high power

Nevus sebaceus

This is a hamartoma of three components: follicular, sebaceous and apocrine glands, and mesenchymal (vessels).

Prepubertal nevus sebaceus

- The surface is flat (the clinical differential diagnosis is aplasia cutis congenita)
- *Immature abortive hair structures* from cords of undifferentiated follicular epithelium (embryonic follicular structures) to "pseudo-vellus" follicles (no hair shaft differentiation)
- Dilated keratin-filled infundibula
- *No* sebaceous glands

Postpubertal nevus sebaceus

- The surface is papillomatous/verrucous
- *Mature and usually hypertrophic sebaceous glands* open directly to the surface **(Figure 5.102)**
- Ectopic and dilated apocrine glands

> NB Most common appendageal proliferations arising in nevus sebaceous after puberty include:
> - Malformed basaloid epithelial proliferations (buds of undifferentiated germinative cells) which simulate basal cell carcinoma (and have previously been regarded as BCC) develop in half of cases
> - Trichoblastoma
> - SCAP

Sebaceous hyperplasia

- Mature large sebaceous lobules are grouped around a central dilated sebaceous duct **(Figure 5.103, Photomnemonic 5.21)**
- The duct opens directly to the surface (which corresponds to the clinical umbilication)
- The mature lobules are lined by a rim of basaloid germinative cells

Sebaceous adenoma

- Contiguous sebaceous lobules connect and *open directly to the surface* **(Figure 5.104A)**
- The lobules replace the normal epidermis at the site of proliferation (look for a collarette)
- Most cells are mature sebocytes (compare to sebaceoma)
- Debris of holocrine pink secretion (sebum) may be present in the cystic ducts
- The stroma is fibrotic

> NB Cystic, ulcerated tumors or with intra/peritumoral lymphocytes: rule out Muir Torre syndrome **(Figure 5.104B)**.

Sebaceoma

- Multinodular masses of smooth-contoured "bluish" lobules **(Figure 5.105)**
- No connection to the epidermis (or only focal)
- Majority of cells (at least 50%) are small blue cells with round nuclei (germinative cells)
- Scattered ducts with debris of holocrine secretion (sebum) and small keratinous cysts are common
- Mitoses are not rare

Differential diagnosis: From basal cell carcinoma with sebaceous differentiation: no palisading, no stromal clefts, sebum, BerEP4-

> NB Overlapping features with sebaceous adenoma may be present in the same lesion.

Sebaceous carcinoma

Aggressive tumor with high risk for local recurrence and distant metastases

> NB Diagnosis of sebaceous carcinoma requires investigation for Muir Torre syndrome (AD syndrome, mutations in the MSH2 and MLH1 genes).

- It looks "bad" when compared to the benign sebaceous tumors
- Multilobular, well-differentiated lobules or sheets invade the dermis (infiltrative pattern) depending on the grading
- Pagetoid spread to the epidermis is possible
- Variable differentiation: 1) undifferentiated cells with prominent nuclear atypia, prominent nucleoli; and 2) atypical sebocytes with oval vesicular nuclei, prominent nucleoli, and abundant bubbly cytoplasm (compare to the well-compartmentalized, vacuolated cytoplasm of normal sebocytes)
- Many mitotic figures
- Tumoral necrosis

CUTANEOUS LYMPHOID NEOPLASMS

> **Definition:** Primary cutaneous lymphomas are neoplastic proliferations of T- and B-lymphocytes which are confined to the skin and persist for more than 6 months after completing staging. Secondary cutaneous lymphomas (metastatic to the skin from usually nodal lymphomas) have similar pathologic findings and complete staging investigation is necessary for the diagnosis.

General concepts

- B-cells are produced in the **B**one marrow.
- T-cells are produced in the bone marrow but mature in the **T**hymus.
- Each T- and B-cell binds to a specific antigen portion called the *epitope*, via a receptor (TCR or BCR) expressed on their surface; the receptor is genetically encoded and exists in thousands of identical copies before the cell ever meets an antigen.
- The "T or B phenotype" of the lymphocytic infiltrate is assessed by immunohistochemical markers called *clusters of differentiation* (CD) (see Chapter 1); the *clonality* of the infiltrate is assessed by analysis of the gene rearrangement for TCR and BCR (known as immunoglobulin heavy chain receptor $J_H R$) with southern blot/PCR.
- A *clone* is a population of cells bearing the same antigen receptor (those cells have identical specificity); benign lymphoid proliferations are polyclonal, malignant proliferations are monoclonal.

> NB Some inflammatory dermatoses rarely show monoclonal pattern and lymphomas may be polyclonal, especially in early stages.

B-CELLS

B-cells do not enter the epidermis.

- **In benign conditions** (*reactive lymphoid hyperplasias/pseudolymphomas*) they aggregate into reactive lymphoid follicles (germinal centers) in the dermis due to persistent antigen stimulation.

- **In malignant conditions** *(B-cell lymphomas)* they infiltrate the dermis by splaying apart collagen bundles and mesenchymal cells.

> NB B-cells displace without invading the adnexal structures; T-cells are "adnexotropic".

The job of B-cells

- Pick up intact soluble antigens from the antigen-presenting cells (macrophages and dendritic cells)
- Express digested portions of the antigen on their surface, recognized then by the TCR of the helper T-cells (Th-cells)
- Naive B-cells multiply and differentiate into plasma cells (after the Th-cells bind them and release cytokines to stimulate them)
- The plasma cells produce a clone of B-cells with identical surface-bound BCR and soluble BCR (antibodies)

T-CELLS

T-cells are divided into two groups based on their TCR type: α/β (betaF1+) and γ/σ (betaF1−).

- **α/β cells** are 95% of the T-cells; they re-circulate between the blood and the lymph nodes and enter the epithelia, including skin

> NB In benign conditions T-cells change the epidermis (spongiosis, acanthosis, apoptosis) whereas in malignant conditions they aggregate "passively" in the epidermis.

- **γ/σ cells** are not studied well; once they enter the epithelia, they stay there "as guardians" and only less than 5% can be detected in the blood
- **NK/T cells** are a type of T-cells which also express some surface antigen molecules for NK cells

> NB NK cells are natural killer cells which are of neither T- nor B-cell lineage and have the ability to directly eliminate cells infected by a virus or cancer).

The job of T-cells

CD4 (helper T-cells, Th):

1. *Involved in cell-mediated immunity:* Bind to antigen presenting cells and secrete lymphokines to attract other cells, resulting in inflammation
2. *Involved in antibody-mediated immunity:* Bind to B-cells to stimulate them to multiply into activated plasma cells which produce antibodies (see above)

CD8 (cytotoxic T-cells, Tc):

Bind to cells expressing foreign antigen material on their surface and destroy them via cytotoxic molecules; these molecules are positive for the immunohistochemical markers TIA-1, granzyme B, and perforin.

On low power

See also Chapter 1

LYMPHOID CELLS

Small cells (smaller size than the nucleus of a histiocyte) **(Figure 5.106)**

- Lymphocyte: an ink-blue cell with scant cytoplasm (see below)
- Centrocyte: a cleaved lymphocyte

Intermediate cells (similar size to the nucleus of a histiocyte)

- Lymphoblast: a convoluted nucleus (like a bisected walnut)

Large cells (larger than the nucleus of a histiocyte)

- Centroblast: irregular vesicular nucleus with prominent nucleoli attached in a Mercedes Benz pattern to the nuclear membrane
- Immunoblast: reddish-blue cytoplasm and an oval vesicular nucleus with a single cherry-colored central nucleolus

LYMPHOID FOLLICULAR STRUCTURES

Secondary follicle (site of lymphocytic activation and proliferation): a layered structure with several components:

Germinal center (pale circle in the middle):

- Contains centroblasts and centrocytes, follicular Th-cells, regulatory T-cell (T-regs) and follicular dendritic cells (FDC, usually seen in clusters: "kissing nuclei")
- Tingible-body macrophages (large empty spaces) with dots of apoptotic debris due to digested and processed antigen material by the macrophages **(Figure 5.107, Photomnemonic 5.22)**

Mantle zone (dark inner rim):

- Tight collection of small B-lymphocytes

Marginal zone (the light zone in the outer rim of the mantle zone):

- Loose collection of small B-lymphocytes with more cytoplasm (memory B-cells derived after T-cell mediated stimulation of naive B-cells)

Immunophenotype: CD20+, CD79+ (B-lymphocytes); CD10+ (early B-lymphocytes in germinal centers), bcl6+ (protein needed for the formation of germinal centers), bcl2- (apoptotic regulator), CD21+ (FDC)

> NB Ki67+ ≥ 90% of the cells in normal germinal centers and ≤ 50% in neoplastic germinal centers.

> NB bc2 expression in primary cutaneous lymphomas: bad prognosis; always rule out nodal lymphoma.

On high power

Only the most common lymphomas are presented below. For more information, see the EORTC-WHO classification from 2005 (www.bloodjournal.com).

CUTANEOUS T-CELL LYMPHOMAS (CTCLS)

Mycosis fungoides (MF)

Immunophenotype: From **T** (betaF1+, CD3+, CD5+) **helper** (CD4+, CD8−) **memory cells** (CD45Ro+); CD4: CD8 ratio is more than 6:1

> NB Compare to benign inflammatory diseases where the CD4:CD8 ratio is less than 2:1.

1. **Patch stage:**
   - Individual haloed lymphocytes aligned at the basal layer like a string of beads
   - Haloed intraepidermal collections of lymphocytes (Pautrier's microabscesses)
   - Disproportionate epidermotropism (epidermotropic lymphocytes without/with mild spongiosis) **(Figure 5.108A)**
   - Lymphocytes in the epidermis are bigger than those in the dermis
   - Expanded papillary dermis with coarse bundle of collagen, polymorphous infiltrate of lymphocytes, eosinophils, plasma cells but *no neutrophils*
2. **Plaque stage:**
   Additional findings:
   - Possible psoriasiform hyperplasia
   - Lichenoid patchy lymphocytic infiltrate (the infiltrate does not obscure the dermoepidermal junction) **(Figure 5.108B)**
   - More prominent epidermotropism
3. **Tumor stage:**
   - Less epidermotropism
   - Diffuse dermal infiltrate of usually large pleomorphic cells
   - Decreased number of reactive lymphocytes
   - *Transformation:* more than 25% of the cells are blasts

> NB The blasts may or may not be CD30+ **(Figure 5.108C, D)**

Variants of MF:
- *Syringotropic MF:* Atypical lymphocytes surround and invade *sweat glands* (glands may show hyperplasia)
- *Folliculotropic MF* (MF with follicular mucinosis): Atypical lymphocytes within and around a follicular infundibulum which is distorted and dilated by mucin deposits **(Figure 5.109)**
- *Granulomatous MF:* Huge giant cells with numerous nuclei and intracytoplasmic lymphocytes (emperipolesis) in sarcoidal granulomas in the upper dermis; elastophagocytosis
- *Granulomatous slack skin:* Similar findings but involve the entire dermis and subcutaneous fat

Pagetoid reticulosis
- Psoriasiform hyperplasia with parakeratosis but also hyperkeratosis **(Figure 5.110)**
- Striking epidermotropism by haloed lymphocytes **(Photomnemonic 5.23)**

> NB The cells may be CD4+CD8− or CD4−, CD8+, CD30+/−.

Sézary syndrome

Immunophenotype: T (CD3+, CD5+), **helper** (CD4+, CD8−) **memory cells** (CD45RO+); the majority of cells are also CD7−, CD26−, and the CD4:CD8 ratio is more than 10:1

The diagnosis is based on:
- Presence of a monoclonal T-cell population in the blood (Sézary cells: more than 1000/mm^3 or more than 20% of circulating lymphocytes)
- Lymph node involvement
- Abrupt onset of erythroderma with palmoplantar keratoderma, alopecia, and ectropion
- *Pathology is indistinguishable from MF (plaque stage):* psoriasiform + spongiotic epidermis + band-like infiltrate

> NB The presence of an identical clone in the blood and the skin is an independent prognostic criterion for a worse prognosis.

Adult T-cell leukemia/lymphoma

A CTCL resulting from infection with the HTLV-1 virus

Immunophenotype: T (CD3, CD5+), **helper** (CD4+) *CD25+*
- Similar to MF *but always involves the dermis*
- Atypical lymphocytes of medium to large size with irregular polylobulated nuclei
- The infiltrate fills the entire dermis in the nodular/tumor stage **(Figure 5.111A)**
- When microabscesses are present, they contain numerous apoptotic fragments (some of which are apoptotic lymphocytes) **(Figure 5.111B, C)**

CD30+ CTCL

CD30 is expressed in individual lymphoid cells in reactive conditions and in *sheets/clusters* of clonally expanded atypical lymphocytes in primary cutaneous CD30+ lymphomas.

Lymphomatoid papulosis (LyP)

Immunophenotype: Activated CD30+ T (CD3+), **helper** (CD4+CD8–) cells releasing **cytotoxic** molecules (TIA-1, granzyme B)

- The surface can be ulcerated or acanthotic
- Wedge-shaped infiltrate of lymphoid cells in the dermis

Type A ("histiocytic type"):

- The most common type
- Wedge-shaped infiltrate of atypical cells but also with many reactive cells: histiocytes, eosinophils, and neutrophils ("inflammatory type") **(Figure 5.112A)**
- The atypical cells are large with ample cytoplasm and sometimes prominent bilobed nuclei **(Figure 5.112B)**
- Increased mitotic activity

Type B (MF-like)

- Epidermotropism: small atypical lymphocytes with cerebriform nuclei (CD30–)
- Some classify it as "a papular variant of MF"
- Distinction from anaplastic large cell lymphoma with small/medium cells requires clinical data

Type C (anaplastic large cell lymphoma-like, ALCL-like)

- The epidermis is spared
- Grenz zone
- The dermis is infiltrated in a nodular pattern by sheets of cohesive atypical large cells, entrapping the collagen as in dermatofibroma **(Figure 5.112C)**
- The infiltrate does not extend into the subdermis; compare to an ALCL (see below)
- The cells are atypical, large (blasts), similar to immunoblasts, and show increased mitoses **(Figure 5.112D)**

NB Distinction from ALCL requires clinical data.

Type D (Epidermotropic CD8+)

- CD30+ CD8+ large cells in the epidermis. (Differential diagnosis: aggressive epidermotropic cytotoxic CD8+ lymphoma is CD30–)

Type E (Angioinvasive)

- Small to medium CD30+ CD8+ atypical lymphocytes surround and invade blood vessels **(Figure 5.112E)**

Anaplastic large cell lymphoma (ALCL)

Immunophenotype: Activated CD30+ **T** (CD3+), **helper** (CD4+CD8-) cells releasing **cytotoxic** molecules (TIA-1, granzyme B); ALK–, EMA– (compared to nodal ALCL which is +)

NB Distinction from LyP (type C) requires clinical data.

- Ulcerated surface with epidermal hyperplasia
- Sheets of cohesive large atypical cells fill the dermis and invade the subdermis **(Figure 5.113)**
- *More than 75%* of the cells are atypical large (blasts) with prominent nucleoli
- The morphology of the large cells includes: epithelioid, multinucleated, immunoblasts, Reed Sternberg (large "owl"-like)
- Small/medium size appearance is also possible
- Reactive neutrophils are possible ("pyogenic" ALCL)

Subcutaneous T-cell lymphoma

Immunophenotype: T (betaF1+, CD3+, CD5+) **suppressor** (CD8+) releasing **cytotoxic** molecules (TIA1+, granzyme B+, perforin+)

- The epidermis and dermis are spared
- Lobular panniculitis (septa are spared) due to infiltration of atypical small to medium-size cells in the fat lobules with reactive small lymphocytes **(Figure 5.114A)**
- The atypical cells rim the adipocytes **(Figure 5.114B, Photomnemonic 5.24)**
- The cells are larger, with pleomorphic, bizarre-shaped nuclei
- Extensive fat necrosis, lipomembranous changes

NB Differential diagnosis: Distinguishing from lupus panniculitis can be very difficult. Look for germinal centers, hyalinization of the fat, plasma cells collections, and usually no atypia of the rimming lymphoid cells in lupus panniculitis.

(Table 5.12)

CUTANEOUS B-CELL LYMPHOMAS (CBCLS)

Primary cutaneous follicle center lymphoma (PCFCL)

NB This is the most common primary CBCL.

Nodal extracutaneous FCL shows follicular pattern due to proliferation of neoplastic germinal centers.

NB PCFCL only rarely shows follicular pattern (mostly in small, early lesions).

Immunophenotype: CD20+, CD79a+, CD10+, *CD21+*, *bcl6+*, *bc2–*, *MUM-1-*

- Three patterns (diffuse, follicular to diffuse, and follicular)
- The epidermis is spared by a Grenz zone
- Diffuse involvement of the dermis (and the subdermis) **(Figure 5.115A)**
- Mixture of: 1) medium to large centrocytes (cleaved lymphocytes), and 2) centroblasts **(Figure 5.115B)**
- In the follicular (nodular) pattern the follicles are abnormal/"naked": reduced mantle zone, no distinct pale and dark areas and no tingible bodies
- "Spill out" of reactive small lymphocytes is possible (early lesions)

Table 5.12 Differential diagnosis of cutaneous cytotoxic T-cell lymphomas

Diagnosis	Subcutaneous TCL	Extranodal NK/T-cell lymphoma	Cutaneous γ/σ lymphoma	Primary cutaneous aggressive epidermotropic CD8+ T-cell lymphoma
Immunophenotype	CD3+ CD4– CD8+ TIA-1 +	CD3+ CD4– CD8– TIA-1+	CD3+ CD4– CD8– (+) TIA-1+	CD3+ CD4– CD8+ TIA-1+
bF-1	+	–	–	+
CD56	–	+	+	–
EBV	–	+	–	–
Epidermotropism	–	+	+	++
Dermal involvement	–	+	+	+
Angiocentric/angiodestructive infiltrate	–	+	+	–

Primary cutaneous marginal zone lymphoma (PCMZL)

Associations: *Borrelia burgdorferi*, tattoo, vaccination
Immunophenotype: CD20+, CD79a+, CD10–, *bcl6–*, *bcl2–*; *CD21+ in the germinal centers*, CD3+ reactive T-cells, *MUM-1-*

- The epidermis is spared by a Grenz zone
- On low power: *Multicentric nodular infiltrate* due to diffuse pattern with residual (germinal) follicles
- The infiltrate extends along hair follicles and sweat glands in the dermis (and subdermis)
- The infiltrate is top-heavy and looks "benign" due to *many reactive cells*: lymphocytes, eosinophils, plasma cells **(Figure 5.116A)**
- The tumor is composed of *marginal zone cells*: cleaved centrocytes, small lymphocytes, plasmocytoid cells, and plasma cells, and only some blasts; eosinophils and granulomatous reaction can be noted in some cases **(Figure 5.116B)**

Primary cutaneous diffuse large B-cell lymphoma (DLBCL)

DLBCL divides into 1) DLBCL leg type, and 2) DLBCL other.

NB "Other" tumors on head, neck, and trunk have a good prognosis but leg tumors have a poor prognosis.

NB DLBCL can be seen in immunocompromised patients.

Immunophenotype: CD20+, CD79+, CD10–, *bc2+*, bcl6+, *MUM-1+* (postgerminal B-lymphocytes), CD30+/–

- Diffuse dense infiltrate fills the entire dermis and subdermis ("dramatic blue tumor replaces the entire skin") **(Figure 5.117A)**
- NB the epidermis can be involved; Grenz zone may be absent
- Large cells: *immunoblasts* and *centroblasts* with frequent mitoses **(Figure 5.117B, C)**
- Absent centrocytes and reactive small lymphocytes (compare to PCFCL and PCMZL)
- Mosaic arrangement of the infiltrate can be present

Differential diagnosis: Merkel cell carcinoma: the cells are uniform blue, non-cohesive as in lymphoma, form cracks, and have many dispersed apoptotic cells ("dots").
(Table 5.13)

Cutaneous pseudolymphoma (CPL; benign lymphoid hyperplasia)

Benign reactive proliferation of predominantly T-lymphocytes with various clinical presentations
Immunophenotype: CD20+, CD79+ (≤ 50% of the cells), CD3+, CD5+ (≥ 50% of the cells), CD21+ (regular distribution), Ki67+ (≥ 90% of the cells), κ +and λ + (polyclonal immunoglobulin light chains), J_HR-

- Diffuse nodular architecture
- The infiltrate is top-heavy and *does not infiltrate* as individual cells among the collagen bundles **(Figure 5.118)**
- Lymphoid follicles (germinal like centers): mature B-lymphocytes, centrocytes
- Tingible bodies (see Figure 5.106)
- Numerous reactive cells: eosinophils, plasma cells
- Mitoses and apoptotic cells may be numerous

(Table 5.14)

Table 5.13 Summary of the main features of the most common PCBCLs

Diagnosis	PCFCL	PCMZL	DLBCL
Cells of origin	Germinal center cells	Marginal zone cells	Postgerminal center cells
Infiltrate pattern	Diffuse, spares the epidermis	Multicentric nodular, spares the epidermis	Diffuse, dense and cohesive, may involve the epidermis
Cell morphology	Centrocytes > centroblasts	Centrocytes and many reactive cells, plasma cells, eosinophils	Centroblasts and immunoblasts
CD20	+	+	+
CD79a	+	+	+
CD10	+	–	–
CD21	+	+ (only in germinal centers)	–
Bcl6	+	–	+
Bcl2	–	–	+
MUM-1	–	–	+
CD30	–	–	+/–

Table 5.14 Summary of the main histologic features of cutaneous pseudolymphomas

T-cell predominant CPL	B-cell predominant CPL	CD30+ CPL
Actinic dermatitis	Lymphocytoma cutis after:	Inflamed molluscum contagiosum
Lymphomatoid contact dermatitis	• *Borrelia burgdorferi*	Orf
Lymphomatoid drug reaction	• medicine leech therapy	Herpes simplex and herpes zoster
Lymphomatoid keratosis	Persistent postscabietic nodules	Arthropod reactions
Lichen aureus	CPL at vaccination site	
Lymphocytic infiltration of skin (Jessner-Kanof)	CPL at tattoo site	
	Acral pseudolymphomatous angiokeratoma (APACHE)	

NEURAL TUMORS

Definition: Neural tumors are derived from the peripheral nerve network in the skin. Malignant neural neoplasms are rare in the skin (except for Merkel cell carcinoma).

General concepts

COLOR AND SHAPE

Most neural tumors have pale color (myxoid stroma) and fascicular pattern (see Photomnemonic 5.7 in Soft tissue tumors).

NB Merkel cell carcinoma is an exception: it is a dark blue cell tumor.

The anatomy of the cutaneous neural network and the helpful immunohistochemical stains is reviewed in Chapter 1.

CLASSIFICATION

1. **Hamartomas of the nerve sheath:** Expanded proliferation of the normal components of the nerve fiber in different proportions:
   - Neuroma
   - Neurofibroma
2. **True nerve sheath tumors:**
   - Schwannoma
   - Nerve sheath myxoma and neurothekeoma
   - Malignant peripheral nerve sheath tumor
3. **Miscellaneous:**
   - Granular cell tumor

- Neuroendocrine carcinomas (Merkel cell carcinoma, MCC)

On high power

HAMARTOMAS

NEUROMAS

Neuromas are hyperplasias of the axons and the associated nerve sheath cells: axons and Schwann cells are arranged in interlacing (tortuous) fascicles.

Extraneural neuromas

Acquired traumatic neuroma

- A circumscribed but not encapsulated dermal proliferation
- Regenerating nerve fibers are organized in a haphazard arrangement **(Figure 5.119A)**
- The stroma is fibrotic

> NB Rudimentary supernumerary digit is an incorrect term as this tumor is in fact a traumatic neuroma; it has the silhouette of an acquired digital fibrokeratoma with regenerating nerve fibers in a haphazard pattern

- A clue to acral skin: thick stratum corneum, sweat glands are present but no hair follicles
- A polypoid lesion with hyperkeratosis **(Figure 5.119B)**
- Loose fibrous stroma
- Small caliber nerve bundles in a haphazard array

Intraneural neuromas

Palisaded encapsulated neuroma (PEN)

A solitary intraneural bulbous expansion of the peripheral nerve

> NB All stains are positive (S100, NSE for Schwann cells, silver stains for axons, and EMA for perineural capsule).

- A clue to facial skin: flat rete ridges and vellus follicles, sebaceous glands
- A round oblong nodule in the dermis **(Figure 5.120A)**
- Tightly woven interlacing fascicles of axons (dots) and Schwann cells (spindled cells with wavy nuclei but no Verocay bodies) in a ratio of 1:1 **(Figure 5.120B)**
- Clefts between the fascicles
- A thin capsule of perineural cells is missing towards the epidermal surface

> NB There is no fibrous stroma (compare to traumatic neuroma).

Multiple spontaneous neuromas

These neuromas share the histologic features of PEN but are non-encapsulated. They are part of the multiple endocrine neoplasia syndrome MEN 2b (Marfanoid body habitus, mucosal neuromas, phaeochromocytoma, and medullary thyroid carcinoma).

NEUROFIBROMAS (NF)

NFs are hamartomatous proliferations of the *entire nerve fiber*: axons, Schwann cells, and endoneurium (fibroblasts, mast cells, and perineural cells) in varying proportions.

> NB As a rule axons do not duplicate and therefore there are fewer of them; Schwann cells are usually the predominant component.

> NB All neural stains are positive in a neurofibroma (S100, NSE, CD57 for Schwann cells, CD34 and F.XIIIa for endoneural fibroblasts, and silver stains for axons).

Extraneural NF (diffuse NF)

Faintly eosinophilic circumscribed but not encapsulated dermal proliferation of:

- Slender serpentine spindled cells with wavy nuclei and pointed ends **(Figure 5.121A)** (see also Photomnemonic 1.5 in Chapter 1)
- Pink collagenous loose stroma of wavy collagen bundles, mucin and mast cells **(Figure 5.121B)**
- Entrapped small nerve twigs are often found

Differential diagnosis: Schwannoma is intraneural, encapsulated, and shows Verocay bodies and hyalinized vessels.

Intraneural NF (a plexiform arrangement of encapsulated extraneural NFs)

This is a circumscribed plexiform tumor in the fibrofat tissue.

- Interlacing bundles and fascicles of markedly expanded nerves are organized in a plexiform architecture (see Photomnemonic 5.4 in soft tissue tumors) **(Figure 5.122)**
- Axons and tightly packed Schwann cells are arranged along the long axis of the nerve; myxoid fibrous matrix of fibroblasts and mast cells
- Each intraneural NF is surrounded by thick perineurium
- The stroma in the dermis is edematous

> NB 5% may transform to malignant peripheral nerve sheath tumors.

NB Diffuse (extraneural) and intraneural neurofibromas can be seen in the same specimen and are called **paraneurofibromas**.

TRUE NERVE SHEATH TUMORS

SCHWANNOMAS

Schwannomas are intraneural encapsulated tumors in the deep dermis made of Schwann cells only, and no axons.

- The Schwann cells proliferate within the nerve fiber and displace the rest of its components to the periphery.
- The displaced axial bundle in the compressed nerve is the cause of the common pain.
- **Antoni A:** Solid proliferation of Schwann cells whose nuclei are arranged back to back in compact fascicles **(Figure 5.123A)**
- Two nuclear palisades and the enclosed cytoplasmic processes form the Verocay body **(Figure 5.123B)**
- **Antoni B:** Cystic myxoid edematous stroma as a feature of degeneration

NB Schwannomas may show dilated congested vessels with fibrinoid necrosis and hyalinized thrombi as well as foamy histiocytes and lymphoid cells.

NB **Clue:** look for nerve origin at the periphery of the lesion.

Differential diagnosis: PEN has axons and clefts among the fascicles and the silver stains are positive.

Types of schwannoma

- **Plexiform**
  - Schwann cells form interconnecting fascicles and nodules in a plexiform arrangement
  - Mimics plexiform neurofibroma but has Antoni A
- **Cellular**
  - Closely packed Schwann cells
  - May show cellular atypia and mitoses (up to two mitoses per high power field)

Differential diagnosis: Leiomyoma (schwannoma is S100-positive, desmin- and SMA-negative)

- **Epithelioid**
  - A zone of sclerosis (collagenous spherulosis) surrounded by a zone of palisading epithelioid cells
- **Glandular** (forming gland-like structures)
- **Psammomatous melanocytic schwannoma**
  - Part of Carney's complex (myxomas of the skin and the heart, lentiginosis, and endocrine over-reactivity)
  - Psammoma bodies and dendritic melanocytes
- **Intraneural microscopic schwannomatosis:** Schwannomas arising in NFs

NERVE SHEATH MYXOMA (NSM) AND NEUROTHEKEOMA (NTK)

These are neuromesenchymal tumors characterized by proliferation of nerve sheath cells in myxoid stroma.

NB The cells are immature with multiple lines of differentiation.

- **NSM:** Hypocellular tumor of slender bipolar cells in ample stroma
- **Cellular neurothekeoma:** Hypercellular tumor of plump cells in scant stroma

NSM

- Well-defined lobules and fascicles of bipolar/stellate cells with hyperchromatic nuclei in a plexiform lobular arrangement **(Figure 5.124)**
- Peripheral fibrous border
- Whorls around vessels
- Lymphocytes may be present
- The stroma is myxoid

The cells can be negative for CD57 and NSE as they are immature; S100+

Cellular NTK

- Non-encapsulated tumor which shows an infiltrative pattern
- Fascicular/nodular/plexiform/nested arrangement of plump epithelioid cells with large ovoid nuclei in scant myxoid stroma **(Figure 5.125)**
- Spindle-shaped and stellate cells are common too

S100- negative, NK1/C3-positive; MART-1 is always negative

MALIGNANT PERIPHERAL NERVE SHEATH TUMOR

Other names include neurofibrosarcoma and malignant schwannoma.

The tumor arises *de novo* or in neurofibromatosis type 1 from plexiform neurofibromas.

It shows mesenchymal differentiation of different phenotypic populations including spindle, epithelioid, osteoid, and rhabdomyoid cells:

- Variable pleomorphism and mitotic activity
- Patterns:
  - *Mesenchymal:* Light and dark fascicles of spindle cells arranged radially/concentrically around vessels; areas of necrosis
  - *Epithelioid/glandular:* Usually in MPNST of high-grade atypia arising *de novo*. Areas of necrosis with concentric palisade of plump epithelioid cells; matrix is scant or absent

Immunohistochemistry: 40–80% are positive for S100; increased expression of Ki67 correlates with decreased survival

Differential diagnosis: Fibrosarcoma, MFH, melanoma, leiomyosarcoma, rhabdomyosarcoma

MISCELLANEOUS

Granular cell tumor

NB The cell of origin is undecided: most argue for Schwann cell origin (previous name granular cell schwannoma).

- A non-encapsulated ill-defined "pale" infiltrating proliferation
- Irregularly arranged sheets of large polyhedral cells which show small hyperchromatic nuclei and coarse granular cytoplasm **(Figure 5.126A)**
- The cytoplasm appears vesicular due to PAS-positive pink granules surrounded by halo (pustulo-ovoid bodies) **(Figure 5.126B)**
- The cells have indistinct cytoplasmic membranes
- They infiltrate the collagen bundles and may surround appendages and nerves
- Pseudoepitheliomatous hyperplasia is possible

Immunohistochemistry: S100+, CD68+, CD57+, NSE+, PGP 9.5+, NKI/C3+

Differential diagnosis: Reticulohistiocytoma is also a pale tumor but the histiocytes have ground glass (homogenous, not granular) cytoplasm.

Merkell cell carcinoma

A primary cutaneous neuroendocrine carcinoma: originates from a primitive epidermal stem cell which differentiates towards neuroendocrine cells and keratinocytes.

Nodules and sheets of round blue cells occupy the dermis and sometimes extend in the fat **(Figure 5.127A)**.

- There are three growth patterns: 1) in sheets, 2) nested, and 3) trabecular **(Figure 5.127B)**
- The cells are usually 2–3 times bigger than a lymphocyte; they show pleomorphism with hyperchromatic nuclei and speckled chromatin (finely granular, "salt-and-pepper") **(Figure 5.127C)**
- Mitotic figures and apoptotic debris give "the starry sky pattern" on low power
- Epidermotropism is possible
- Coexistence with SCC (*in situ* or invasive) is possible

Immunohistochemistry: CK20 positive (a perinuclear dot); TTF1 negative (this combination differentiates from metastatic small cell lung carcinoma). Other positive stains: NSE, CD57, chromogranin, synaptophysin. S100 negative

NB Features associated with worse prognosis:

- Small cell size
- >10 mitoses/single high power field
- Angiolymphatic invasion
- CD44+

CUTANEOUS METASTASES

Andrew Miner and Mariya Miteva

Definition: Malignant cells in the skin originating from an internal cancer. In most cases skin metastases appear in patients with a history of known primary internal malignancy and late in the course of the disease (metachronous metastases).

General concepts

- The most common skin metastasis in men before the age of 40 is melanoma and after the age of 40 is lung cancer followed by colon cancer.
- The most common skin metastasis in women of any age is breast cancer followed by colon cancer.
- Cutaneous metastases are most common on the head and neck, trunk, and upper extremities, and least common on lower extremities. Recent research found that sites with more frequent metastases contain a higher density of regulatory T-cells and a lower density of CD8+ T-cells.
- Skin metastases are found usually in the vicinity of the primary tumor.

NB Note, however, that only the breast and the umbilicus have shown co-localization with the primary cancer.

On low power

- Skin metastases usually resemble the primary malignancy but they tend to be more anaplastic and poorly differentiated.
- There is usually a Grenz zone.

NB Melanoma, breast cancer, and extramammary Paget's disease are epidermotropic

- Immunohistochemical studies are utilized for the diagnosis (see below and Chapter 1).

- Several pathologic patterns exist:
  - *Infiltrative (Indian file):* The cells are usually dyscohesive and arranged in a single line between the collagen bundles.
  - *Intravascular/intralymphatic invasion:* Cancer cells are detected inside the vascular lumina
  - *Nodular:* Compact masses of neoplastic cells in the dermis are separated by a Grenz zone.
  - *Diffuse:* There are sheets or columns of neoplastic cells among the collagen bundles.

On high power

ADENOCARCINOMA

Adenocarcinoma is a malignancy from epithelial tissue with glandular origin, glandular characteristics, or both, and is the most common cutaneous metastasis (60%). **(Table 5.15)**

Lung cancer

See below

Breast cancer

- Common metastasis to skin
- Angular (cuboidal) cells with pale cytoplasm commonly arranged in nests, cords, and single files **(Figure 5.128A)**
- Sheets or large clusters of tumor cells in the dermis **(Figure 5.128B)**
- Ductal structures sometimes visible in metastatic ductal carcinoma
- In inflammatory breast cancer, tumor cells plug cutaneous lymphatics (D2-40 highlights the lymphatics) **(Figure 5.128C, D)**

Immunohistochemistry:

- Mammaglobin, GCDFP-15, and GATA3 positivity strongly supports the diagnosis
- ER, PR are of low specificity but together with HER-2/neu guide treatment and prognosis

Ovarian cancer

- Very rare metastasis to skin
- Well-differentiated adenocarcinoma with ductal formation involves the dermis
- Signet ring formation is possible

Prostate cancer

- Very rare metastasis to skin (when present typically late-stage finding with widespread disease already known)
- Undifferentiated cells partially arranged in glands, strands, and cords **(Figure 5.129)**
- Single files
- Necrosis

Colon cancer

- Rare metastasis to skin
- Ductal formation
- "Dirty" necrosis with abscess formation **(Figure 5.130)**

Table 5.15 Immunohistochemical patterns in the most common metastatic adenocarcinomas

Cutaneous metastasis	Histologic features	Positive immunohistochemical stains	Negative immunohistochemical stains
Lung	Non-specific in skin Ductal structures in non-small cell adenocarcinoma	CK7, CEA, TTF-1, Cam5.2	CK20, CK5/6
Breast	Single file Ductal structures	CK7, GATA3, mammaglobin, GCDFP-15 ER and PR (+/–) CEA	CK20, CK5/6
Prostate	Often poorly differentiated in skin	PSA, proPSA, NKX3.1	CK7, CK20
Colon	"Dirty" necrosis and abscess formation Ductal formation	CK20, CEA, CDX2	CK7
Ovarian	May have signet ring cells (eccentric nuclei compressed by the cytoplasm)	CA125, CK7, CEA, PAX8	CK20 (except for mucinous variant)
Gastric	May have signet ring cells	CEA, EMA, CDX2	CK20 (about 60% negative)
Pancreas	Non-specific in skin	CEA, CK7, CA19.9	CK20

SQUAMOUS CELL CARCINOMA (SCC)

This is malignancy of the epithelial cells or cells showing particular cytological or tissue architectural characteristics of squamous-cell differentiation such as lips, mouth, lung, esophagus, urinary bladder, prostate, and others.

Most common cutaneous metastases are from: 1) head and neck cancer, and 2) primary cutaneous SCC metastatic to skin.

Main histologic features:
- Lack of connection to overlying epidermis **(Figure 5.131A)**
- Atypical large angulated eosinophilic cells with prominent nucleoli (if well-differentiated)
- Increased nuclear:cytoplasmic ratio **(Figure 5.131B)**

Immunohistochemistry is often essential in more poorly differentiated spindle cell metastases.

OTHER METASTASES

Small cell lung carcinoma

- 30% of cutaneous lung metastases
- Small round blue cell tumor
- The neoplastic cells are arranged in nests or in a trabecular pattern **(Figure 5.132)**

Immunohistochemistry helps to distinguish from primary or metastatic Merkel cell carcinoma (MCC):
- Positive for keratin (AE1/3)
- About 90% positive for thyroid transcription factor-1 (TTF-1)
- Negative for CK20
- Negative for Merkel cell polyomavirus (MCPyV)

Melanoma

- Skin is a common metastatic site for melanoma
- Lack of overlying connection to epidermis common

Renal Cell Carcinoma (Rcc)

- Rare metastases to skin (in 8%); scalp is a common site
- Most carcinomas develop from the proximal tubular epithelium
- Clear cell changes due to content of glycogen and lipids **(Figure 5.133)**
- Prominent vessels ("chicken-wire" vasculature), red blood cell extravasation, and hemosiderin deposition **(Photomnemonic 5.25)**

Immunohistochemistry:
- PAX8 positive (but also positive in ovarian and uterine cancers)
- CD10 (up to 100% expression)
- RCC-Ma (monoclonal antibody against a proximal tubule antigen is highly specific for RCC and is positive in about 60–70% of cases)

Soft tissue sarcomas

- Rare metastases to skin (2–3%)
- Undifferentiated pleomorphic sarcoma:
  - Atypical infiltrate often with bizarre nuclear features, atypical mitoses, and spindled areas **(Figure 5.134)**
  - Lack of immunohistochemical stains or specific markers allowing for precise diagnosis

Differential diagnosis includes pleomorphic dermal sarcoma (similar features to atypical fibroxanthoma but deeper invasive growth pattern).

Leiomyosarcoma

- Important to differentiate from primary cutaneous leiomyosarcoma (atypical intradermal smooth muscle neoplasm)
- Metastatic leiomyosarcoma is typically more atypical, deeper, and larger than its primary cutaneous counterpart (See Figure 5.53)

Metastatic neural tumors

- Malignant peripheral nerve sheath tumor
- Diffuse S-100 positivity
- Differential diagnosis includes melanoma
- Precursor plexiform neurofibroma helps make the diagnosis

Mimickers of metastatic tumors

Omphalomesenteric duct remnant

- Goblet cells and other features of intestinal or gastric mucosa with adjacent epidermis (sometimes acanthotic)
- Duct formation
- Formerly mistaken for the so-called Sister Mary Joseph node, representing metastatic adenocarcinoma to the umbilicus

KERATINOCYTIC TUMORS (TUMORS OF THE EPIDERMIS)

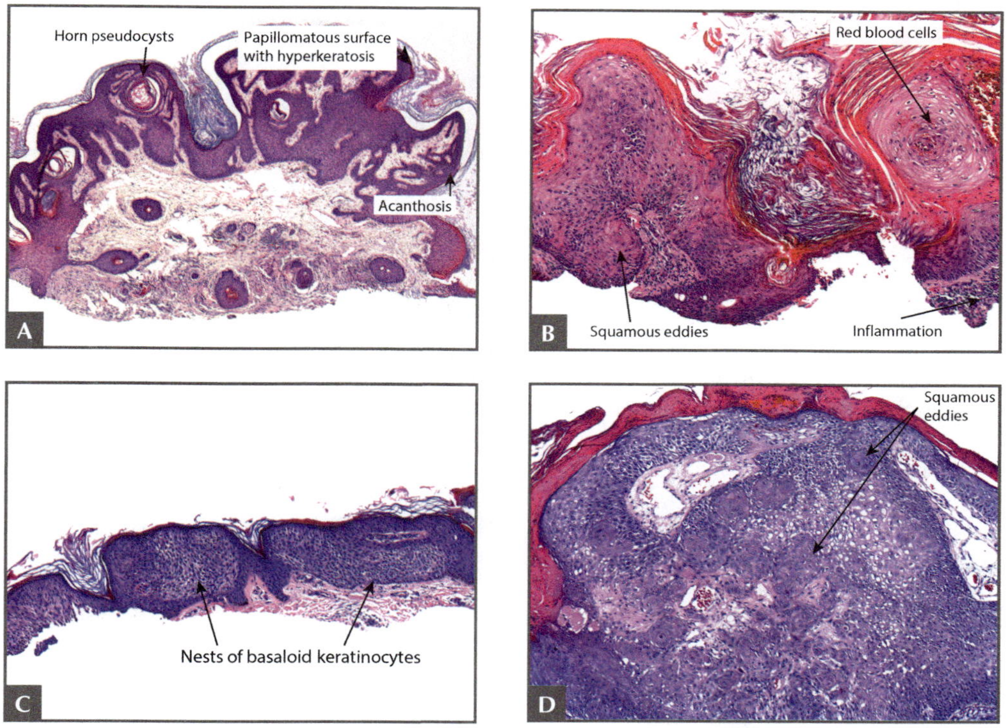

Figure 5.1 Seborrheic keratosis (SK). **A** Acanthotic SK. Note the polypoid papillomatous silhouette. **B** Inflamed SK. Note the presence of inflammation, squamous eddies, hemorrhage. **C** Clonal SK. **D** Inverted follicular keratosis. Note the endophytic growth and the presence of many squamous eddies.

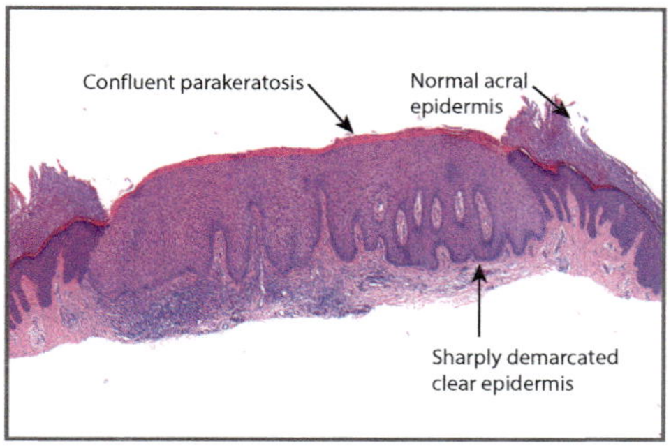

Figure 5.2 Clear cell acanthoma. The lesion stands out as a sharply demarked area of pale epidermis.

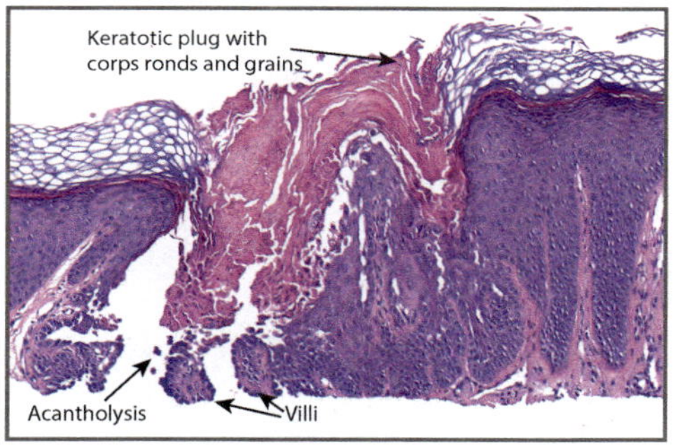

Figure 5.3 Warty dyskeratoma. There is a cystic cavity filled with hyperkeratosis and parakeratosis and lined by epithelial layer showing suprabasal acantholysis and villi.

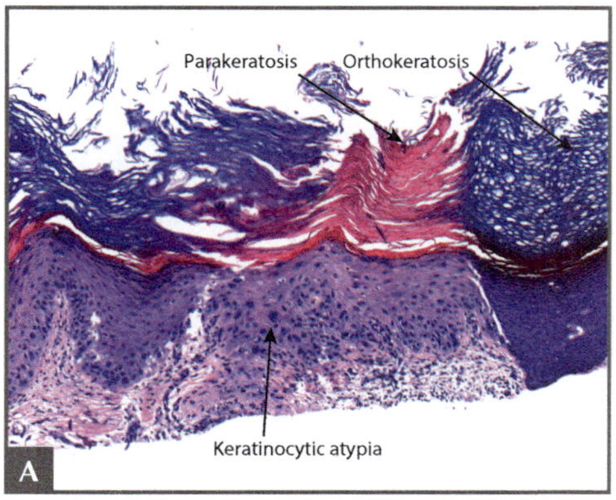

Figure 5.4 Actinic keratosis. **A** Note the keratinocytic atypia and the pink and blue pattern.

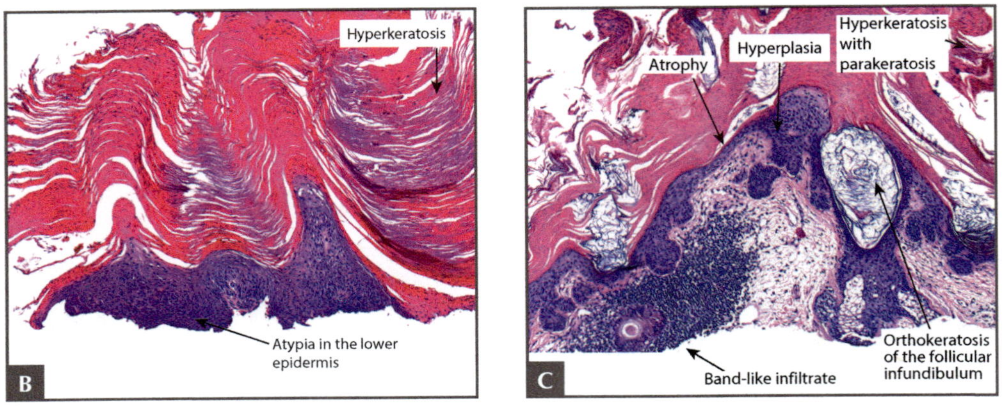

Figure 5.4 Actinic keratosis. **B** Hypertrophic actinic keratosis. **C** Note the band-like infiltrate and the loss of cellular polarity in the lower epidermis (disorganized teardrop-like keratinocytes). There is alternating epidermal atrophy and hyperplasia.

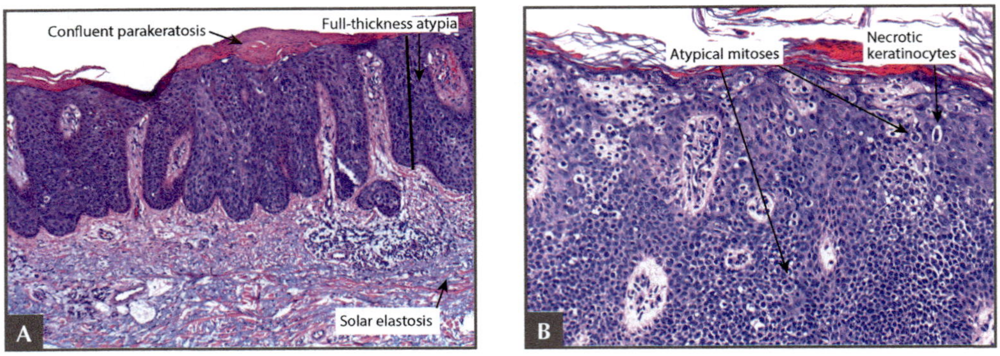

Figure 5.5 Bowen's disease. **A** Epidermal hyperplasia with transepidermal cytologic atypia. **B** Note the full thickness atypia and the increased mitotic rate.

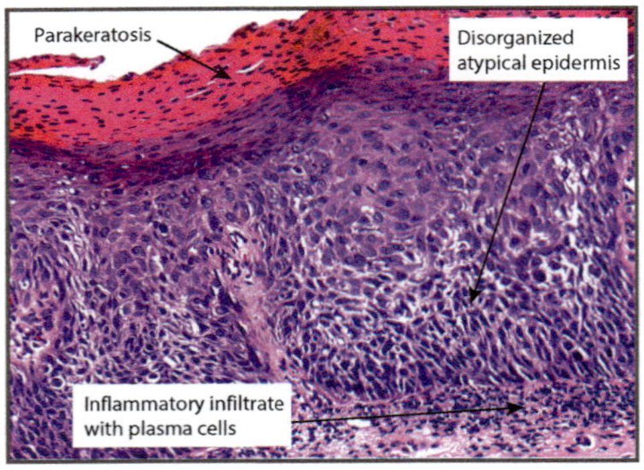

Figure 5.6 Erythroplasia of Queyrat. The features are similar to Bowen's disease.

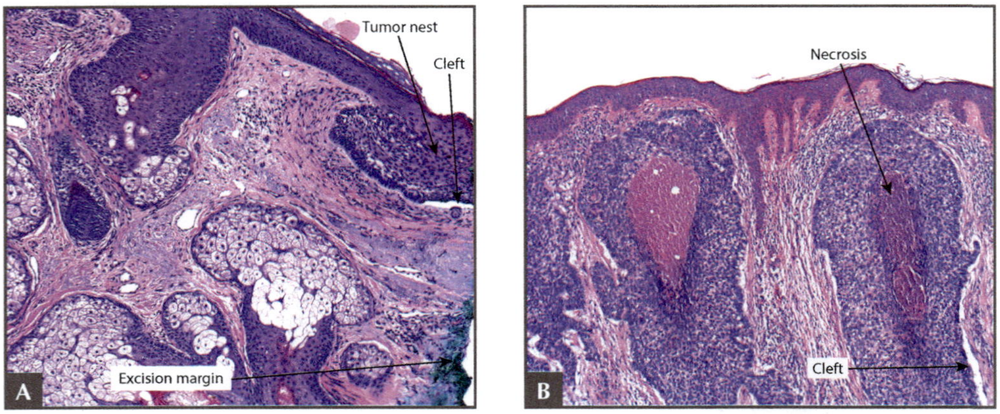

Figure 5.7 Basal cell carcinoma. **A** Superficial BCC involving the excisional margin. **B** Nodular BCC. Note the central necrosis in the big tumor islands.

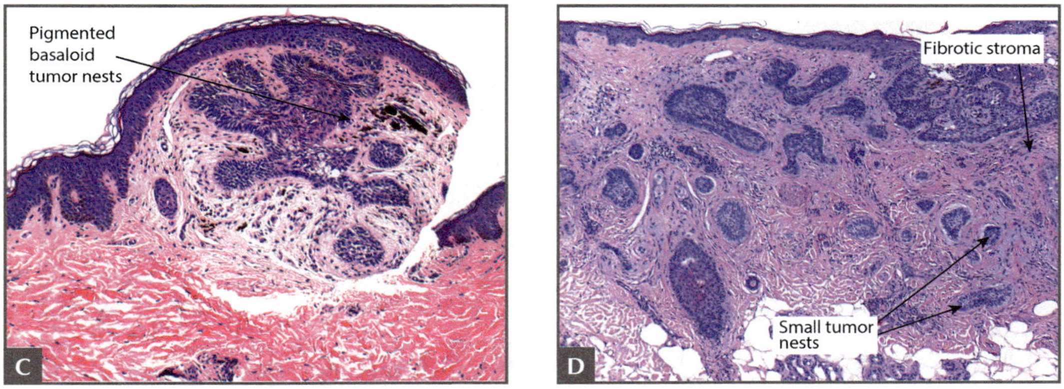

Figure 5.7 Basal cell carcinoma. **C** Pigmented polypoid nodular BCC in a child with basal cell nevus syndrome. **D** Micronodular BCC. Note the small round tumor nests infiltrating the dermis. The stroma is fibrotic.

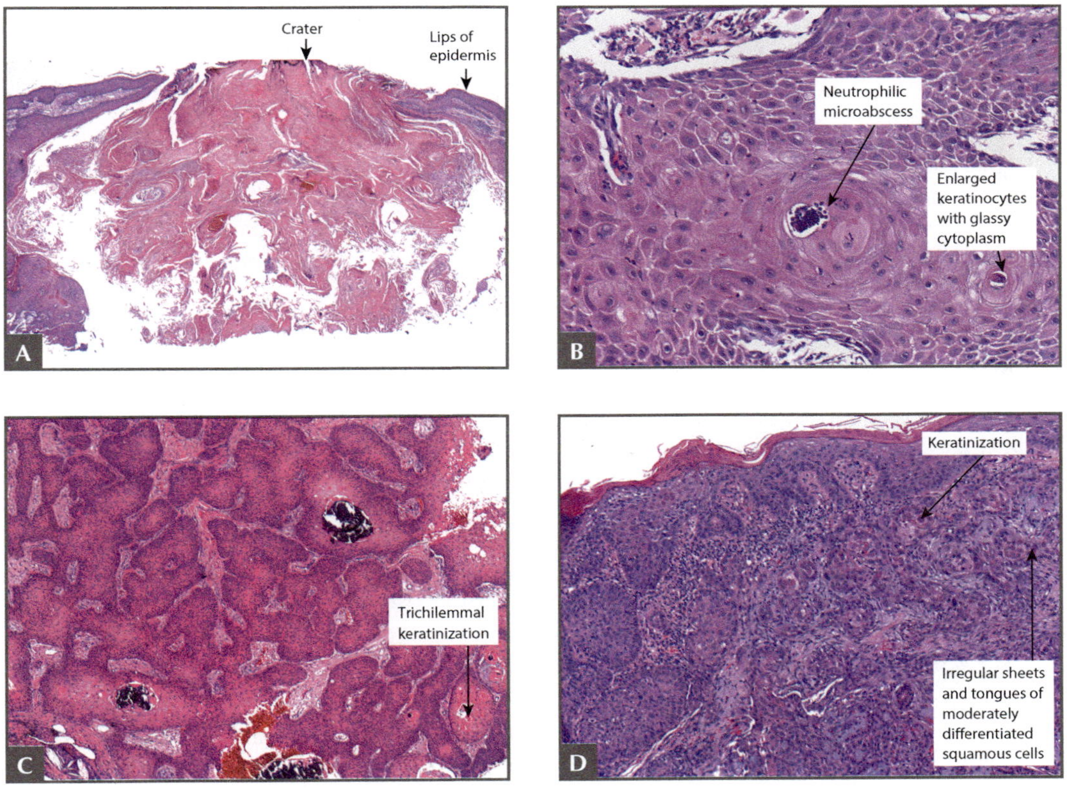

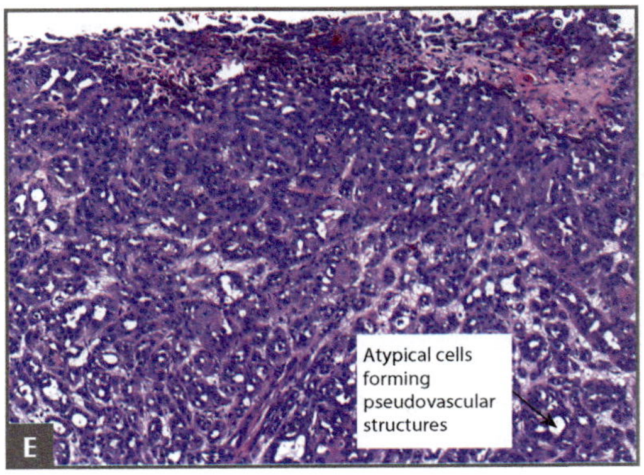

Figure 5.8 Keratoacanthoma-like SCC. **A** Note the crateriform silhouette. **B** Atypical keratinocytes with glassy cytoplasm in the dermis. **C** Well-differentiated SCC. Note the uniform "pink" irregular tongues of well-differentiated squamous cells and foci of keratinization. **D** Moderately differentiated SCC. The tumor shows only focal keratinization. **E** Adenoid/pseudovascular SCC. There are no features of keratinization. The tumor arrangement mimics angiosarcoma.

CYSTS

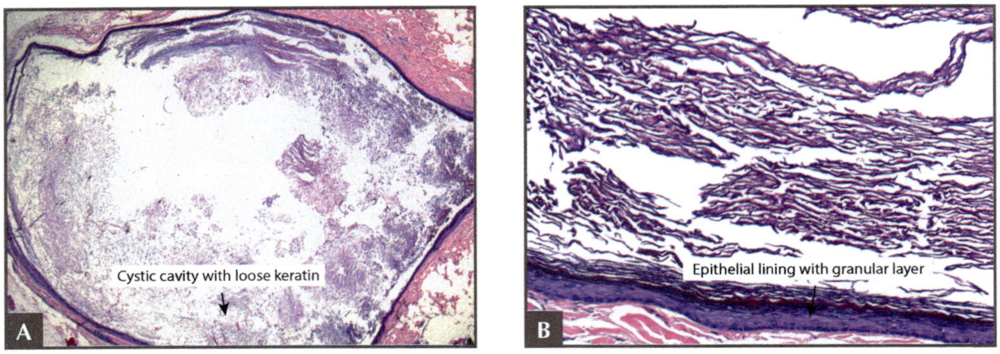

Figure 5.9 Epidermoid cyst. **A** Note the dilated cavity with loose keratin. **B** The wall of the same cyst shows stratified epidermal lining with preserved granular layer.

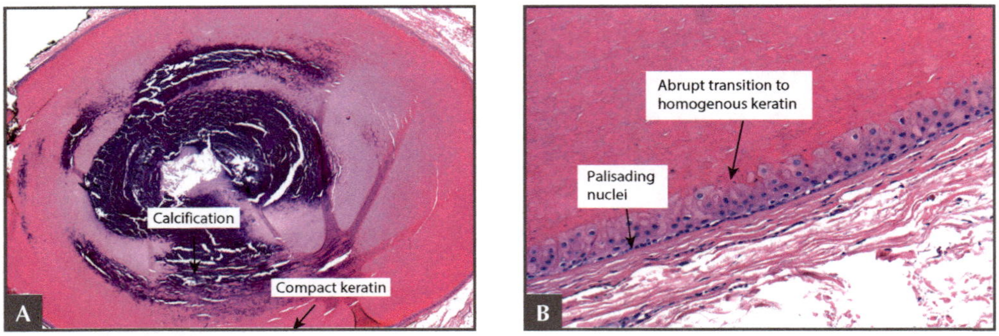

Figure 5.10 Trichilemmal cyst. **A** Homogenous pink keratin with focal calcification. **B** The wall of the same cyst shows abrupt keratinization without a granular layer.

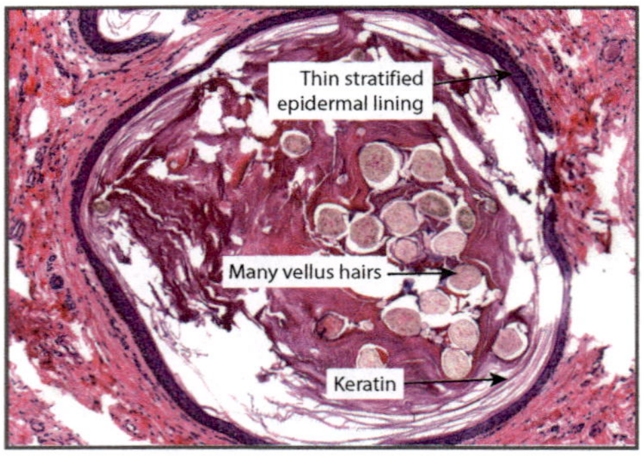

Figure 5.11 Vellus hair cyst.

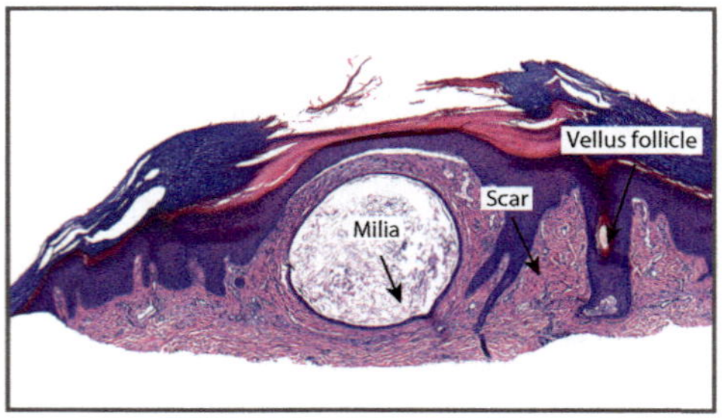

Figure 5.12 Milia on acral skin. This milia has developed secondarily within a scar in a patient with epidermolysis bullosa.

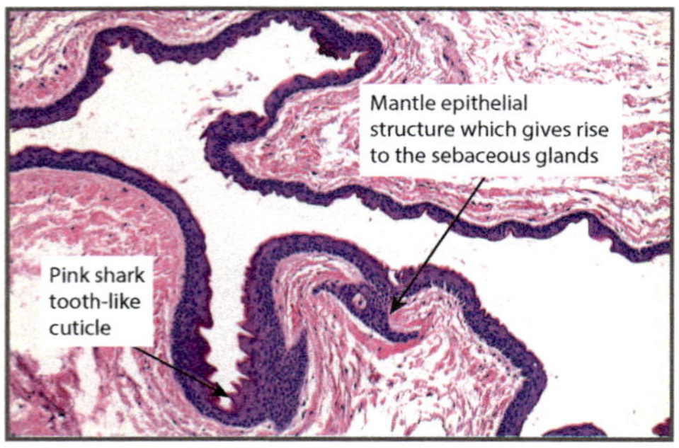

Figure 5.13 Steatocystoma simplex. Note the peculiar serpiginous silhouette compared to the round shape of the epidermoid cyst, the milia, and the vellus hair cyst.

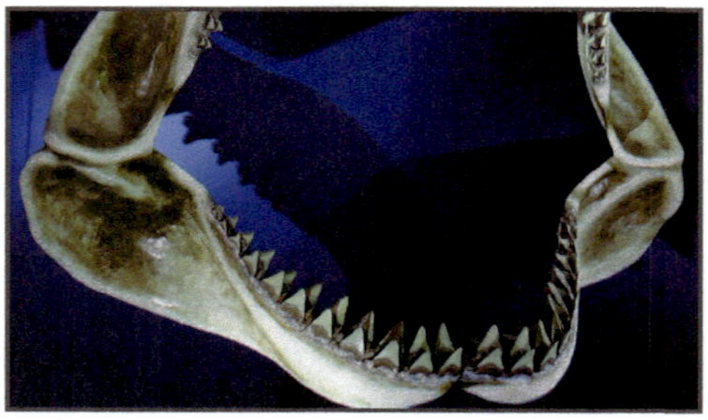

Photomnemonic 5.1 The cuticle in steatocystoma is similar to the sharp teeth in the shark's mouth.

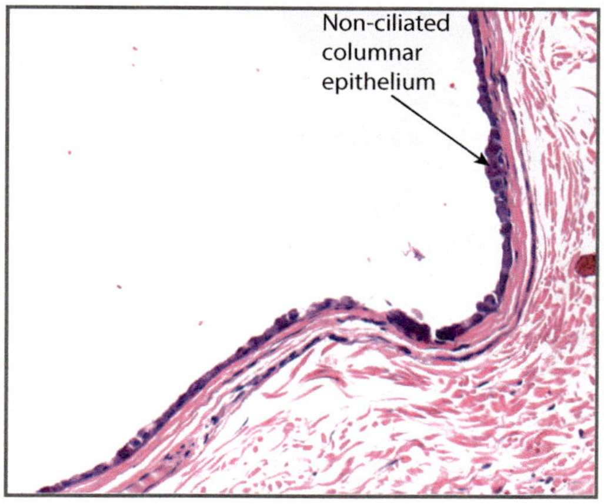

Figure 5.14 Bronchogenic cyst.

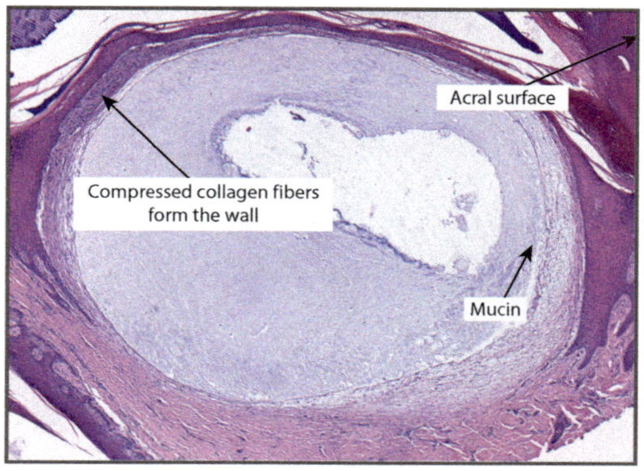

Figure 5.15 Digital mucous cyst: a cystic cavity lined by thin collagen fibers and filled with mucin.

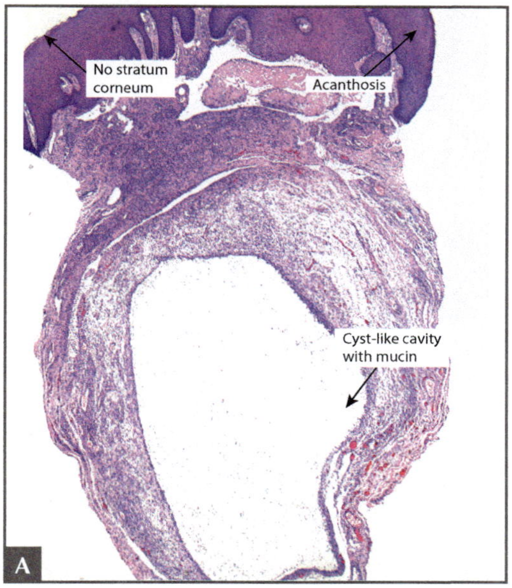

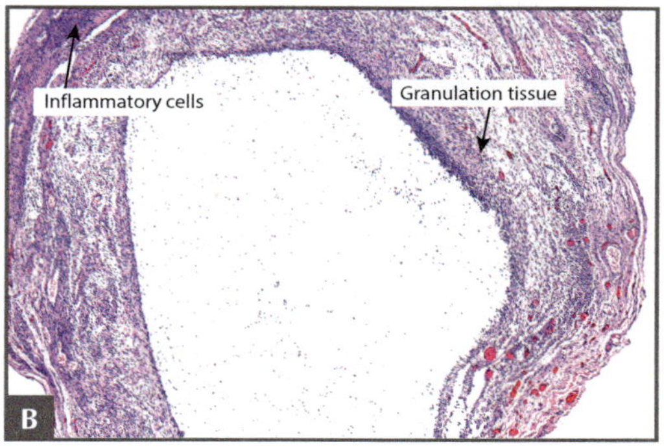

Figure 5.16 Mucocele. **A** Note the mucosal surface and presence of a cyst-like cavity with mucin in the dermis. **B** The wall of the same lesion is lined by granulation tissue and is surrounded by inflammatory cells.

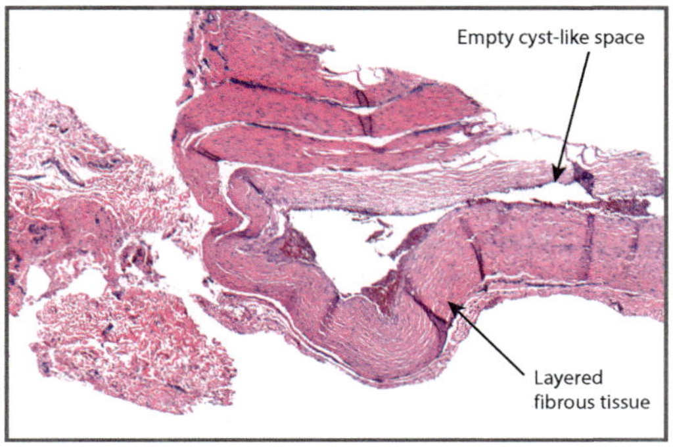

Figure 5.17 Ganglion cyst. Note the thick fibrous tissue surrounding an empty cyst-like space.

SOFT TISSUE TUMORS

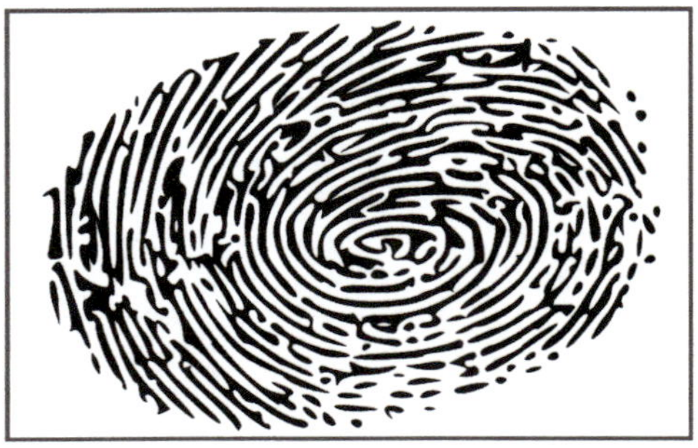

Photomnemonic 5.2 The whorled pattern resembles the concentric arrangement of the dermatoglyphs.

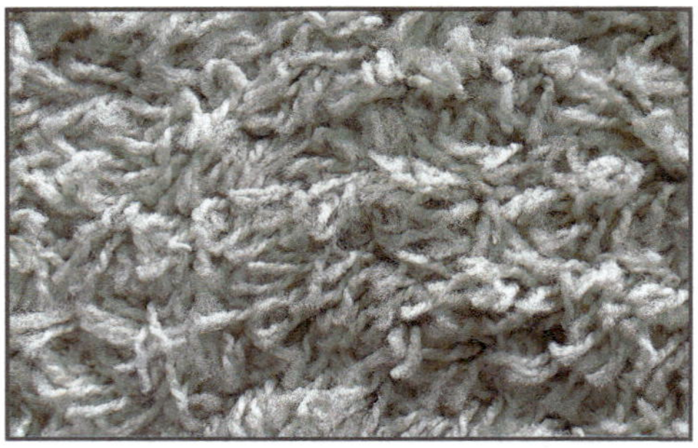

Photomnemonic 5.3 The storiform pattern shows the irregular, chaotic arrangement of the fascicles, like in this rug.

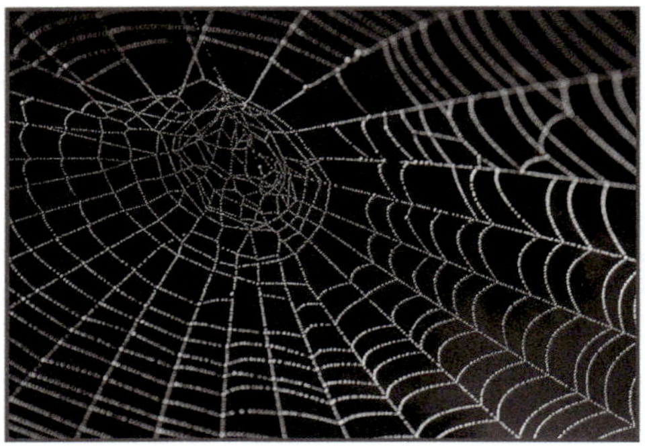

Photomnemonic 5.4 The plexiform pattern resembles the fiber arrangement in a web.

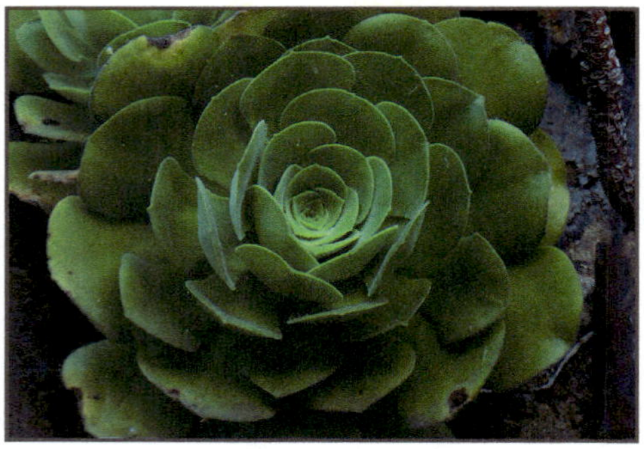

Photomnemonic 5.5 In a rosette-like pattern the cells are arranged in layers in a concentric pattern, as in this *Sempervivum*.

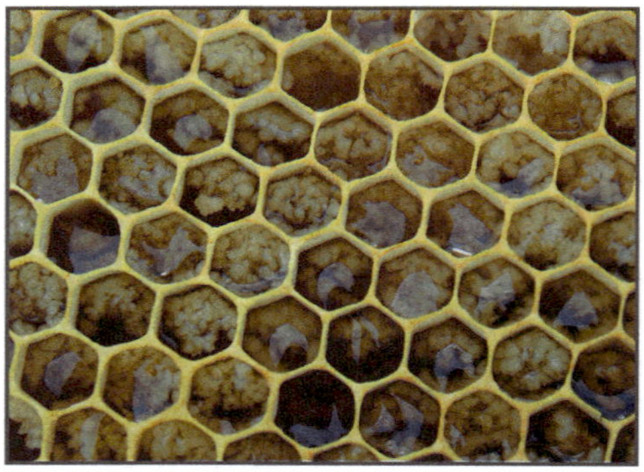

Photomnemonic 5.6 Honeycomb pattern: the cells resemble the adipocytes.

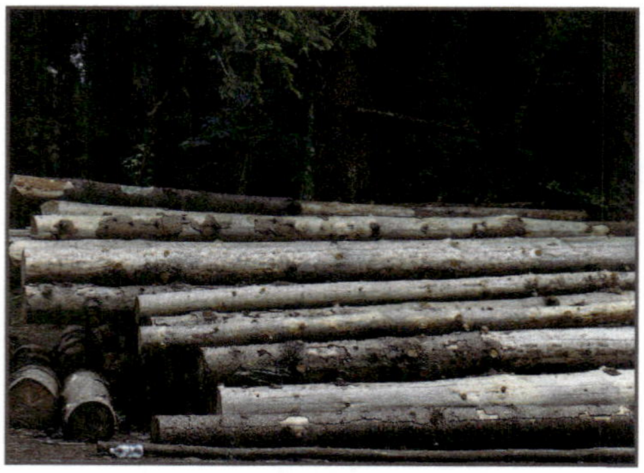

Photomnemonic 5.7 The fascicular pattern resembles a stack of logs.

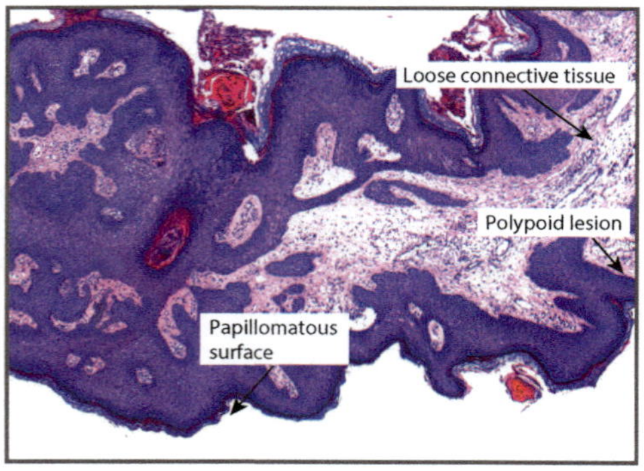

Figure 5.18 Acrochordon.

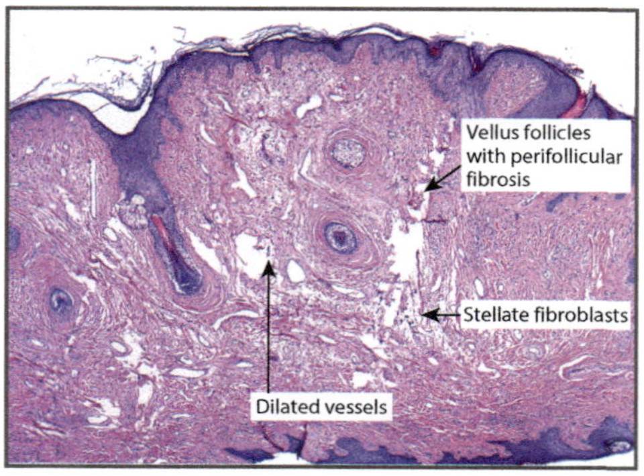

Figure 5.19 Fibrous papule.

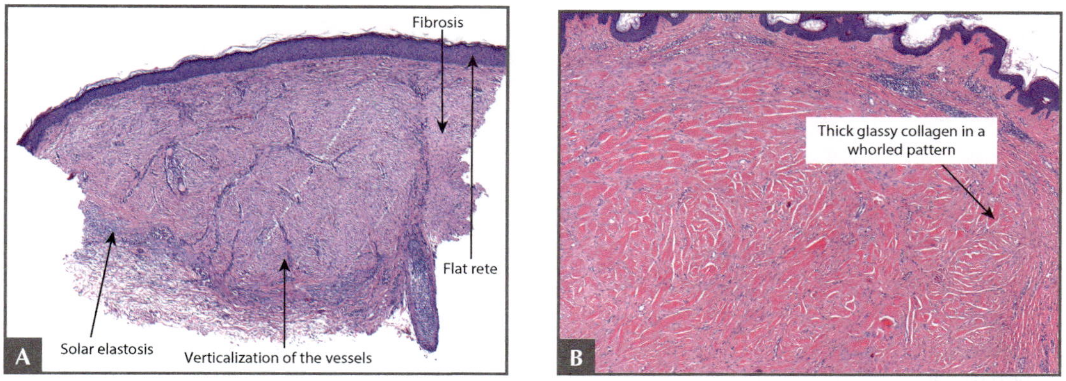

Figure 5.20 A Hypertrophic scar. Note the whorled pattern and the predominant fibrosis over collagen in the dermis which pushes the solar elastosis down and to the side. **B** Keloid. Note the hypocellular thick collagenous stroma. No vessels are noted.

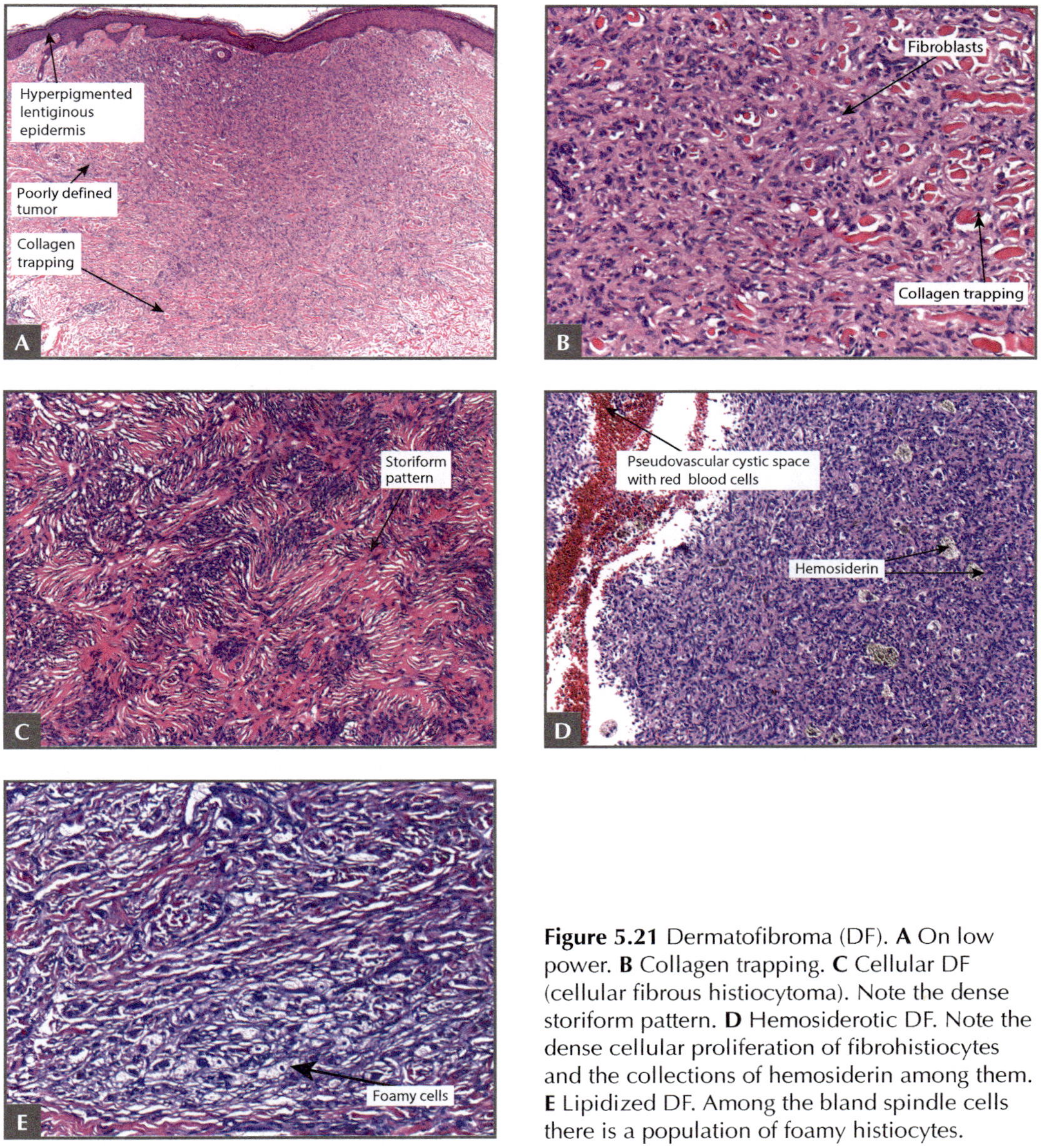

Figure 5.21 Dermatofibroma (DF). **A** On low power. **B** Collagen trapping. **C** Cellular DF (cellular fibrous histiocytoma). Note the dense storiform pattern. **D** Hemosiderotic DF. Note the dense cellular proliferation of fibrohistiocytes and the collections of hemosiderin among them. **E** Lipidized DF. Among the bland spindle cells there is a population of foamy histiocytes.

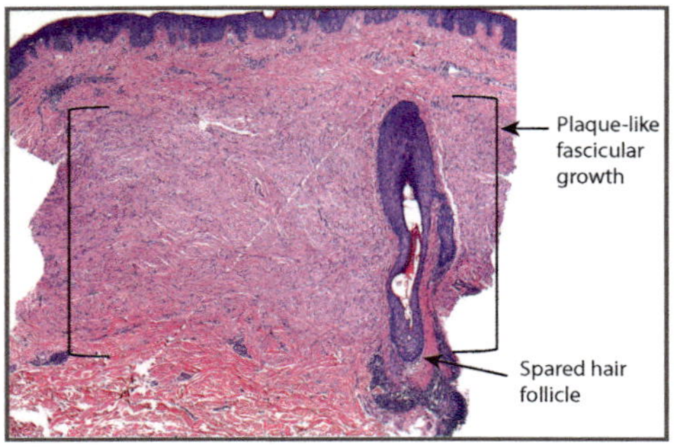

Figure 5.22 Dermatomyofibroma. Note the horizontal plaque-like proliferation of spindle cells.

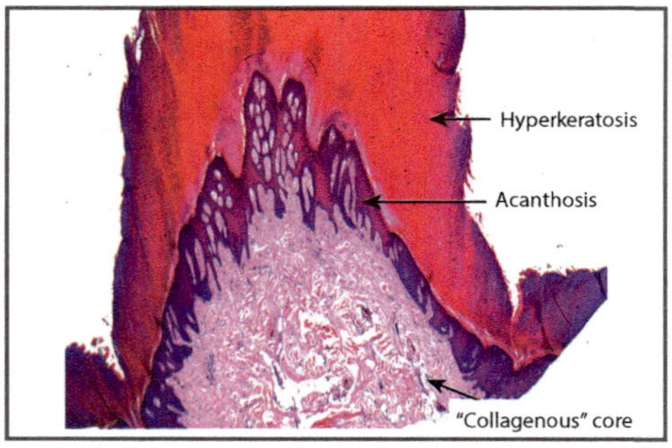

Figure 5.23 Dome-shaped lesion of acquired digital fibrokeratoma (ADFK) on acral skin with collagenous core.

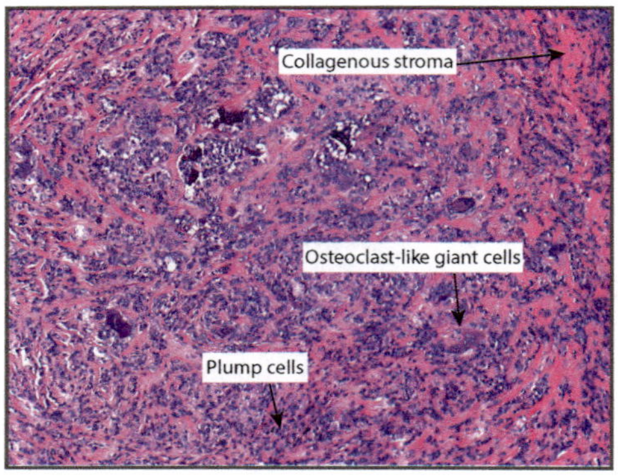

Figure 5.24 Giant cell tumor of the tendon sheath. Note the osteoclast-like giant cells.

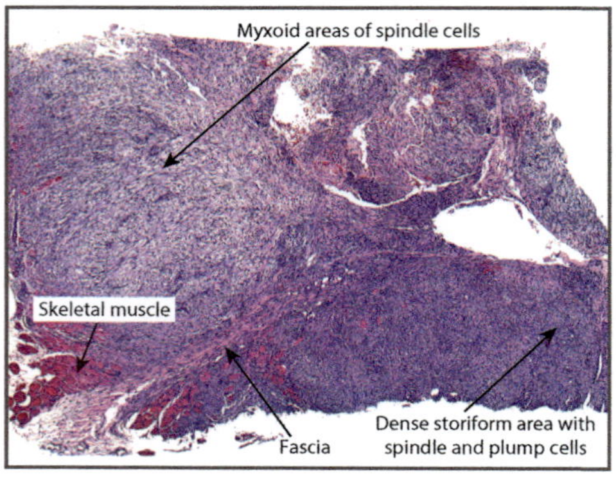

Figure 5.25 A case of proliferative fasciitis. Note the poorly demarcated subcutaneous fibrohistiocytic proliferation.

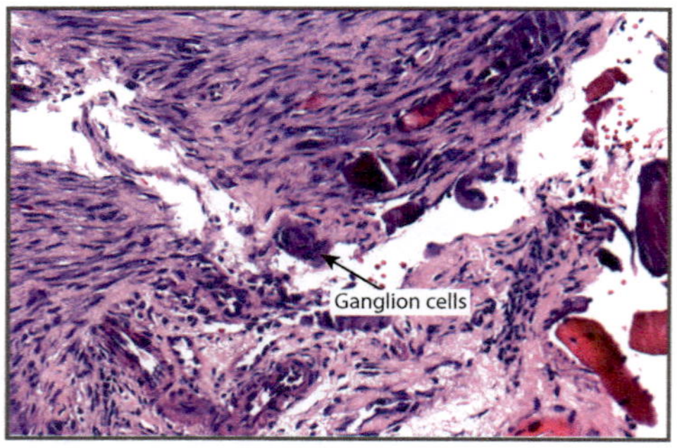

Figure 5.26 Ganglion-like cells on high power in the same case of proliferative fasciitis as Figure 5.25. No mitoses and no atypia can be seen.

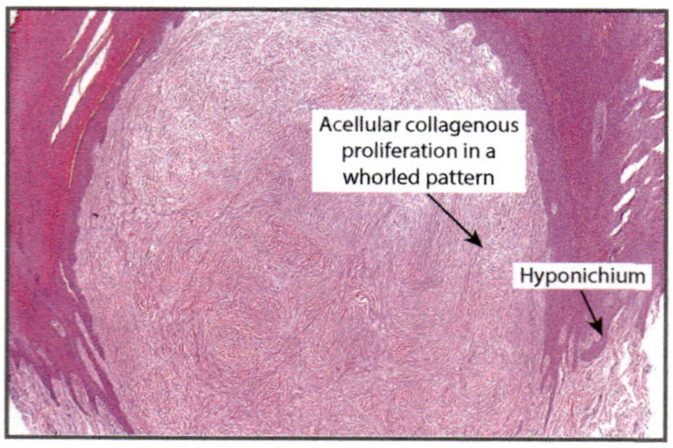

Figure 5.27 Subungual sclerotic fibroma presenting as an acellular eosinophilic mass.

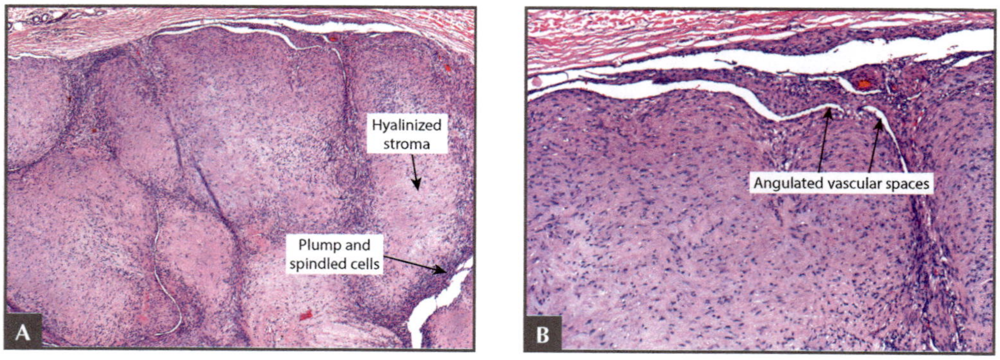

Figure 5.28 Myofibroma. **A** Note the lobular plexiform pattern. The lesion is pale due to the hyalinization of the collagen in the lobules surrounded by more cellular proliferation at the periphery. **B** Hemangiopericytoma area.

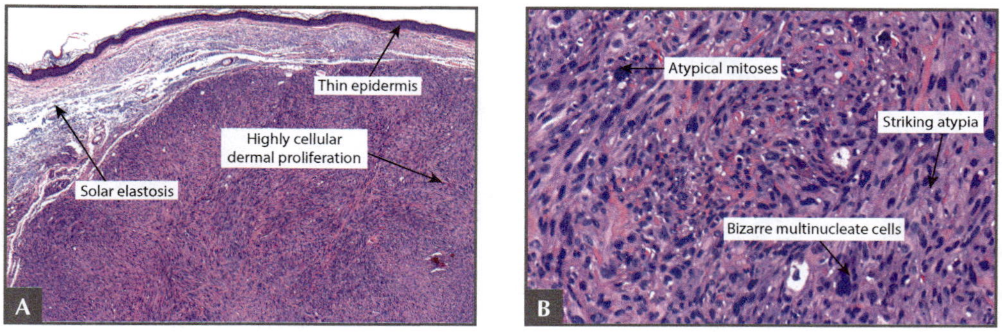

Figure 5.29 Atypical fibroxanthoma. **A** Note the circumscribed cellular proliferation of storiform pattern on sun-damaged skin. **B** Note the striking atypia and increased mitotic rate.

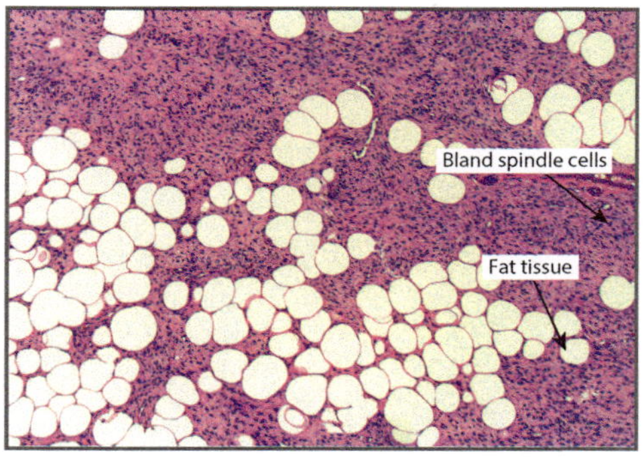

Figure 5.30 Dermatofibrosarcoma protuberans: honeycomb pattern.

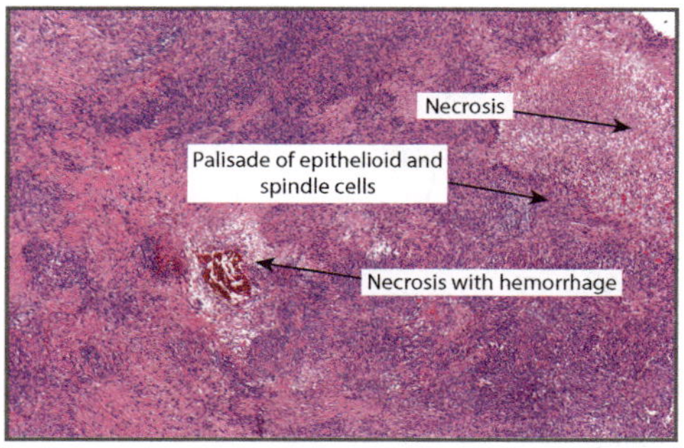

Figure 5.32 Epithelioid sarcoma. Note the geographic necrosis surrounded by fascicles of epithelioid and spindled cells.

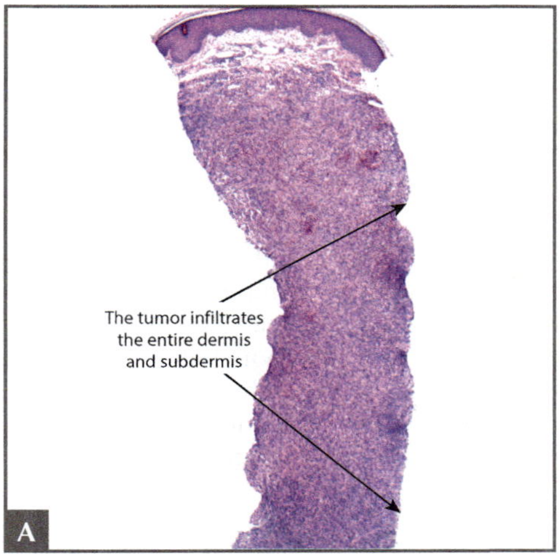

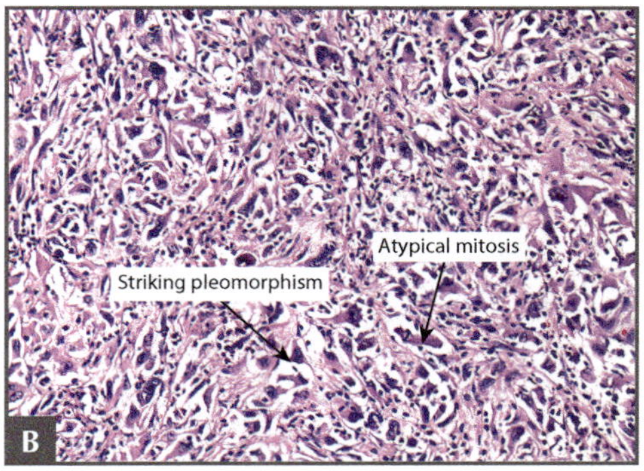

Figure 5.31 Pleomorphic dermal sarcoma (PDS). **A** Note the deep extension of the tumor. **B** Striking atypia and atypical mitoses.

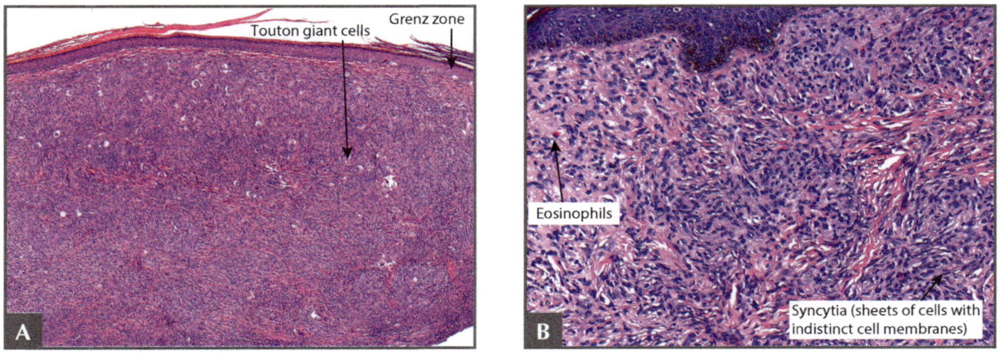

Figure 5.33 Xanthogranuloma. **A** There are numerous Touton giant cells. **B** A close-up view: note the presence of eosinophils.

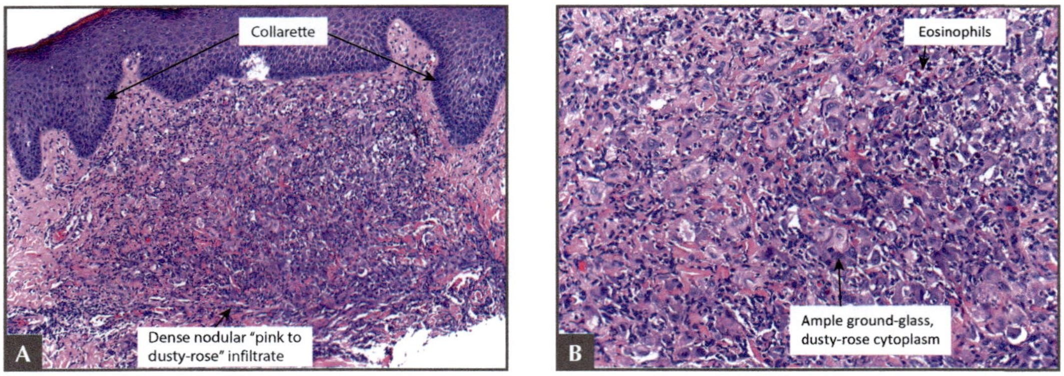

Figure 5.34 Reticulohystiocytoma. **A** Note the pink-to-dusty-rose color of the tumor. **B** A close-up view of the tumor cells: note the presence of eosinophils.

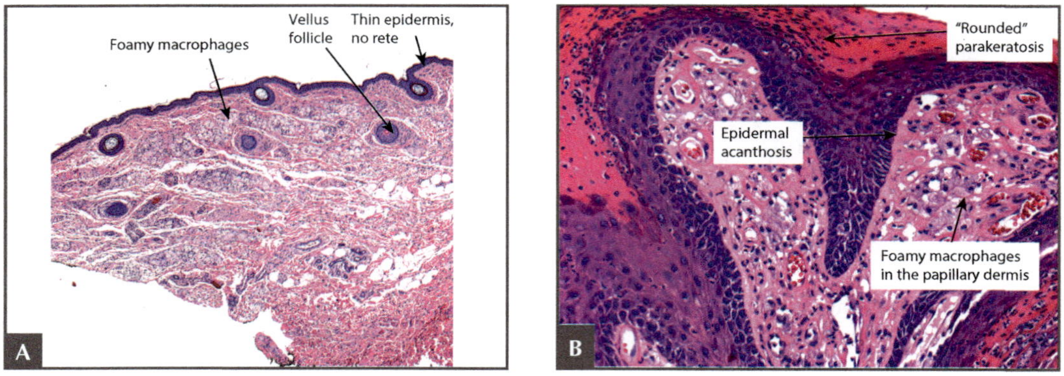

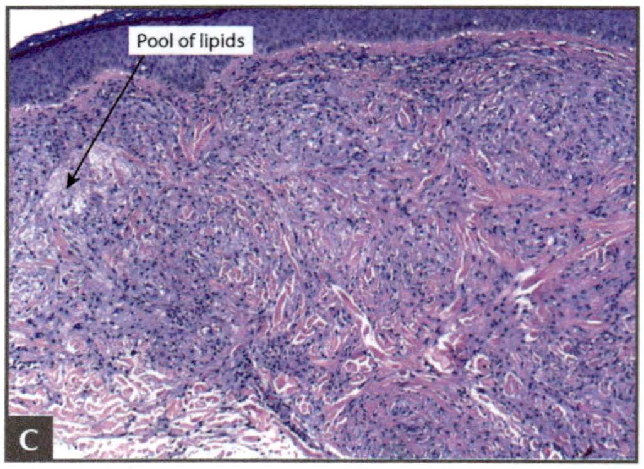

Figure 5.35 Xanthoma. **A** Xanthelasma. The thin epidermis devoid of rete, the vellus follicles, and the thin dermis are a clue to eyelid location. There are sheets of pale foamy macrophages in the dermis. **B** Verruciform xanthoma. This mucosal lesion shows a verruciform silhouette with collection of foamy macrophages foiling the papillae. **C** Eruptive xanthoma. The lesion appears pale due to accumulation of histiocytes. There is a pool of lipids in the dermis. This, together with the absence/decreased number of foamy macrophages, is a clue to the fast/eruptive nature of the lesion.

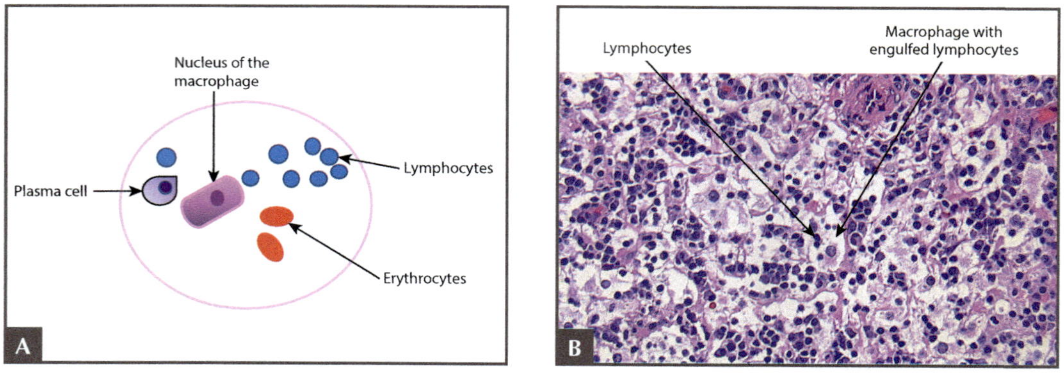

Figure 5.36 Rosai-Dorfman disease. **A** Emperipolesis in Rosai-Dorfman disease: intact cells within the cytoplasm of a macrophage. **B** Intact cells within the cytoplasm of a macrophage (Image courtesy of Gabriel Villada, MD).

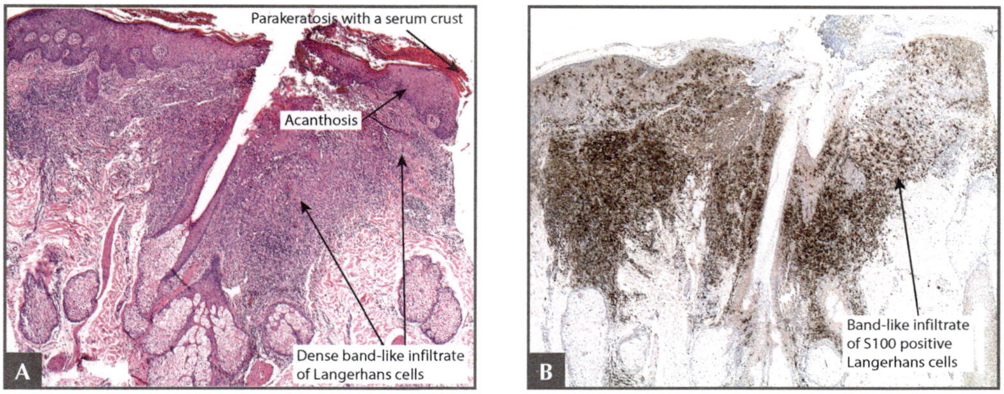

Figure 5.37 Langerhans cell histiocytosis (LCH) of the scalp. **A** Note the band-like infiltrate of Langerhans cells. (Image courtesy of Liliana Muñoz Garcia, MD.) **B** The same case stained with S100. The Langerhans cells can be found also in the epidermis. (Image courtesy of Liliana Muñoz Garcia, MD.)

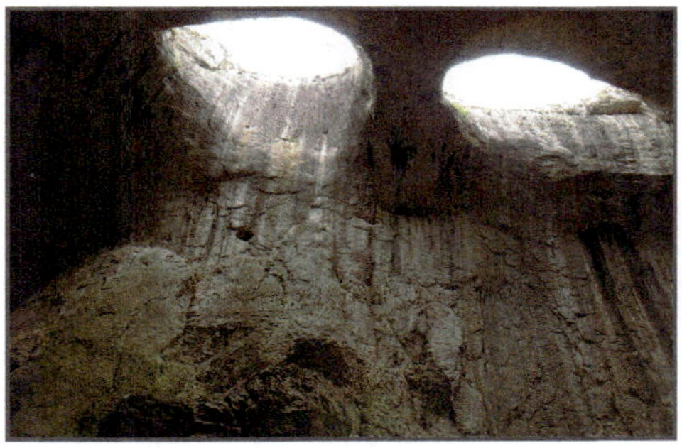

Photomnemonic 5.8 A cavernous (hole-like) pattern is seen in vascular tumors. God's eyes cave in Prohodna, Bulgaria.

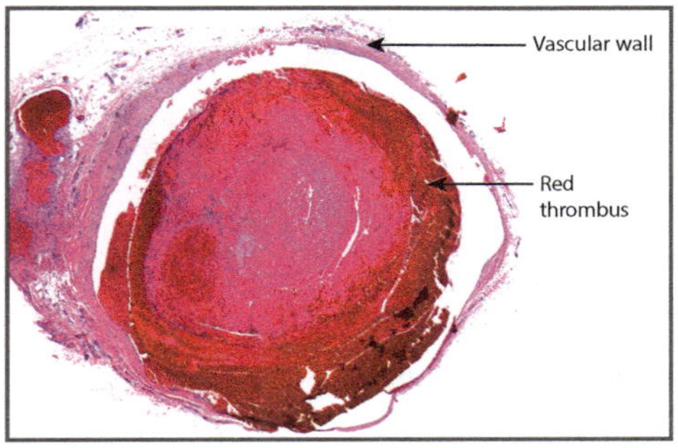

Figure 5.38 A thrombosed lumen of a vein. This thrombus is red as it is made predominantly of red blood cells.

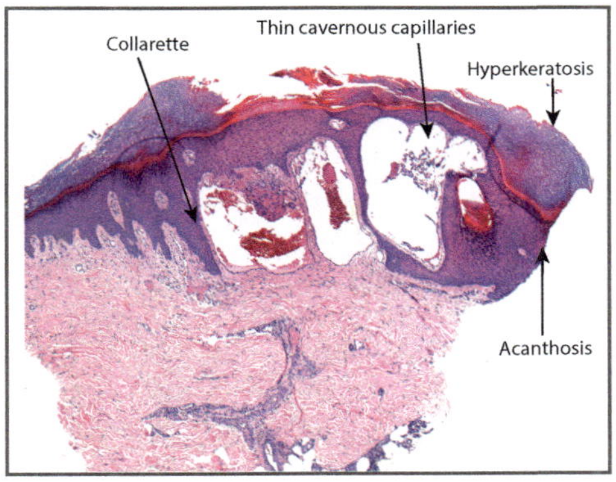

Figure 5.39 A solitary angiokeratoma.

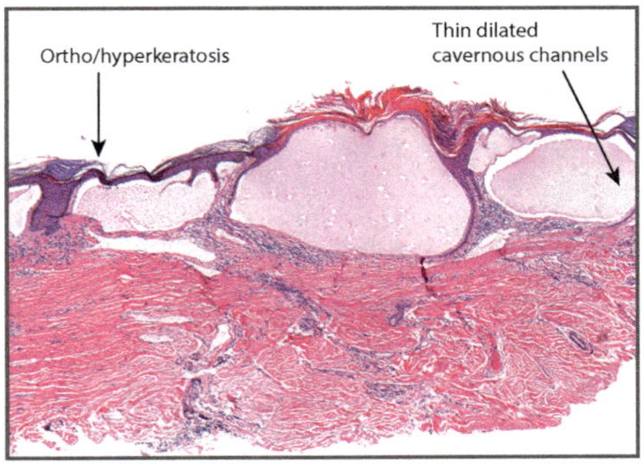

Figure 5.40 Lymphangioma. Note the pink proteinaceous material in the dilated lumina.

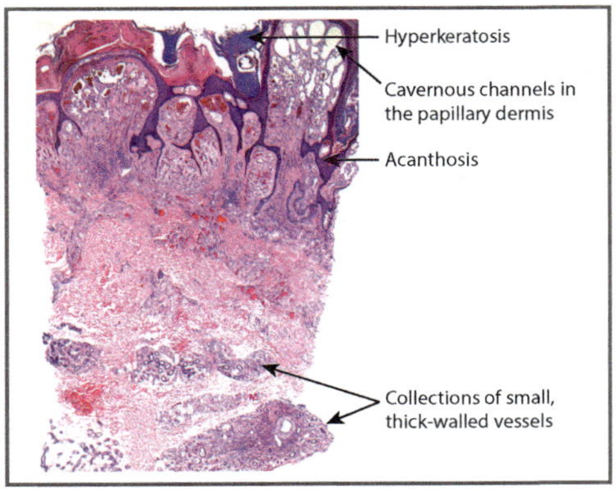

Figure 5.41 Verrucous hemangioma is a combined malformation. Note the angiokeratoma-like surface with the collections of small vessels throughout the entire dermis and the subdermis.

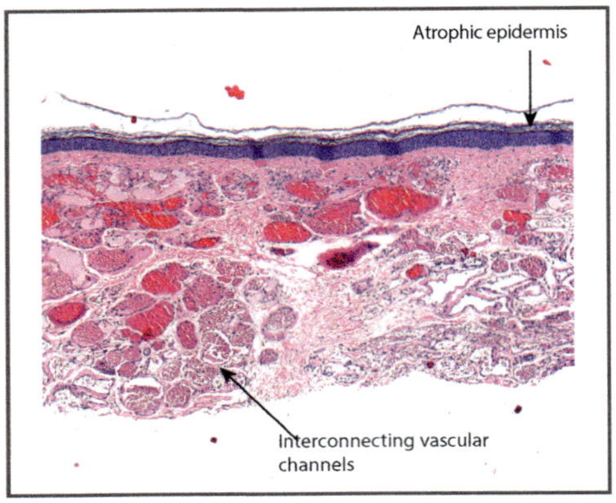

Figure 5.42 Cherry angioma.

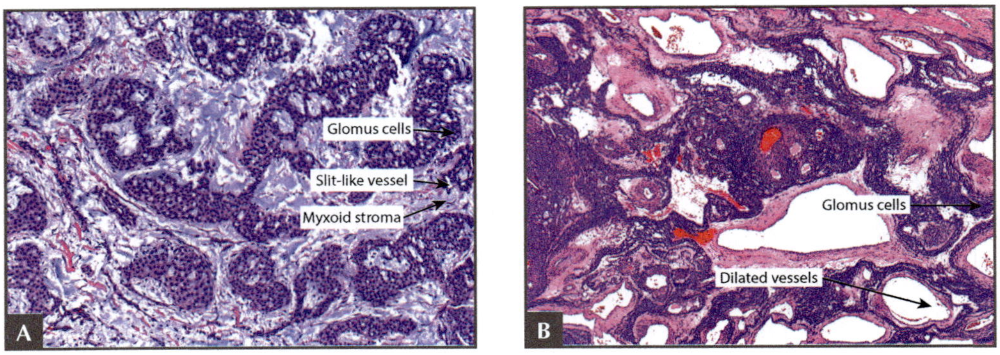

Figure 5.43 A Subungual glomus tumor. Note the collections of uniform "punched-out" blue cells organized in sheets with cribriform pattern in this particular case. The stroma is filled with mucin. **B** Glomangioma. There is a pronounced vascular component. The vessels are dilated and angulated in shape.

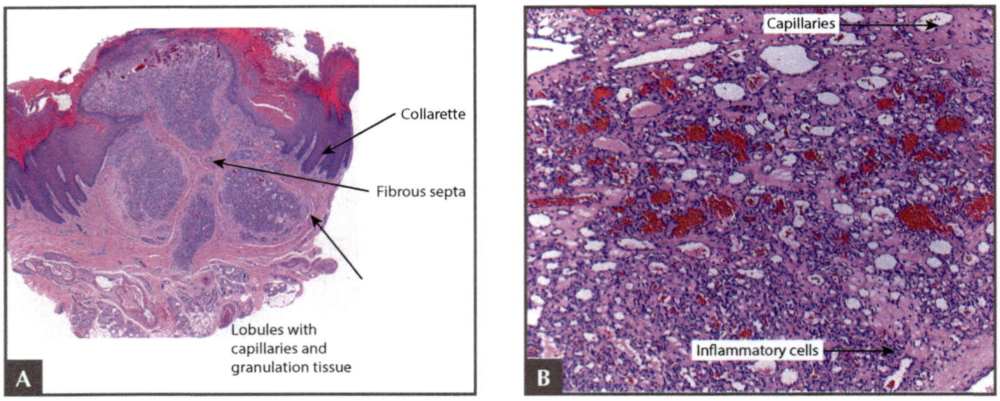

Figure 5.44 Pyogenic granuloma. **A** The pattern is lobular and separated by fibrous septa. **B** Pyogenic granuloma. The "structure" of a lobule on high power shows many small dilated capillaries among the loose stroma with inflammatory cells (granulation tissue).

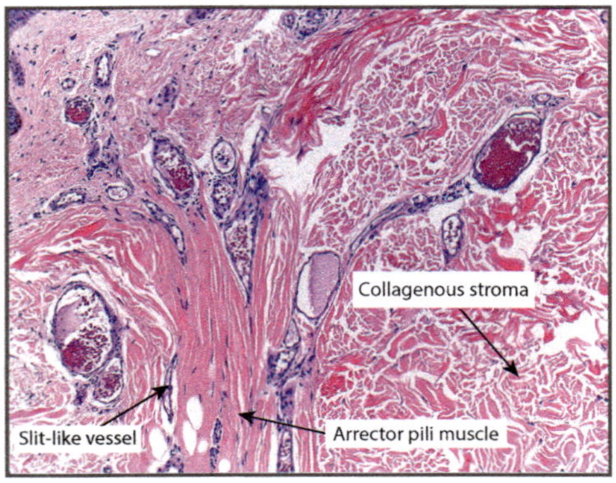

Figure 5.45 Microvenular hemangioma. In this case there is involvement of the arrector pili muscle by slit-like or more dilated venules.

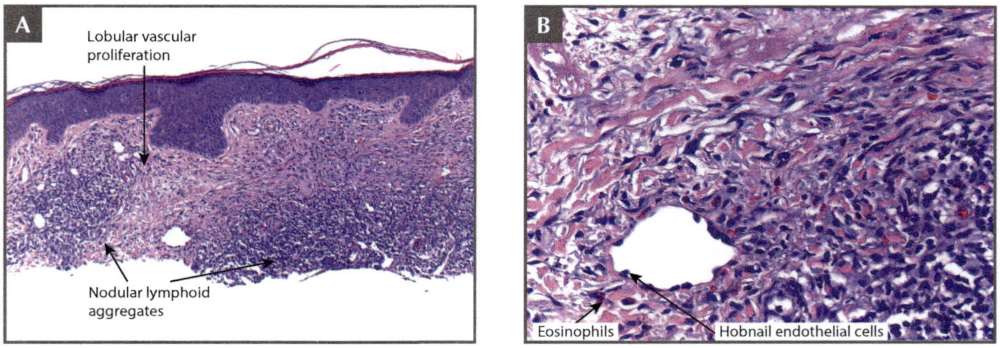

Figure 5.46 Angiolymphoid hyperplasia with eosinophilia. **A** Note the superficial lobular vascular and lymphoid nodular pattern. **B** The same lesion on high power demonstrates the hobnail-like endothelial cells protruding in the lumina and the presence of eosinophils in the infiltrate.

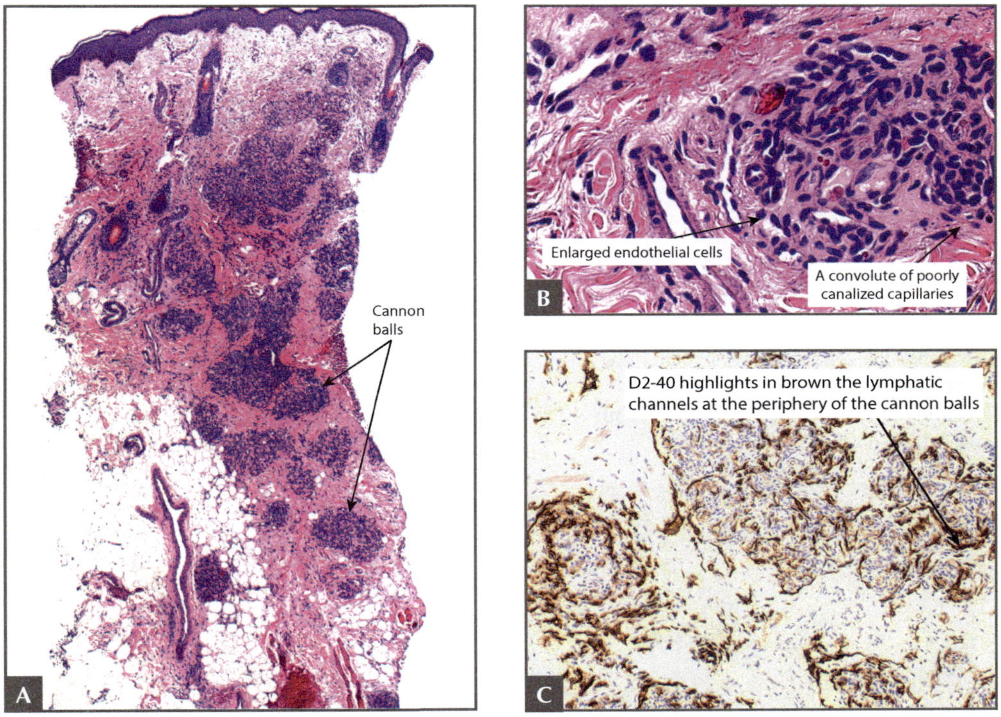

Figure 5.47 Tufted angioma. **A** The lower power is characteristic with these tight convolutes of closely set, poorly canalized capillaries in the dermis resembling cannon balls. **B** The same case shows on high power the enlarged endothelial cells. **C** D2-40 stains the lymphatic channels at the periphery of the cannon balls. Note the negative core of the cannon balls which contains endothelial cells and pericytes.

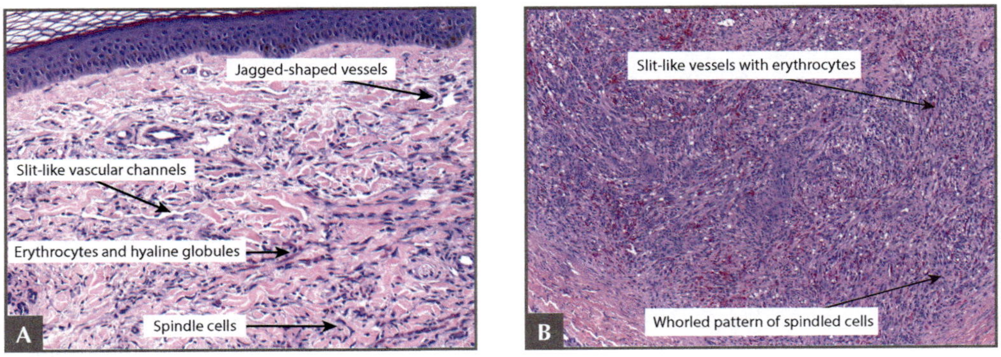

Figure 5.48 Kaposi's sarcoma. **A** Plaque stage. **B** Tumor stage. Note the whorled pattern of dense spindled cells.

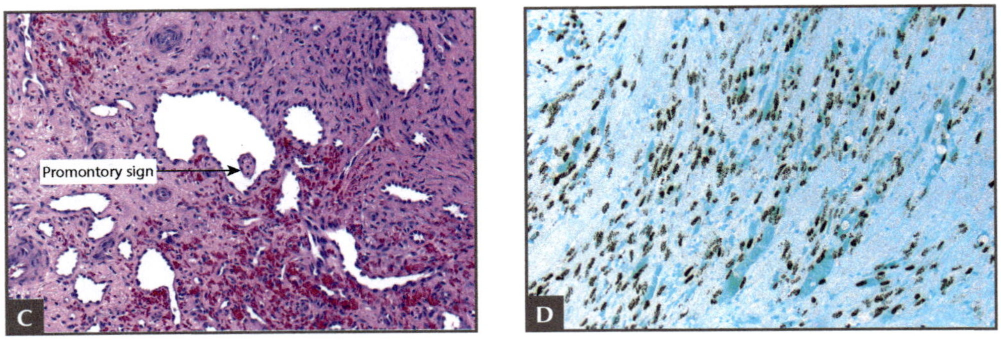

Figure 5.48 Kaposi's sarcoma. **C** Promontory sign. **D** HHV8 nuclear staining is detected in the spindle cells and endothelial cells of the vascular channels in about 80% of cases.

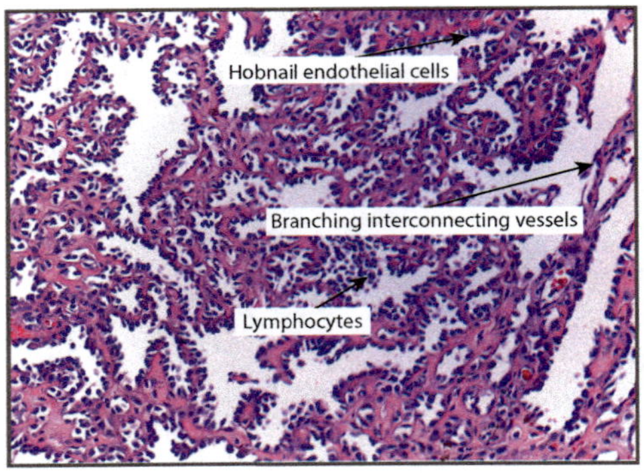

Figure 5.49 Retiform hemangioendothelioma. The pattern resembles rete testis. There are branching blood vessels with hobnail endothelial cells and lymphocytes both within lumina and in the dermis.

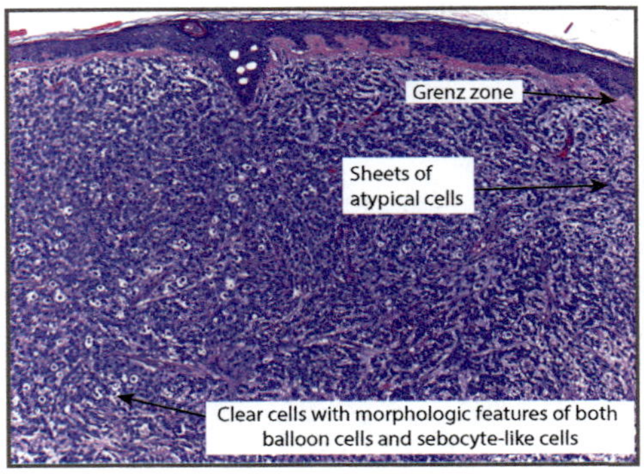

Figure 5.50 Poorly differentiated angiosarcoma. Note the epithelioid morphology of the endothelial cells organized in sheets. There are also atypical cells which appear like clear cells with features simulating balloon cells and sebocytes. Immunohistochemistry is necessary for the diagnosis.

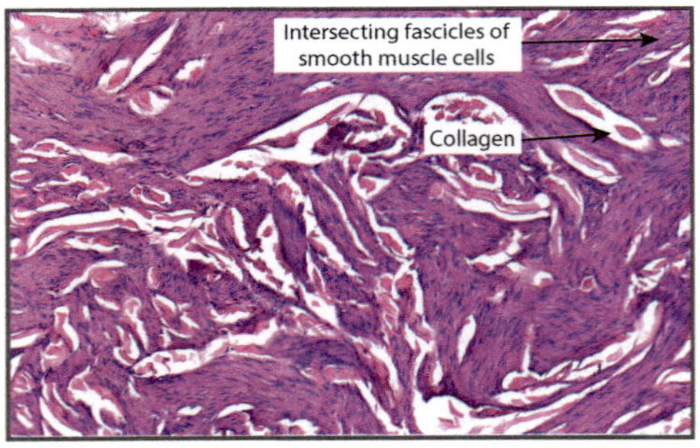

Figure 5.51 Piloleiomyoma in a dog. Note the whorled pattern of interlacing fascicles of smooth muscle cells.

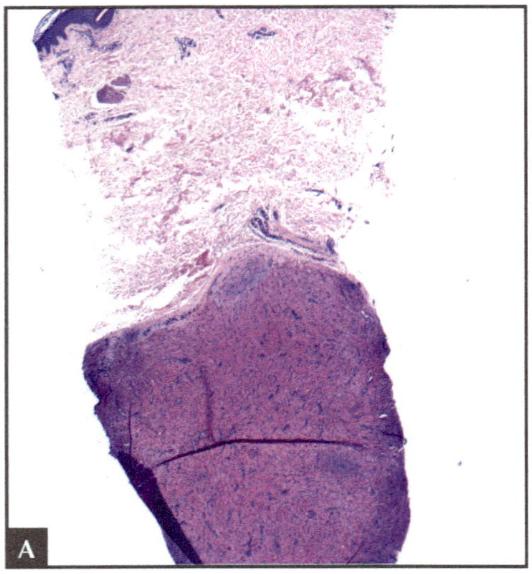

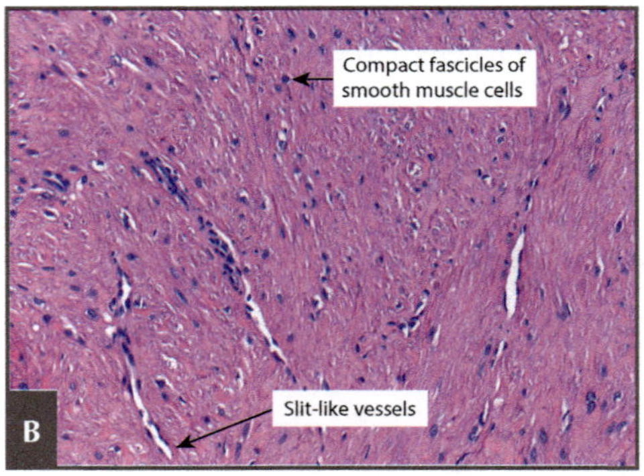

Figure 5.52 Angioleiomyoma. **A** There is a well-circumscribed, very compact eosinophilic tumor with a fibrous capsule in the subdermis. **B** The same case shows the solid pattern of angioleiomyoma on high power: a compact proliferation of interlacing fascicles of smooth muscle cells.

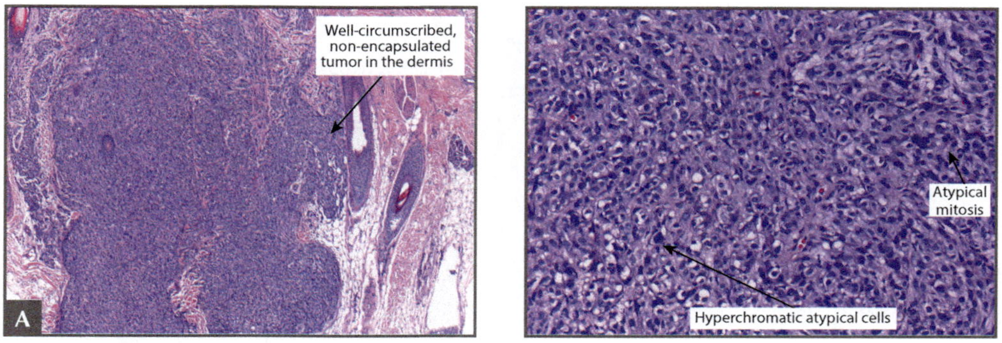

Figure 5.53 Leiomyosarcoma (metastatic uterine leiomyosarcoma to the scalp). **A** Circumscribed non-encapsulated lesion in the dermis. **B** The same case on high power reveals epithelioid morphology. Note the bizarre cells and the atypical mitoses.

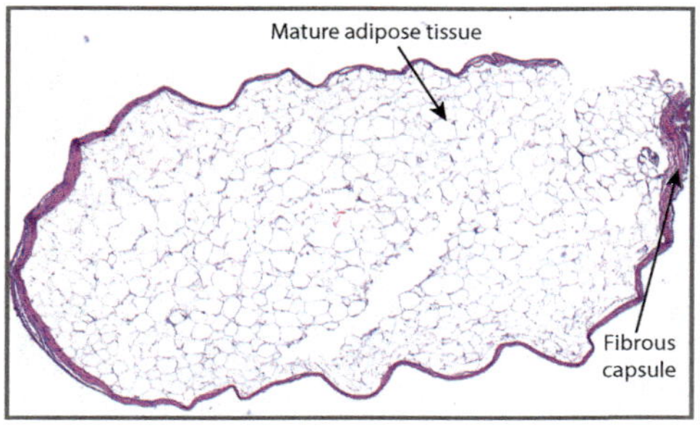

Figure 5.54 Mobile encapsulated lipoma.

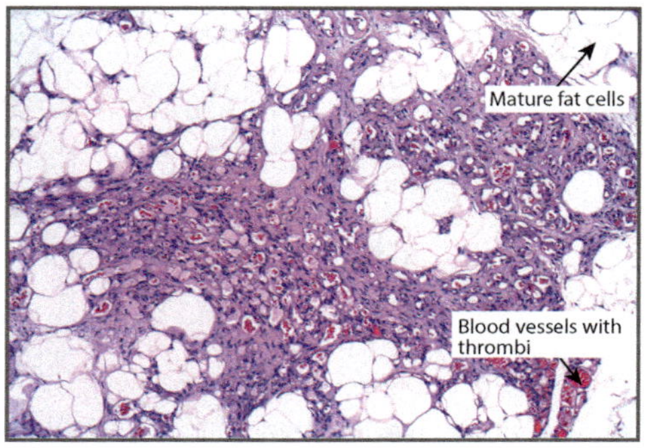

Figure 5.55 Mature fat with numerous mature-looking blood vessels, some thrombosed.

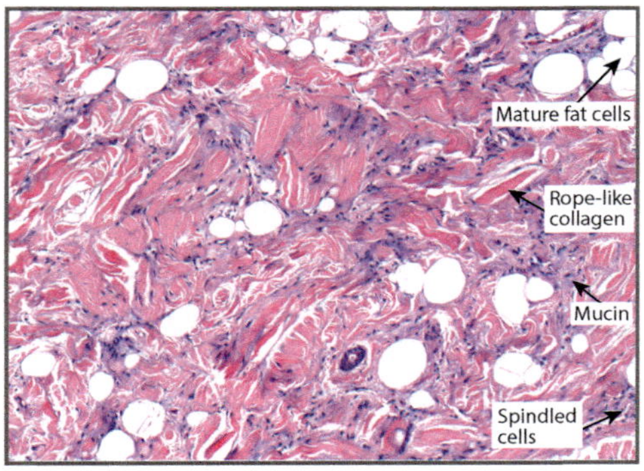

Figure 5.56 Spindle cell lipoma. Note the spindled cell component and the myxoid stroma.

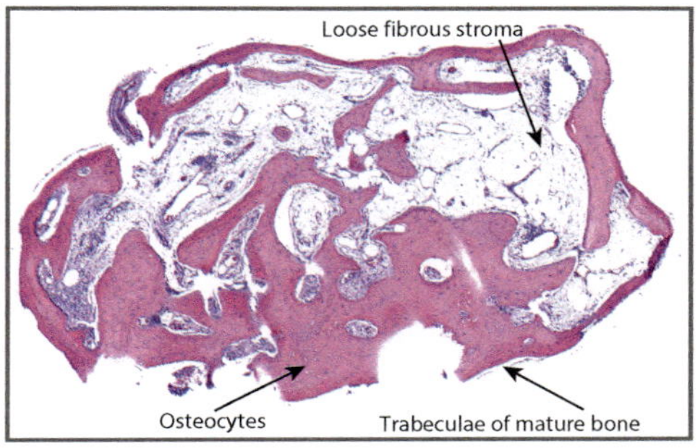

Figure 5.57 Osteoma cutis.

MELANOCYTIC TUMORS

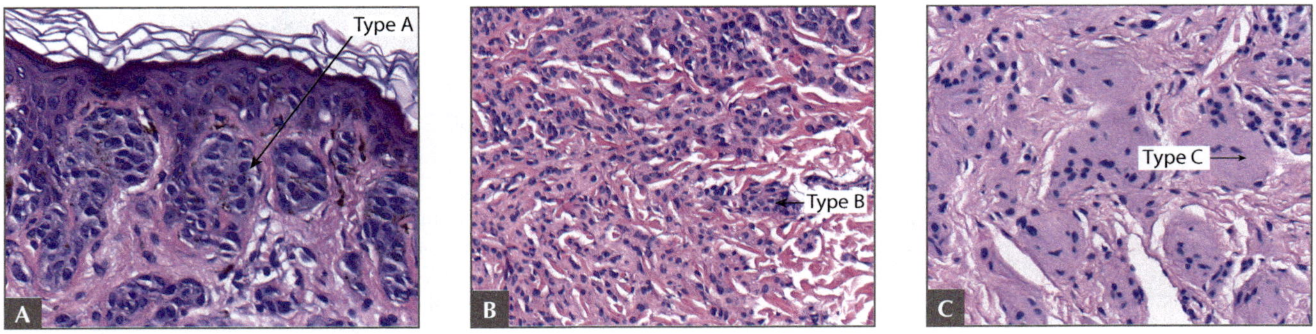

Figure 5.58 Nevus cells. **A** Type A: epithelioid with large pale nucleus and more cytoplasm (a case of a compound nevus). **B** Type B: lymphoid-like cells with blue nuclei and scant cytoplasm in strands (a case of congenital nevus). **C** Type C: elongated, with spindled nuclei (a case of neurotized dermal nevus).

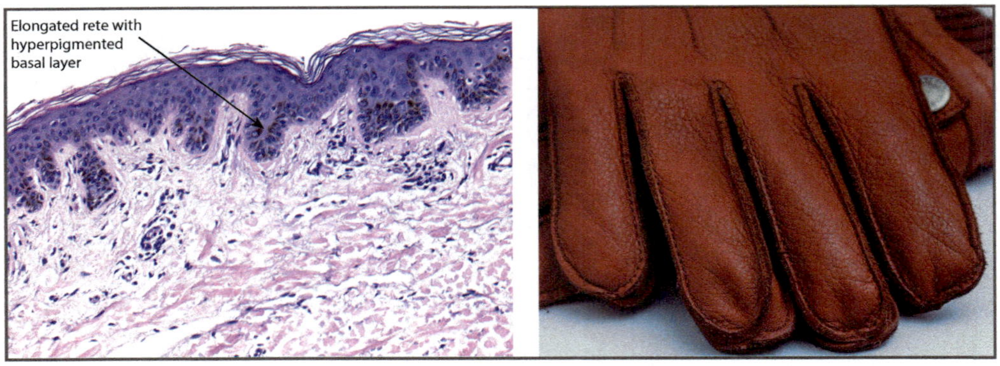

Figure 5.59 and **Photomnemonic 5.9** Lentigo simplex. Note the elongated hyperpigmented rete ridges with melanophages in the upper dermis. The elongated hyperpigmented rete ridges of a lentigo resemble the separate sheaths for the fingers of a brown glove.

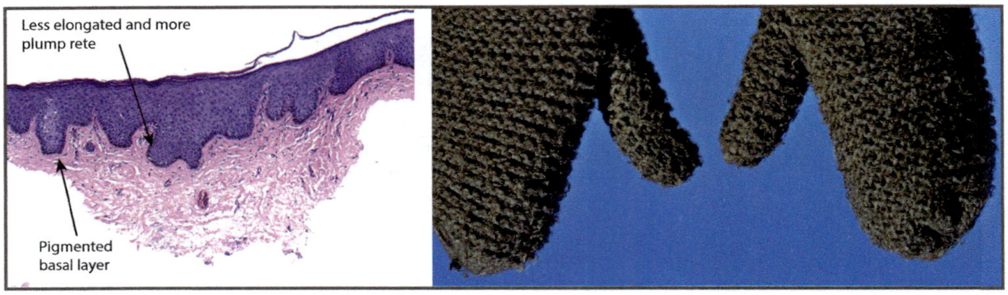

Figure 5.60 and **Photomnemonic 5.10** Labial melanotic macule. Note the absence of a cornified layer. There are plump rete ridges with pigmented basal layer. The plump rete ridges with basal hyperpigmentation resemble a green fingerless glove.

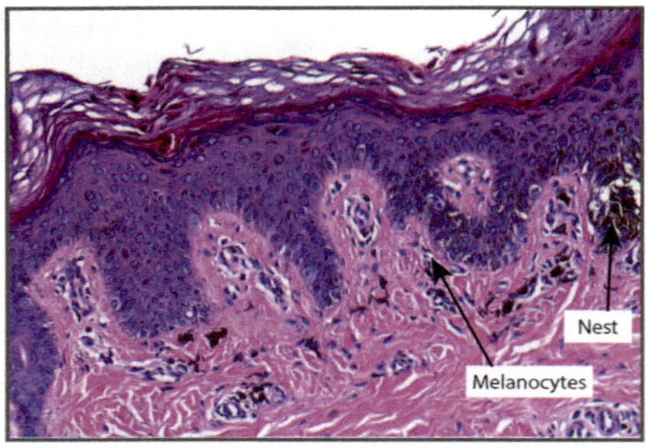

Figure 5.61 Lentiginous junctional nevus on acral site. Note the elongated rete with an increased number of melanocytes and small nests at the dermoepidermal junction.

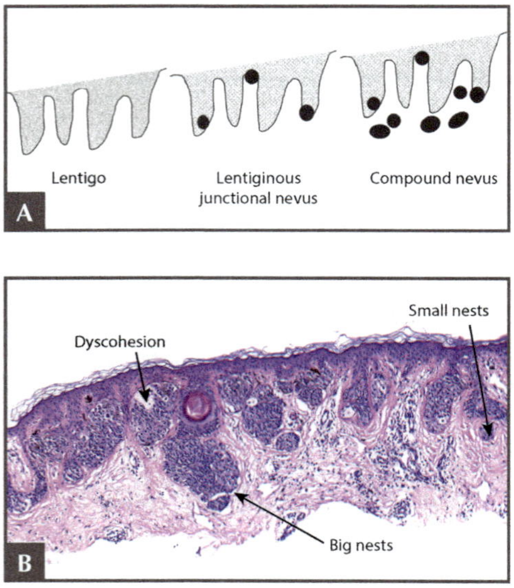

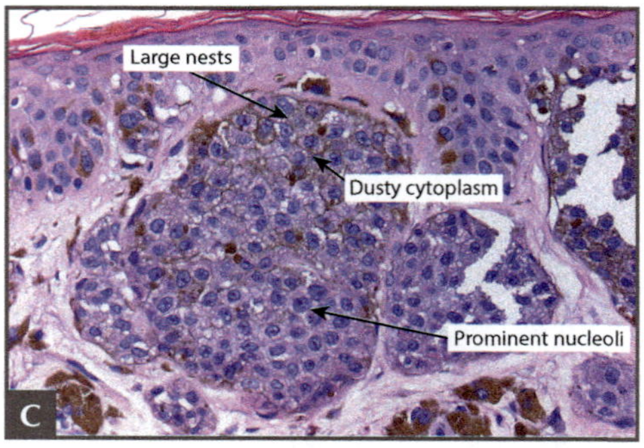

Figure 5.62 Compound nevus. **A** Schematic presentation of the compound nevus type compared to lentigo and lentiginous junctional nevus. **B** Compound nevus of special site (breast). Note the poor lateral circumscription, the variability in the size and shape, as well as the confluence of the nests. **C** Another case of a nevus on the breast demonstrates on high power large nests with ample dusty cytoplasm and prominent nucleoli.

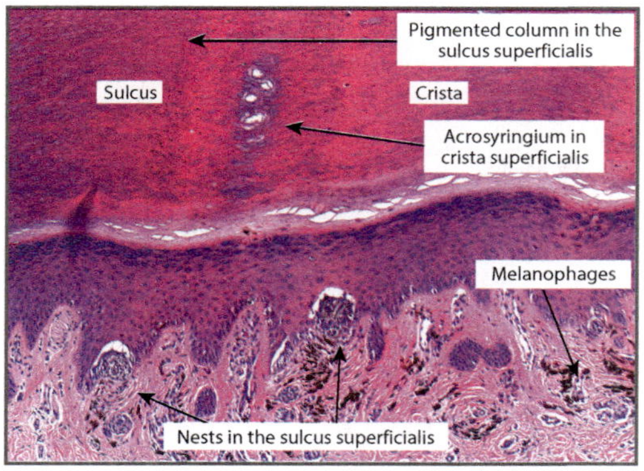

Figure 5.63 Compound nevus of acral site: note the distribution of the nests and the columns of pigment in the furrows (sulcus superficialis). The ridges (crista superficialis) are spared.

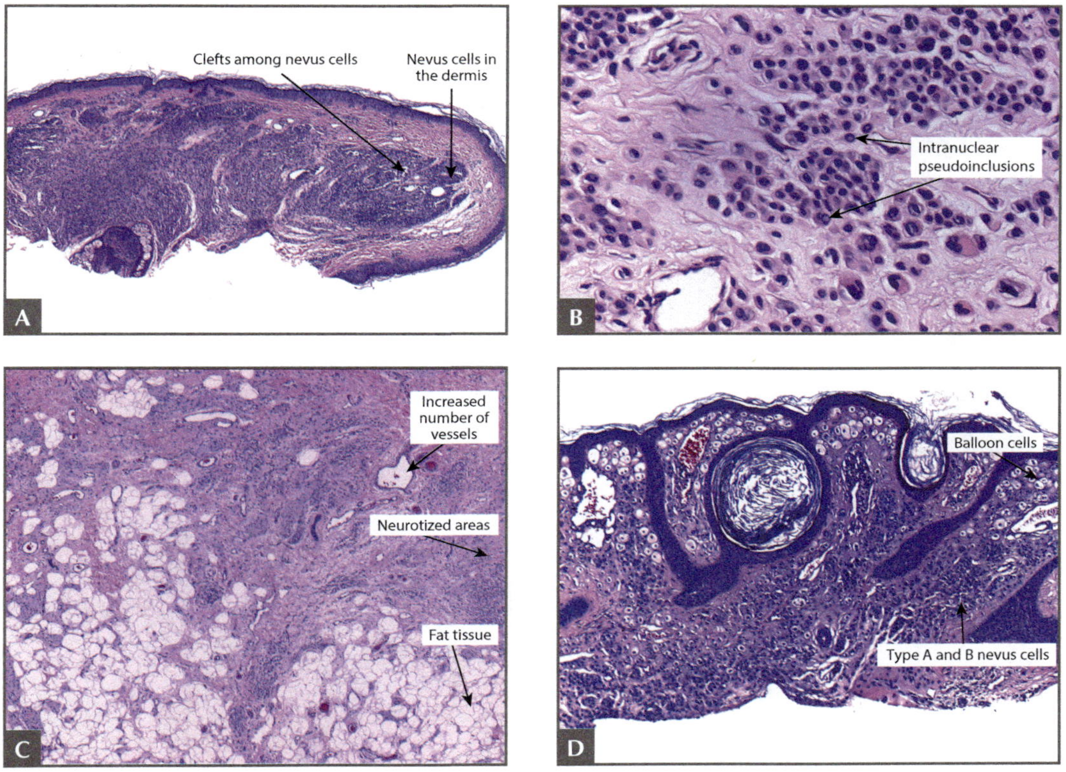

Figure 5.64 Intradermal nevus. **A** Nevus cells are confined to the dermis. **B** Intranuclear pseudoinclusions. **C** Ancient nevus. There is adipose tissue, neurotized strings of spindled cells resembling nerve fibers, and also an increased number of vessels. **D** Balloon cell nevus. Note the pale cells with centrally located nuclei among bland dermal nevus cells.

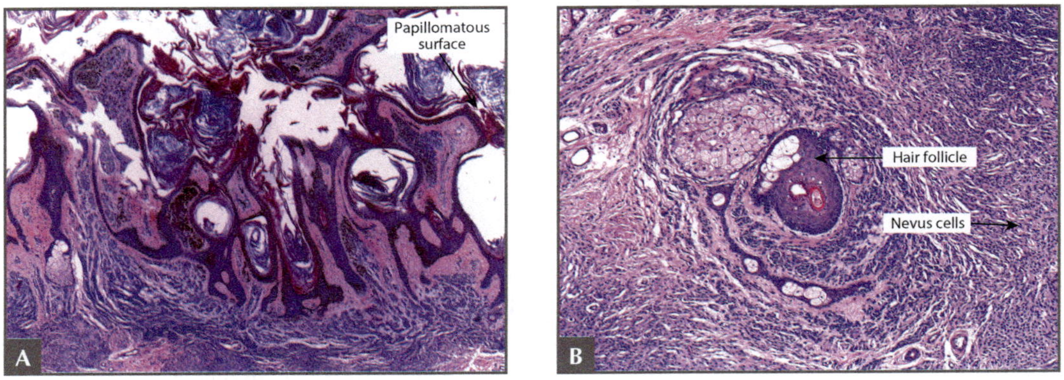

Figure 5.65 Congenital nevus. **A** Note the papillomatous surface mimicking seborrheic keratosis. **B** Congenital nevus. In the lower dermis note the bland nevus cells organized in nests and in strands around the adnexal structures.

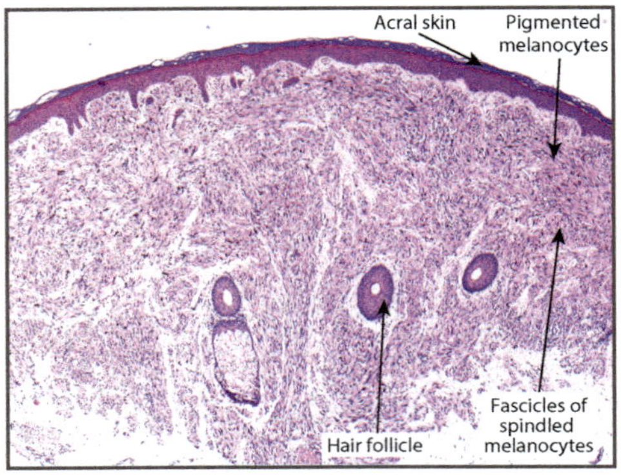

Figure 5.66 Deep penetrating nevus. Note the inverted pyramidal shape. This lesion is sometimes considered a subtype of a blue nevus.

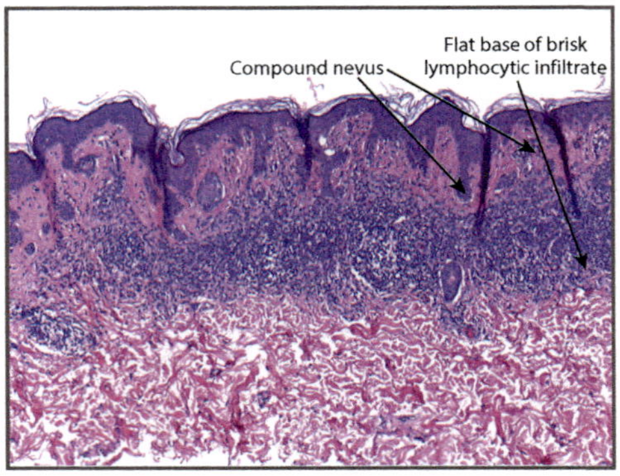

Figure 5.67 Halo nevus. Note the flat base of lymphocytes among which are nevus nests.

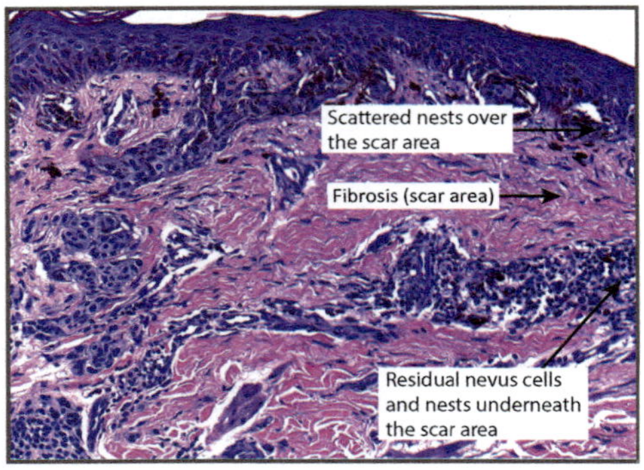

Figure 5.68 Recurrent nevus. Note the zonal arrangement in the dermis.

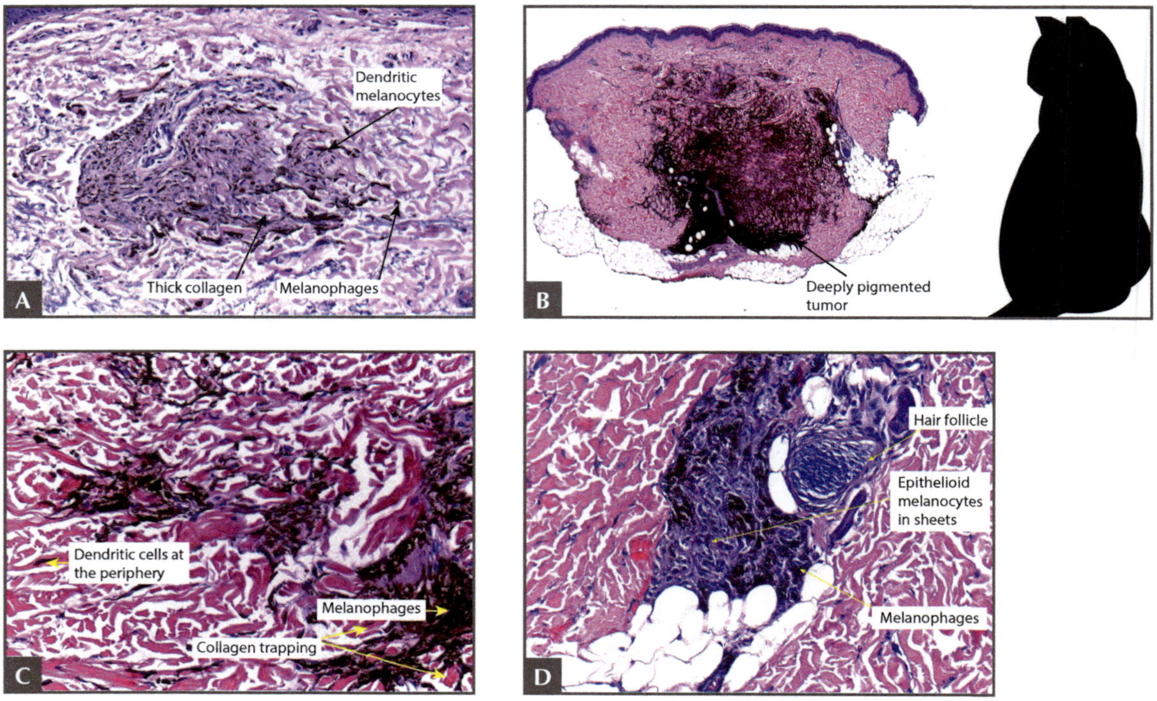

Figure 5.69 and Photomnemonic 5.11 Blue nevus. **A** Small common blue nevus. There are slender dendritic cells among thickened collagen bundles and melanophages. **B** Cellular blue nevus. A deeply pigmented highly cellular tumor in the dermis with its convex bottom silhouette resembles the rear profile of a sitting black cat. **C** Cellular blue nevus: dendritic melanocytes at the periphery of the tumor bulk. **D** Another case of a cellular blue nevus demonstrates the epithelioid component. Note the extension of the nevus cells along the hair follicle into the adipose tissue.

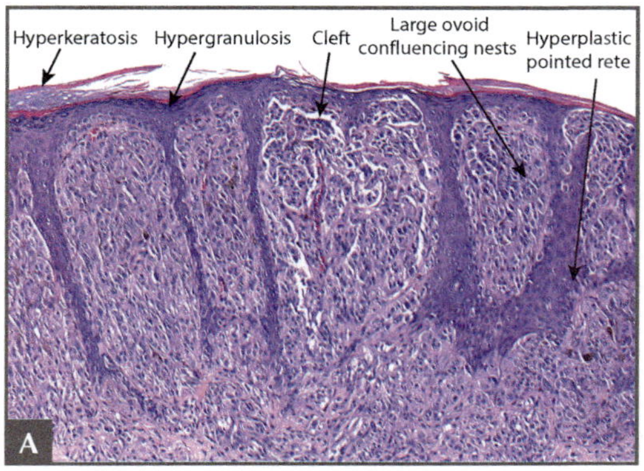

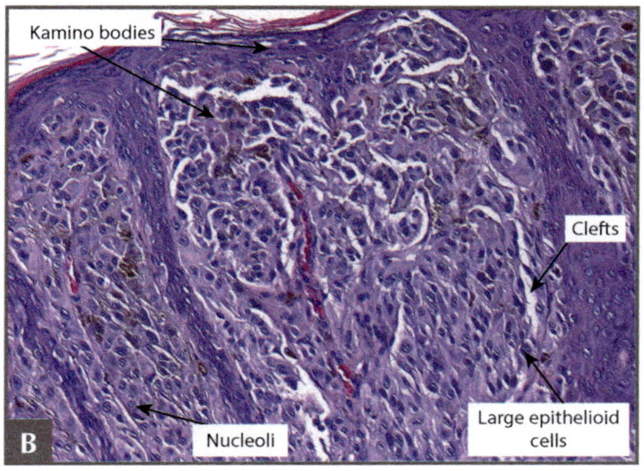

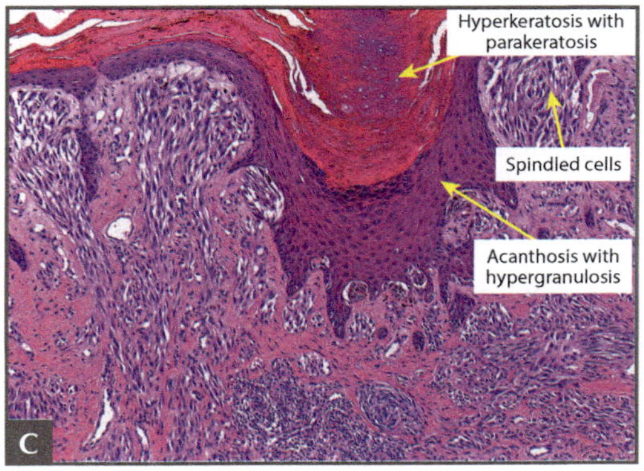

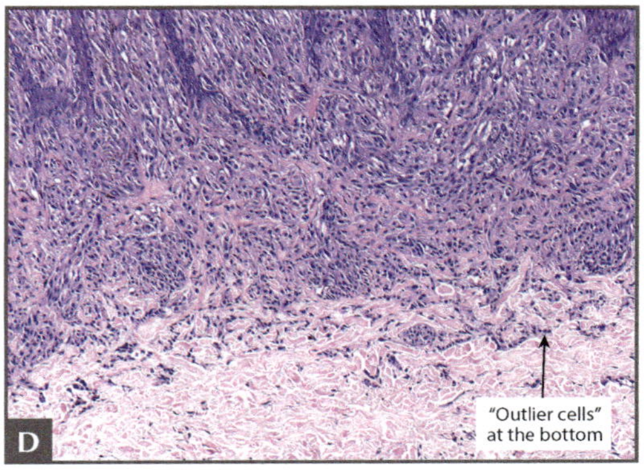

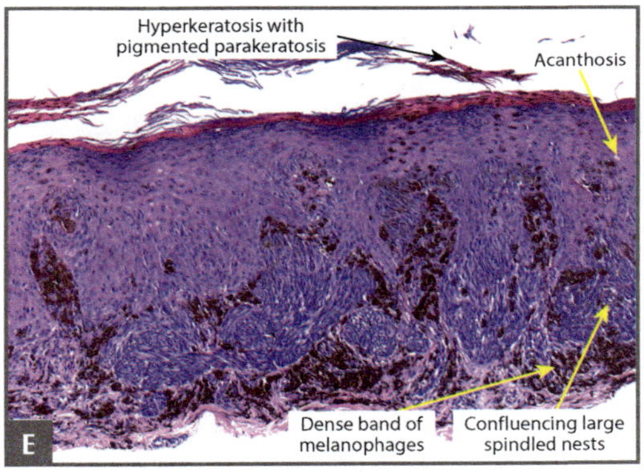

Figure 5.70 Spitz nevus. **A** Note the characteristic silhouette of large-sized nests of epithelioid cells among the elongated rete ridges. **B** Note the large epithelioid cells, in some of which the nucleoli can be seen. The Kamino bodies are pink globules at the dermoepidermal junction. **C** Another case demonstrates the spindled morphology of the cells. **D** Single epithelioid "outlier cells" at the bottom of the lesion in the dermis. **E** Spindle cell nevus of Reed. Note the large vertically oriented nests of spindled cells at the dermoepidermal junction and the band of melanophages in the papillary dermis.

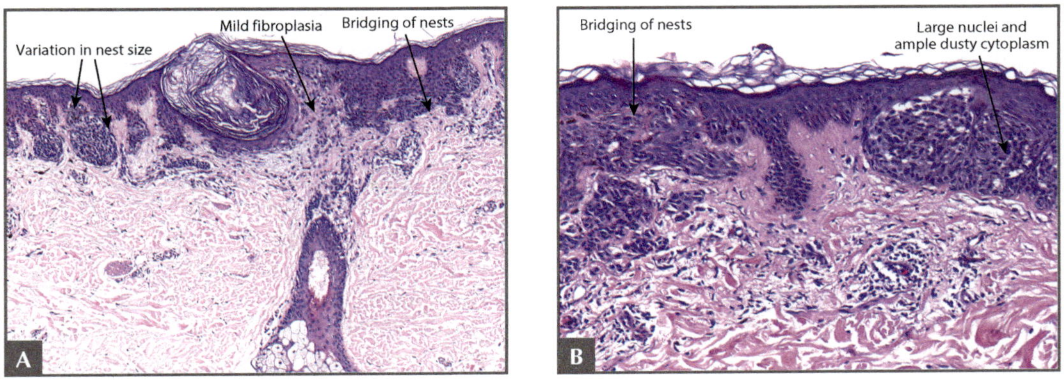

Figure 5.71 Atypical nevus. **A** This is a compound melanocytic nevus, slightly asymmetric. It shows variation in the size and position of the nests with bridging among some. **B** Note the random cytologic atypia by comparing the cells on the right and left side.

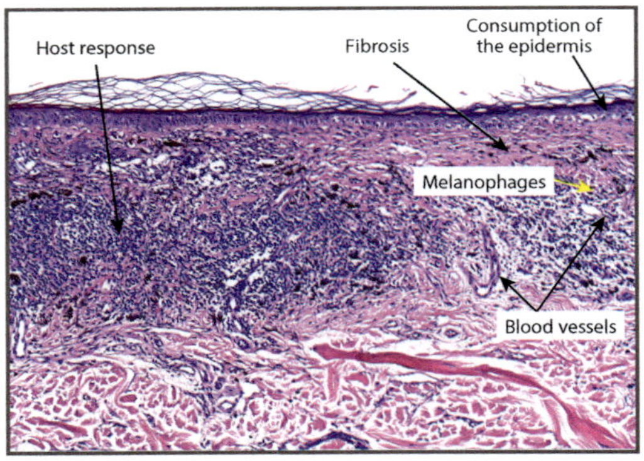

Figure 5.72 Regression in melanoma: note the flat, thin epidermis with features for melanoma in situ. The tumor portion has disappeared and replaced by a zone of fibrosis, melanophages, lymphocytic infiltrate, and increased number of vessels.

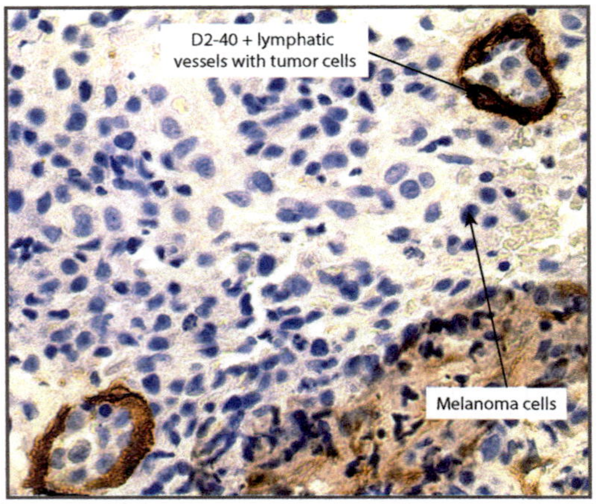

Figure 5.73 Lymphovascular invasion in a case of acral melanoma. D2-40 highlights the lymphatics.

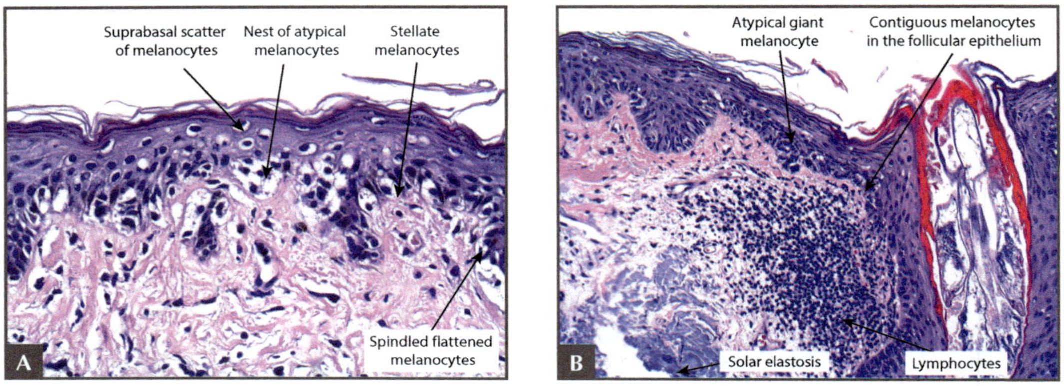

Figure 5.74 A Melanoma in situ. There is a contiguous proliferation of atypical melanocytes at the dermoepidermal junction and suprabasal spread of melanocytes. **B** Lentigo maligna. Note the extension of atypical melanocytes in the follicular epithelium.

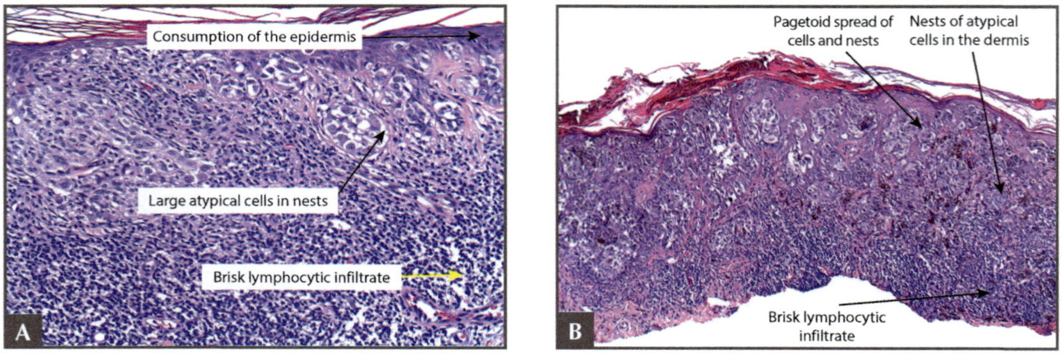

Figure 5.75 Superficial spreading melanoma. **A** Radial growth. There is lentiginous and nested proliferation of atypical pale melanocytes along the dermoepidermal junction. The dermis shows individual melanoma cells and a brisk host response. **B** Vertical growth. Note the nests of atypical melanocytes in the dermis.

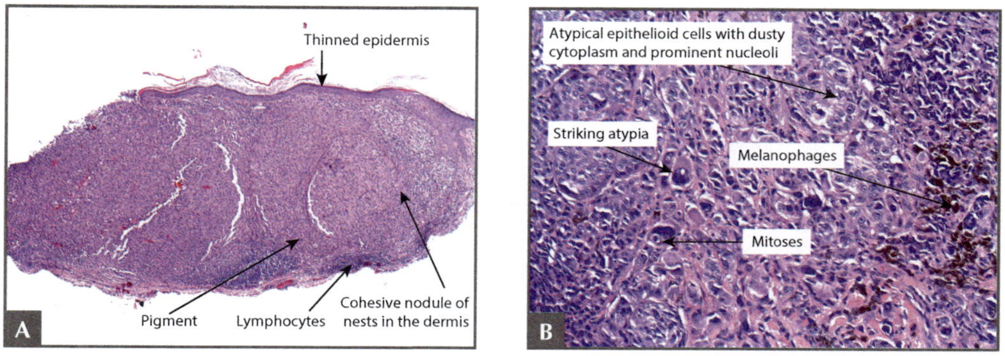

Figure 5.76 Nodular melanoma. **A** Note the overall symmetric nodular proliferation of cohesive sheets of atypical melanocytes in the dermis. Such lesions require immunohistochemical confirmation. Presence of melanin/melanophages is a clue to the melanocytic nature. **B** High-power view demonstrates cohesive nests of strikingly atypical cells in the dermis as well as increased mitotic rate.

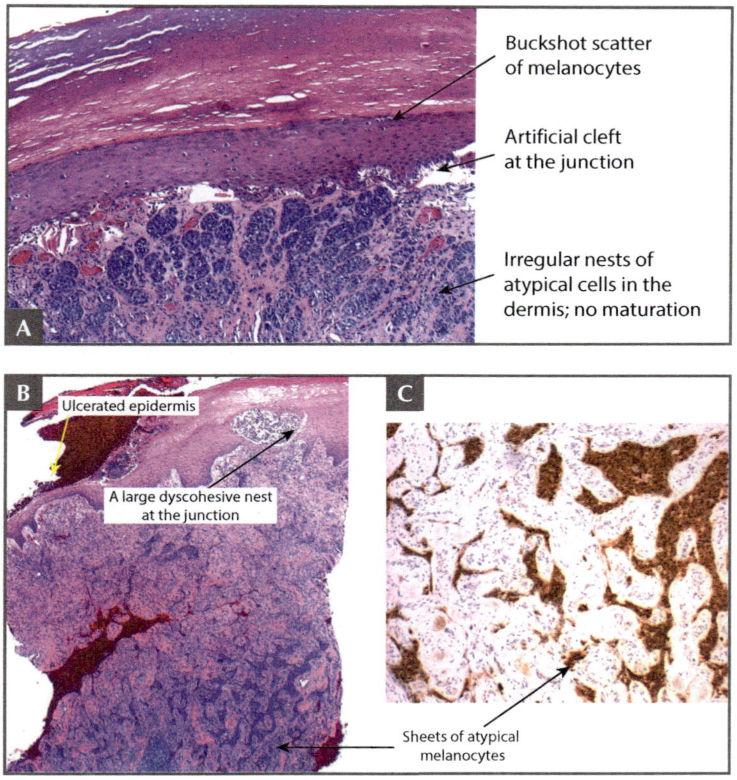

Figure 5.77 **A** Acral lentiginous melanoma (ALM). Compare to acral nevus (Figure 5.61) the diffuse scatter of atypical melanocytes and pigment in the epidermis and in the cornified layer as well as the diffuse proliferation of nests along the entire junction (involving the ridges) and in the dermis. **B** Acral lentiginous melanoma presenting as a chronic ulcer. Note the junctional cavitation (large nest of dyscohesive melanocytes). **C** The same case of acral lentiginous melanoma shows strong MART-1 expression.

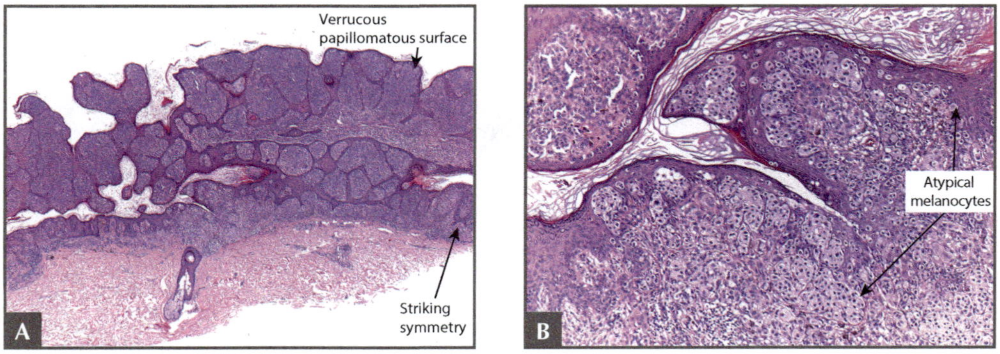

Figure 5.78 Nevoid melanoma. **A** Note the banal appearance of this lesion, which simulates congenital nevus on low power (compare to Figure 5.65A). The architecture is verrucous and with symmetric outlines and sharp circumscription. **B** Careful inspection on high power is necessary for the diagnosis.

ADNEXAL TUMORS

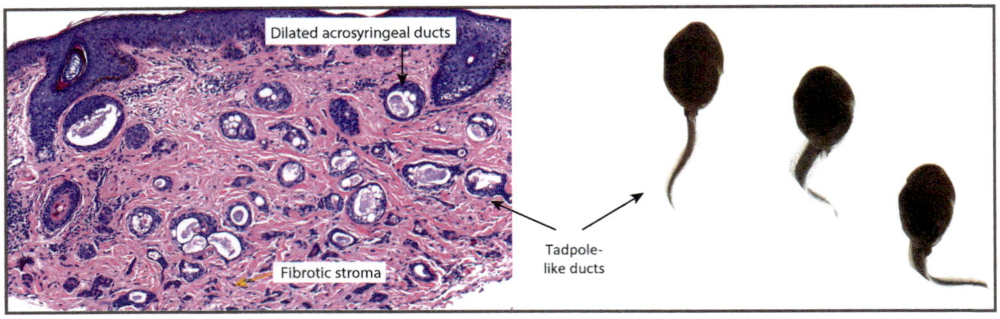

Figure 5.79 and Photomnemonic 5.12 Syringoma. The tumor consists of dilated acrosyringeal ducts with two layers of epithelial lining and pink debris in the lumen. Note that some ductal structures have elongated comma-like tails and resemble tadpoles.

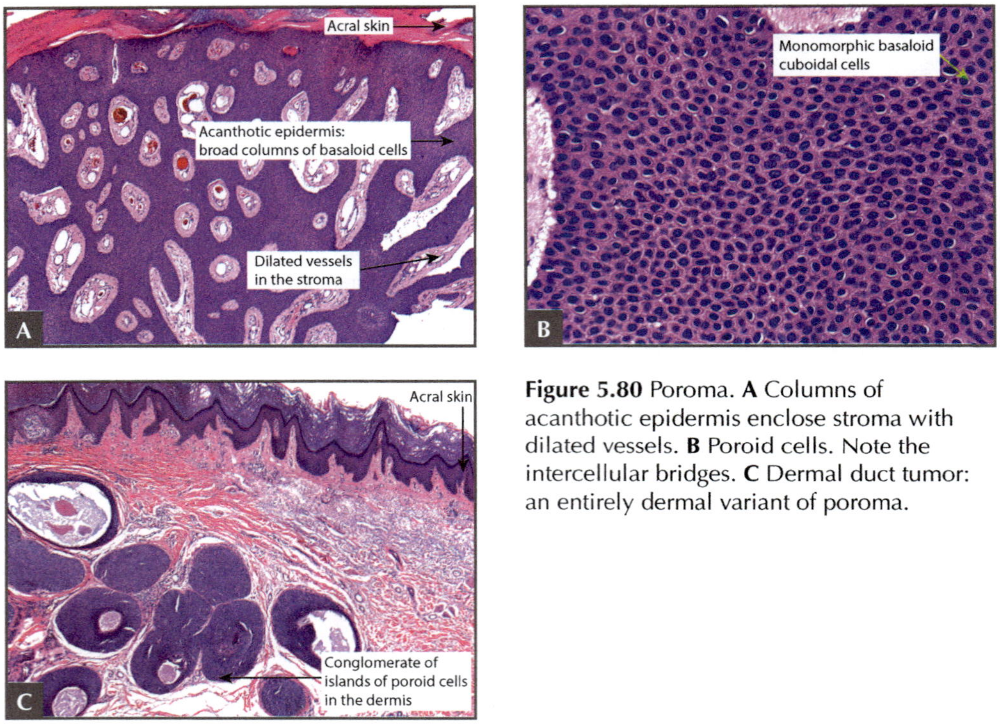

Figure 5.80 Poroma. **A** Columns of acanthotic epidermis enclose stroma with dilated vessels. **B** Poroid cells. Note the intercellular bridges. **C** Dermal duct tumor: an entirely dermal variant of poroma.

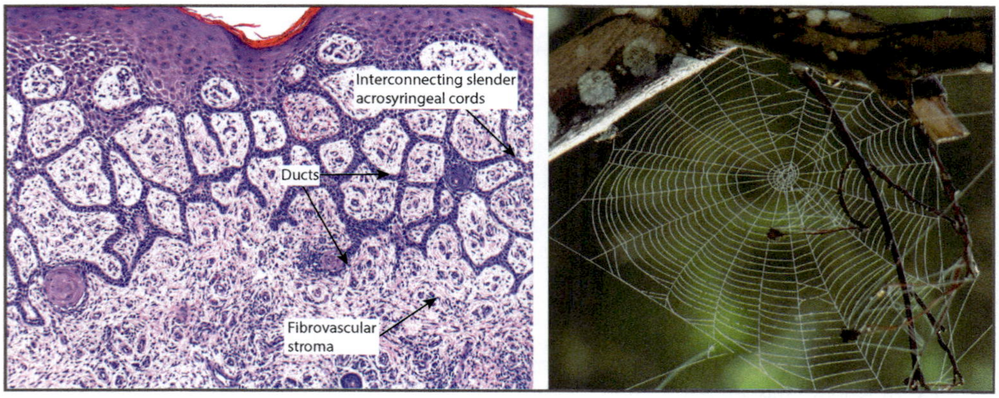

Figure 5.81 and Photomnemonic 5.13 Syringofibroadenoma. Note the network of fine interconnecting slender acrosyringeal cords in the dermis. Syringofibroadenoma resembles a spider web hanging from a tree.

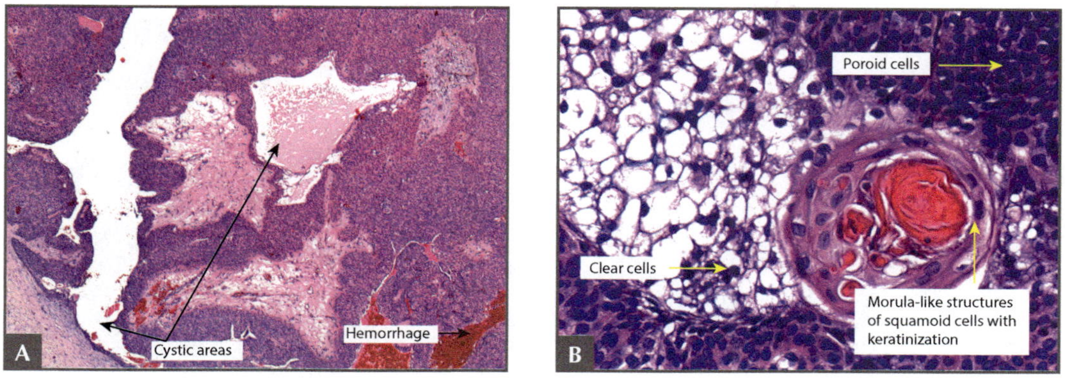

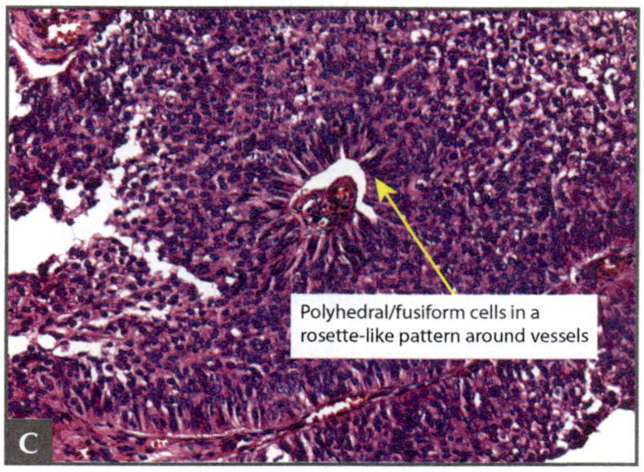

Figure 5.82 Nodular hidradenoma. **A** Lobular non-encapsulated dermal tumor with cystic areas and hemorrhage. **B** Note the different types of cells. **C** Rosette-like arrangement of fusiform cells is a clue.

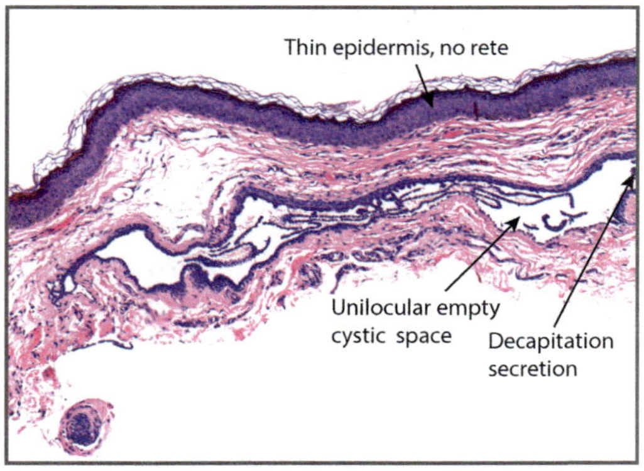

Figure 5.83 Apocrine hidrocystoma arising from the apocrine glands of Moll.

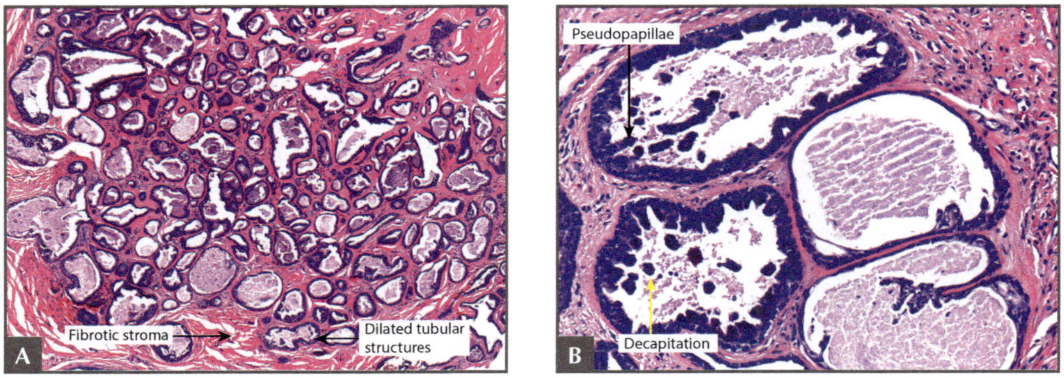

Figure 5.84 Tubular apocrine adenoma. **A** Lobular dermal and subcutaneous tubular apocrine structures encased by fibrous stroma. **B** The same case on high power.

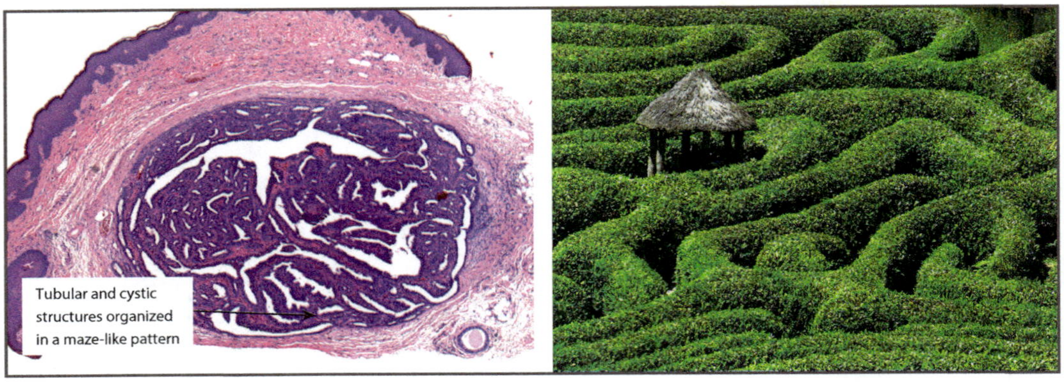

Figure 5.85 and Photomnemonic 5.14 Hidradenoma papilliferum. Note the characteristic pattern of tubular and cystic structures organized in a maze-like pattern. Hidradenoma papilliferum resembles a maze-like proliferation like the maze at Glendurgan Garden in England.

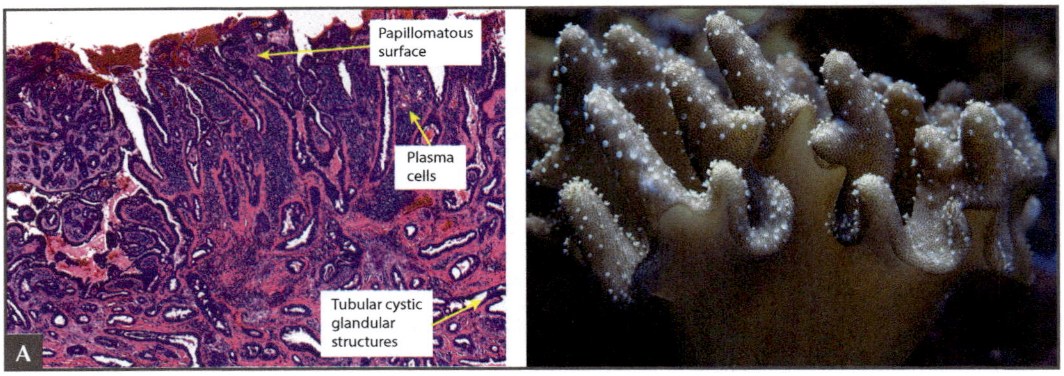

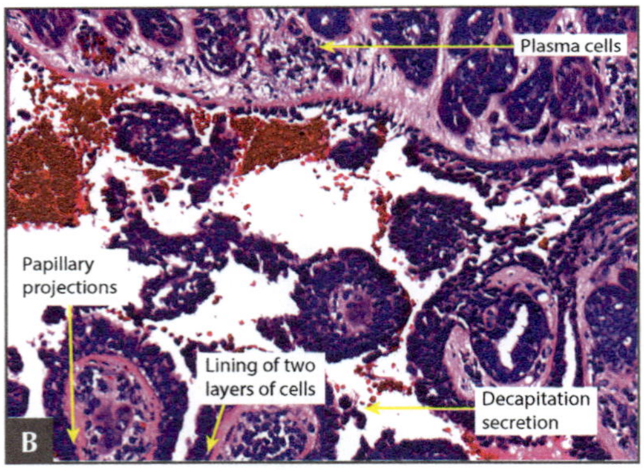

Figure 5.86 Syringocystadenoma papilliferum (SCAP). **A** Note the cystic tubular structures connecting to the surface with papillary projections creating a verrucous surface resembling the undulating surface of a coral. **B** The same case on high power demonstrates that the glands are lined by two layers of cells and show decapitation.

Photomnemonic 5.15 The verrucous surface of syringocystadenoma papilliferum (SCAP) resembles coral.

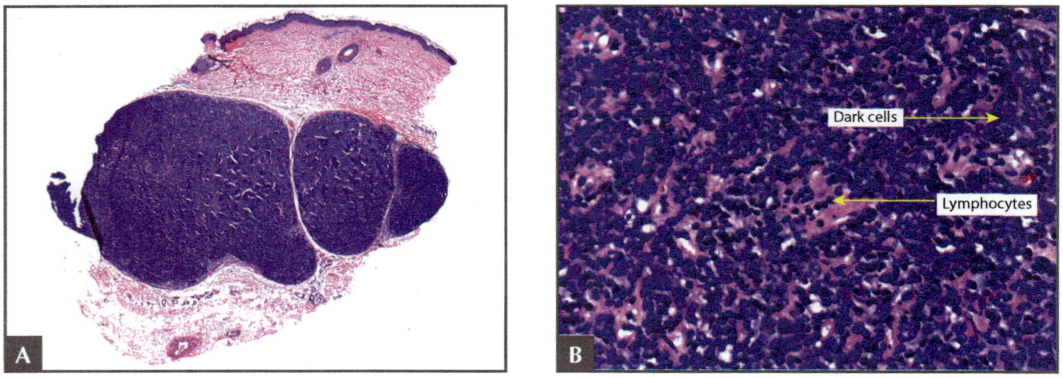

Figure 5.87 Spiradenoma. **A** On low power: the tumor presents as blue ball(s) in the dermis. **B** High power shows the highly cellular blue tumor: dark blue cells and lymphocytes are identified in this case.

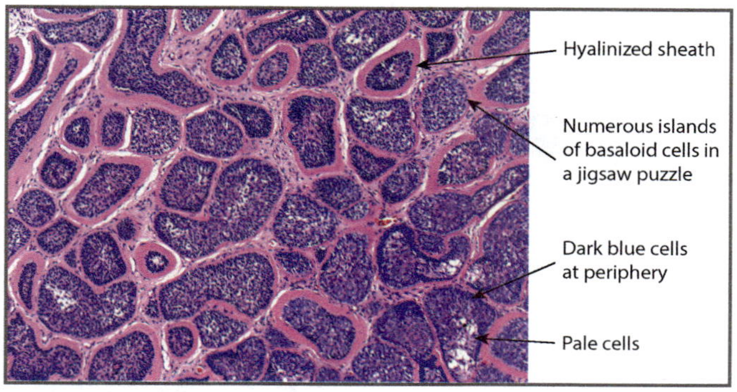

Figure 5.88 Cylindroma. Note the characteristic jigsaw puzzle pattern. The islands show two types of cells: with pale nuclei in the center and with dark nuclei at the periphery.

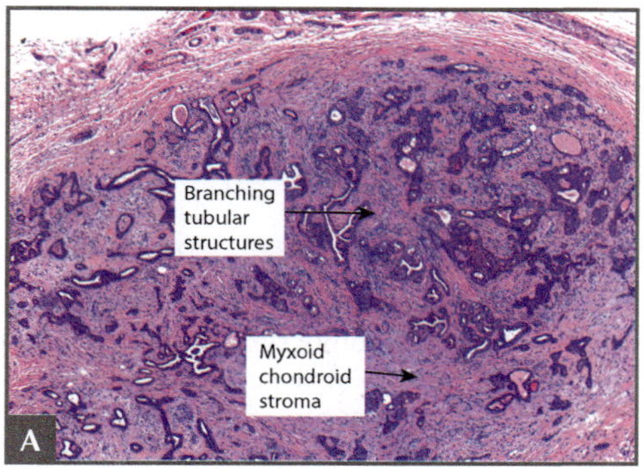

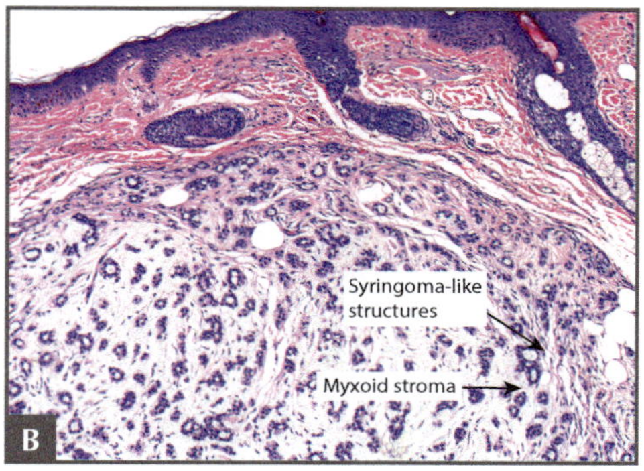

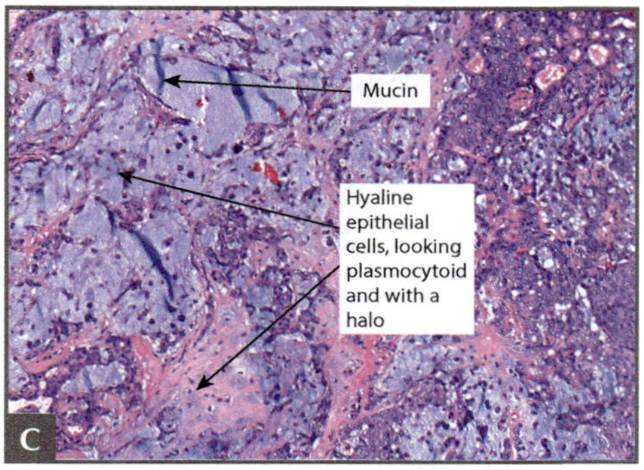

Figure 5.89 Mixed tumor (chondroid syringoma). **A** The overall color is pale-bluish due to the myxoid chondroid stroma. Note that one of the types is made of slender tubular branching glandular structures. **B** The second type is made of small non-branching round dilated structures similar to syringoma. **C** The chondroid stroma in mixed tumor contains hyaline epithelial cells and myxoid matrix.

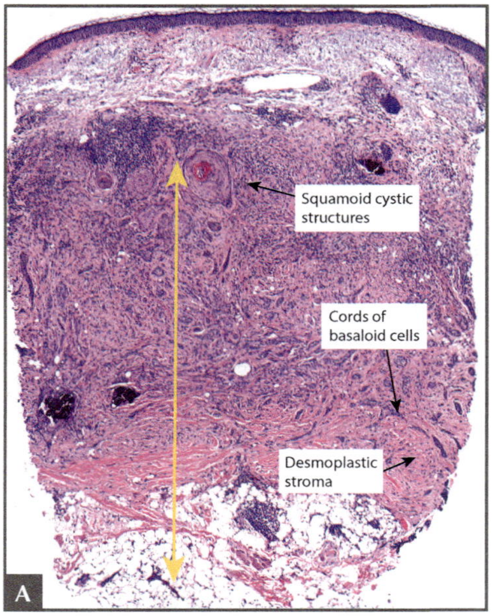

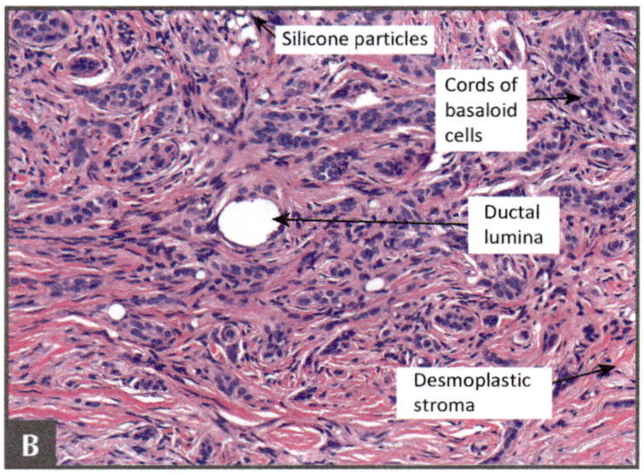

Figure 5.90 Microcystic adnexal carcinoma (MAC). **A** This tumor is poorly circumscribed and shows deep infiltrating growth from the top to the bottom of the specimen (as shown with the yellow arrow). **B** MAC on high power: note the small ducts lined by 1–2 layers of cuboidal cells, which infiltrate the stroma throughout the tumor. In this particular case the MAC was found on the upper lip and the patient had a prior injection of silicone in the same area.

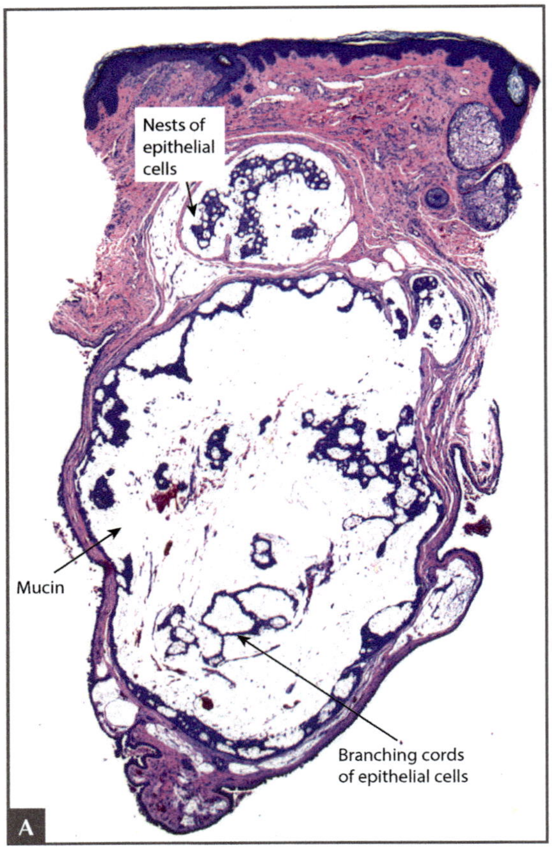

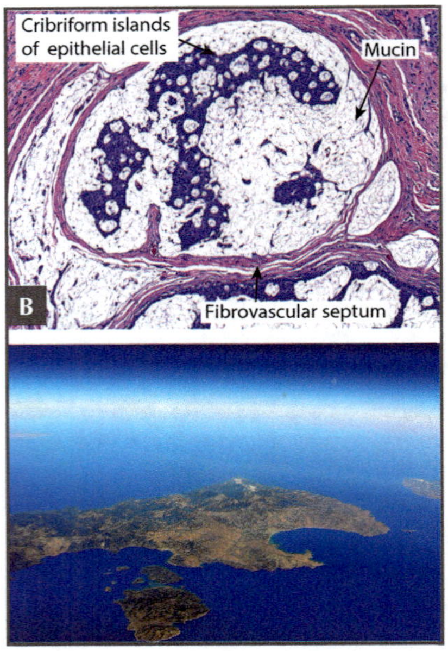

Figure 5.91 Mucinous eccrine carcinoma (MEC). **A** On low power the tumor shows a honeycomb pattern due to aggregates of epithelial cells floating in pools of mucin. **B** The tumor nests are composed of glandular epithelium and show only minimal atypia. They float in the mucin resembling an archipelago in the sea.

Photomnemonic 5.16 The tumor nests of mucinous eccrine carcinoma (MEC) look like an archipelago in the sea.

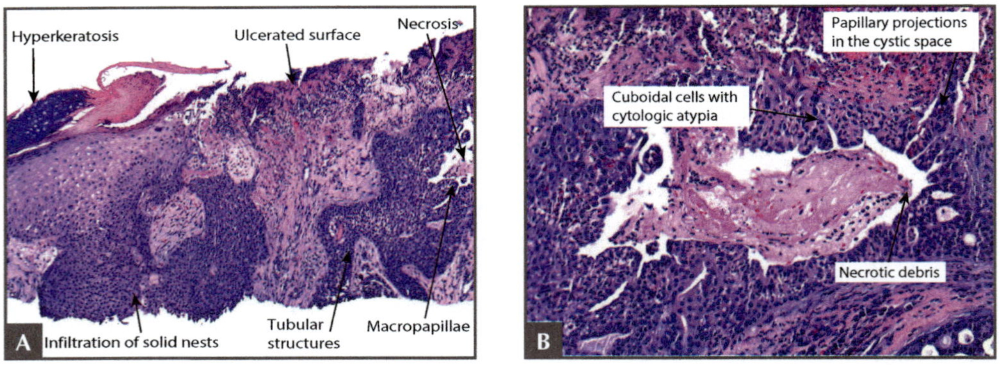

Figure 5.92 A Aggressive digital papillary adenocarcinoma (ADPA). Note the acral location and the infiltrative pattern of solid, tubular, and cystic masses of cuboidal cells with areas of necrosis and papillary projections. **B** ADPA: note the cytologic atypia and the presence of macropapillae in the cystic lumen.

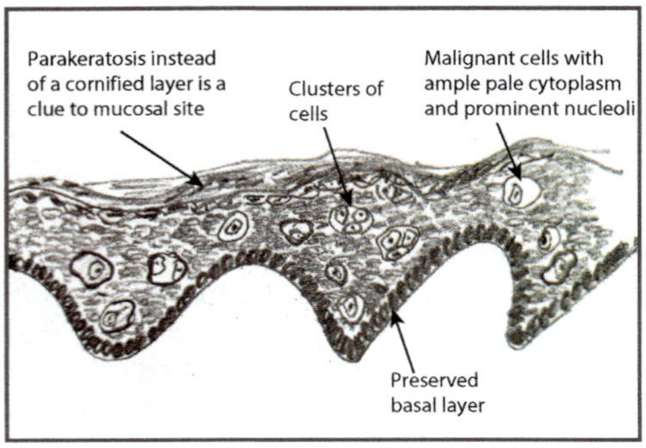

Figure 5.93 Extramammary Paget's disease: schematic presentation of the large pale cells with ample cytoplasm and prominent nucleoli which invade all layers of the epidermis except for the basal layer. Note that the cells are not connected by intercellular bridges with the surrounding cells.

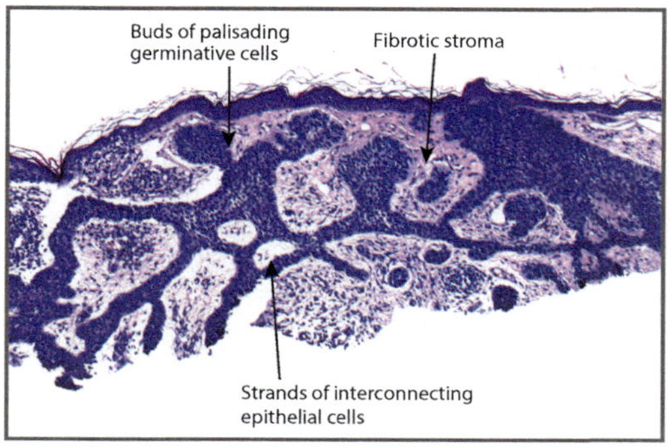

Figure 5.94 Fibroepithelioma of Pinkus: note the fenestrated pattern of branching strands of epithelial cells which interconnect and show buds of germinative cells along their length.

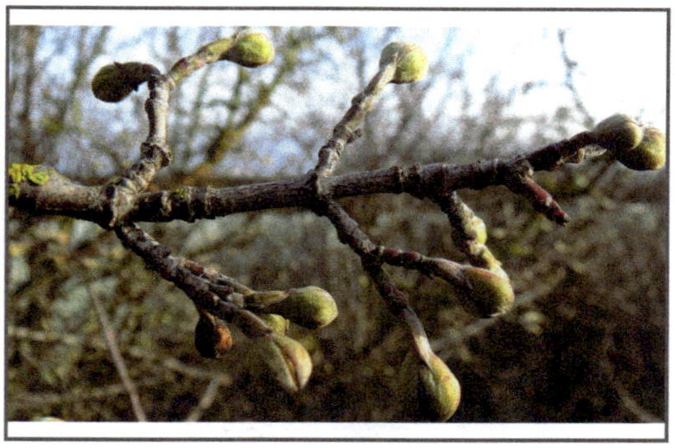

Photomnemonic 5.17 The budding of germinative cells in fibroepithelioma of Pinkus resemble slender cherry tree branches with buds.

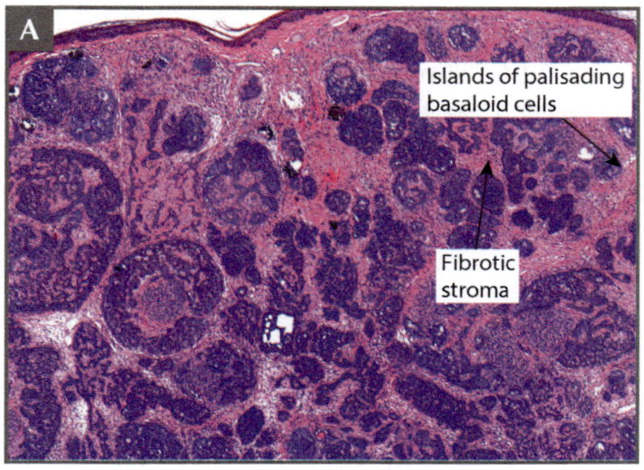

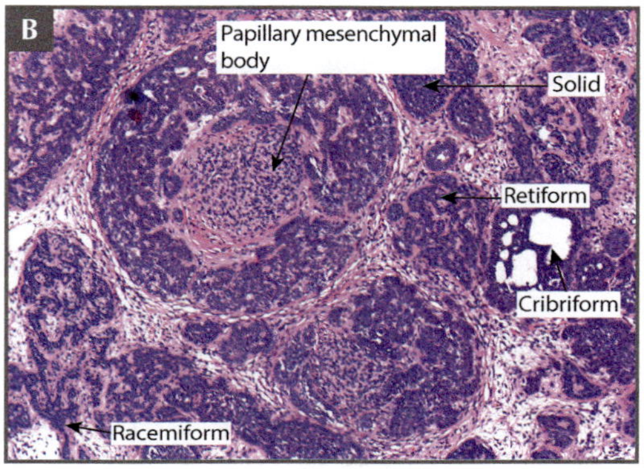

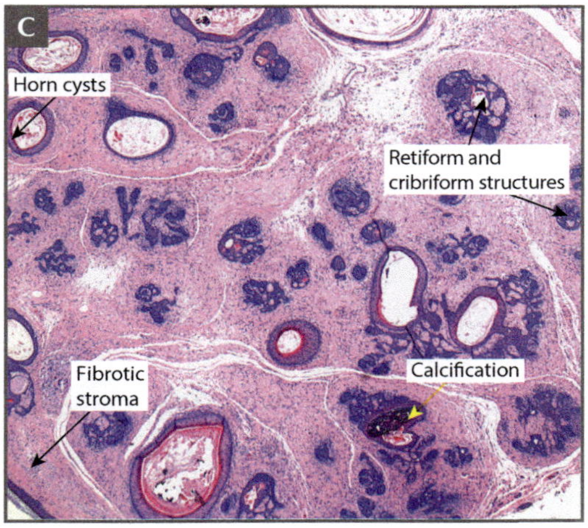

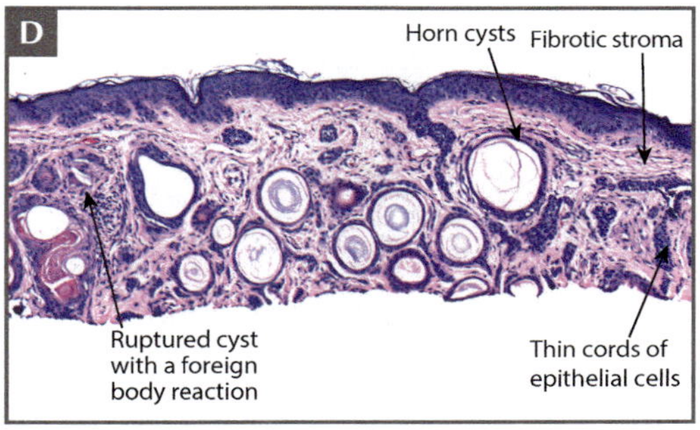

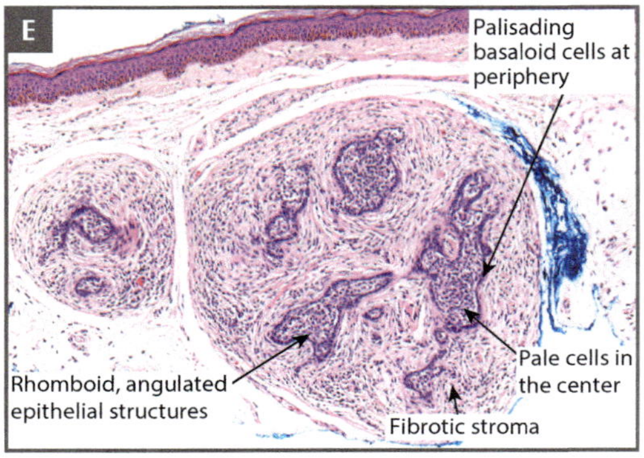

Figure 5.95 Trichoblastoma and trichoepithelioma. **A** Trichoblastoma: note the variously shaped islands of basaloid cells embedded in the fibrotic stroma without surrounding clefts and without connection to the epidermis. **B** Papillary mesenchymal bodies in trichoblastoma: a core of plump or spindle fibroblasts attempts to form papillary mesenchyme. **C** Trichoepithelioma (TEP). Note the cribriform and retiform epithelial structures embedded in a fibrotic stroma. There are also horn cysts and calcifications. **D** Desmoplastic TEP: note the presence of blue cords of epithelial cells among horn cysts in a desmoplastic stroma. **E** Lymphadenoma. Note the rhomboid epithelial structures of central pale cells surrounded by a rim of palisading blue cells. The stroma is fibrotic, and there are no clefts between the tumor and the stroma.

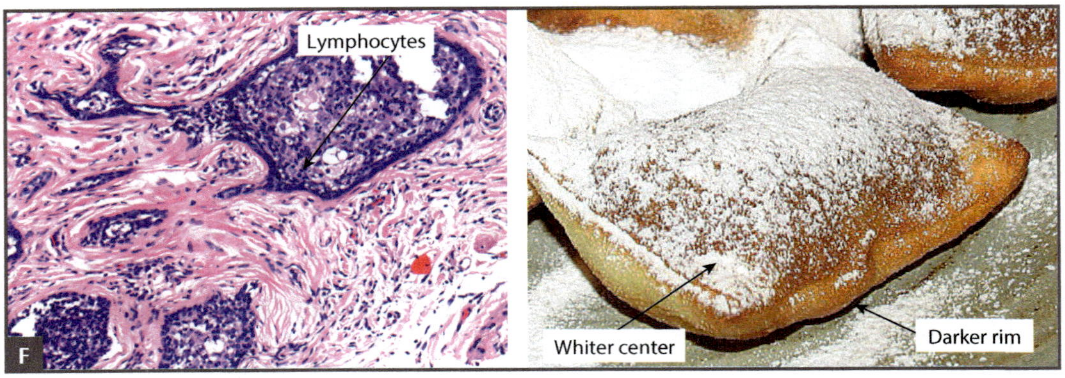

Figure 5.95 Trichoblastoma and trichoepithelioma. **F** Lymphadenoma: on high power the small blue dots within the central pale area are lymphocytes (Images E & F are courtesy of Rossitza Lazova, MD).

Photomnemonic 5.18 Epithelial structures in lymphadenoma resemble beignets with powdered sugar.

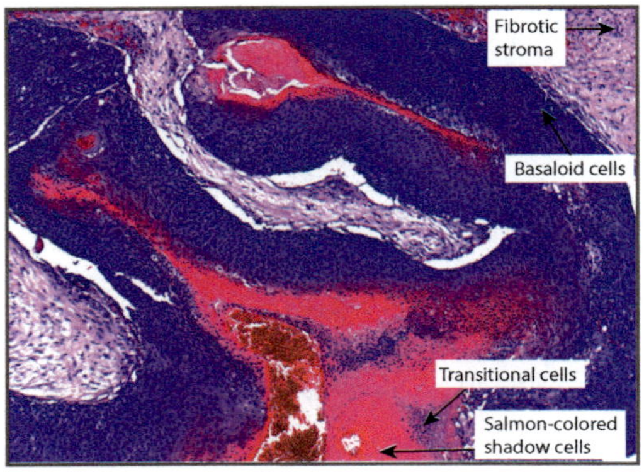

Figure 5.96 Pilomatricoma: this tumor is "tri-colored": note the three types of cells intermingled in epithelial masses.

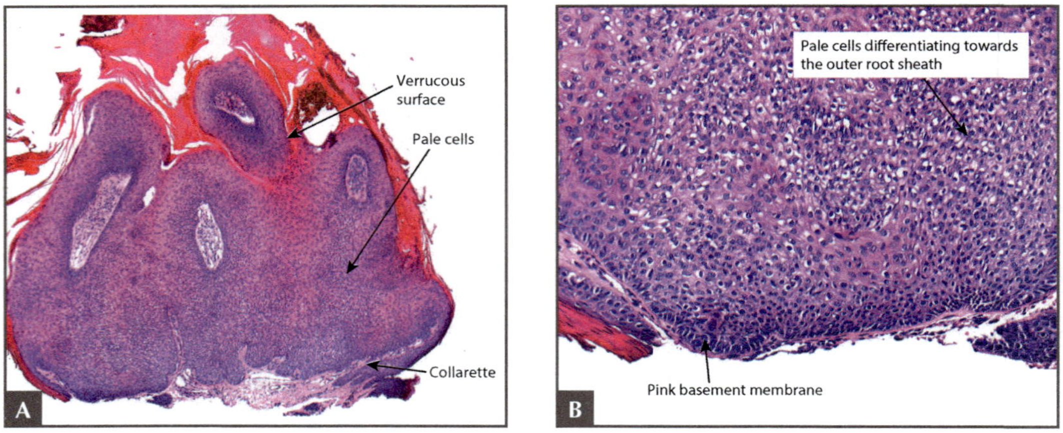

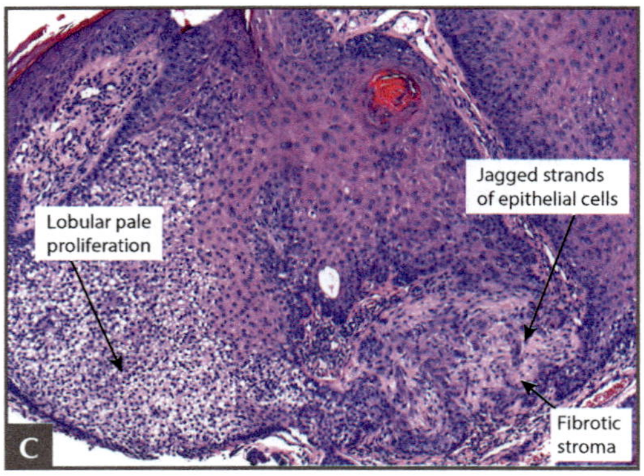

Figure 5.97 Trichilemmoma. **A** The tumor is multilobular with a verrucous surface and of pale color. **B** High power demonstrates the pink thin basement membrane. **C** Desmoplastic trichilemmoma: there is a focal area of strands of epithelial strands embedded in fibrotic stroma.

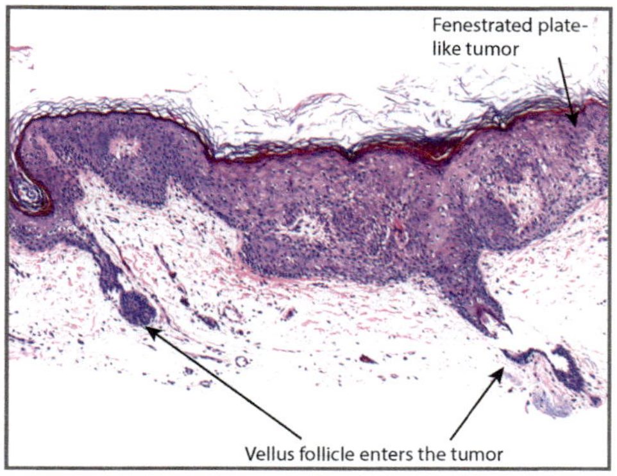

Figure 5.98 Tumor of the follicular infundibulum. The tumor is horizontal and plate-like with fenestrated pattern. Note the pale pink color.

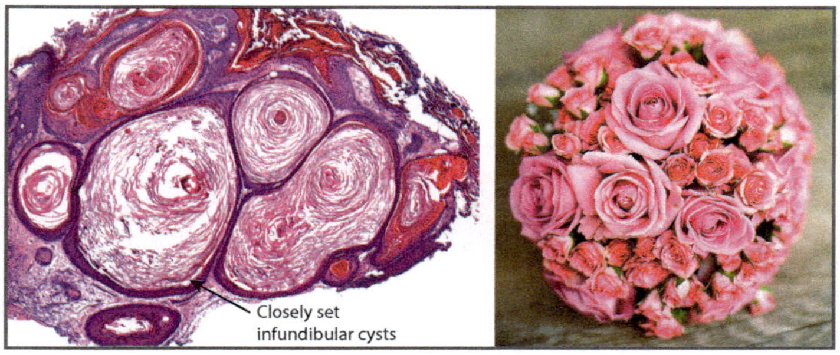

Figure 5.99 and Photomnemonic 5.19 Trichoadenoma. Note the "crowded specimen" of closely set infundibular cysts which resemble a compact bridal bouquet of pink roses.

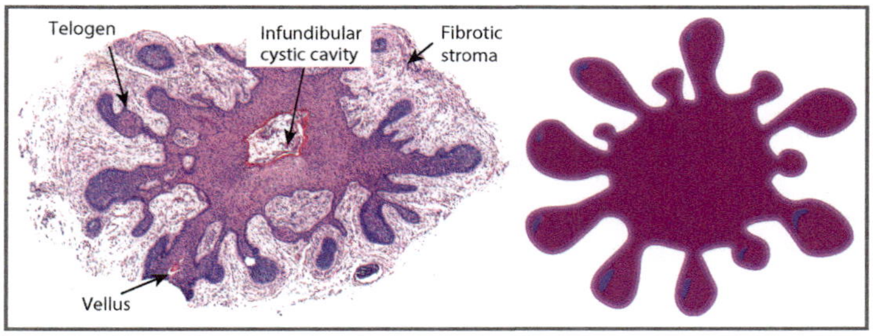

Figure 5.100 and Photomnemonic 5.20 Trichofolliculoma is a highly organized follicular tumor with a silhouette that resembles a purplish pink splash.

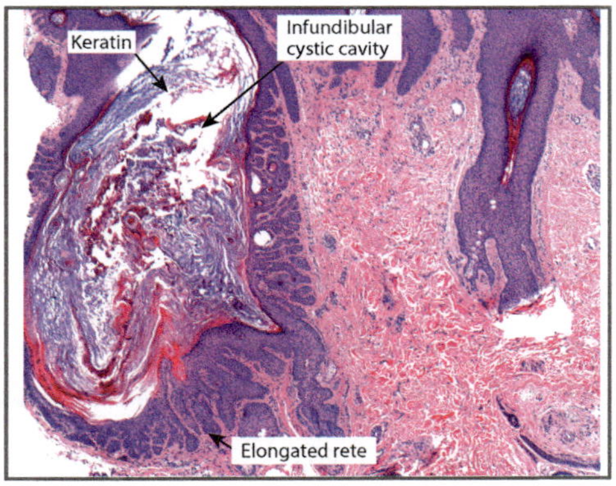

Figure 5.101 An infundibular cystic cavity filled with keratin opens to the surface; elongated rete emanate from the cyst in the dermis.

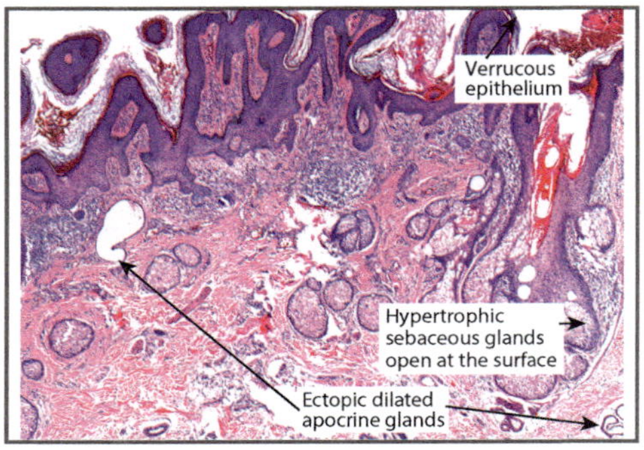

Figure 5.102 Nevus sebaceus. In the postpubertal variant, which is more commonly biopsied, there is verrucous surface. Note the hyperplastic sebaceous glands and the ectopic dilated apocrine glands.

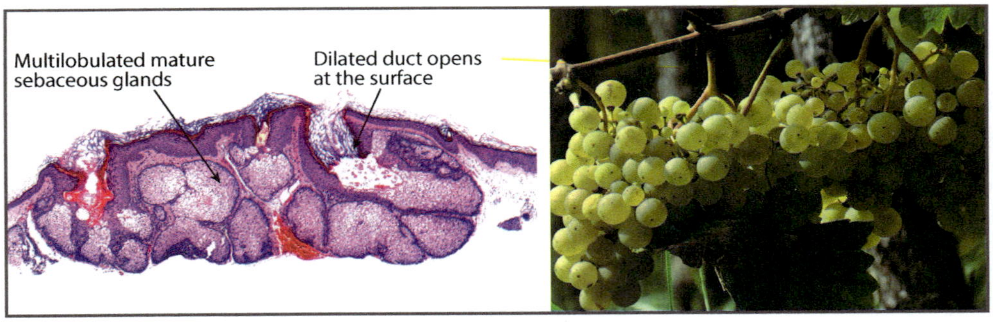

Figure 5.103 and Photomnemonic 5.21 Sebaceous hyperplasia: mature sebaceous lobules grouped around a dilated duct which opens directly at the surface resemble hanging clusters of grapes.

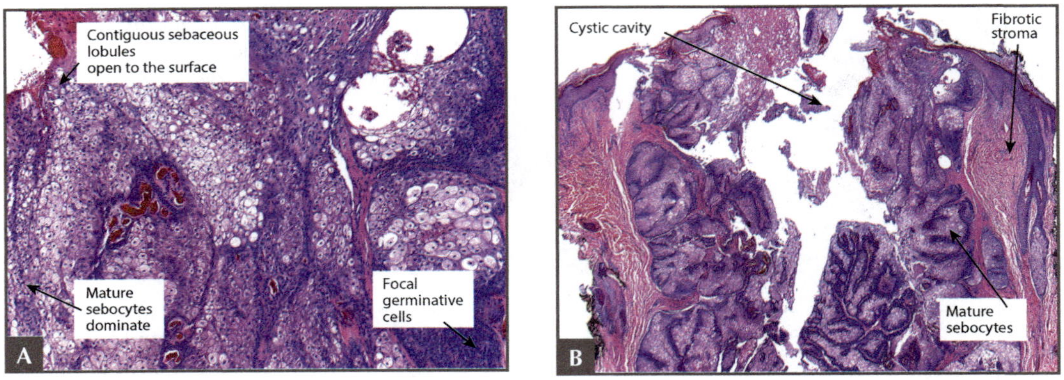

Figure 5.104 Sebaceous adenoma. **A** The sebaceous lobules of predominantly mature sebocytes connect and open directly to the surface. **B** Cystic sebaceous adenoma.

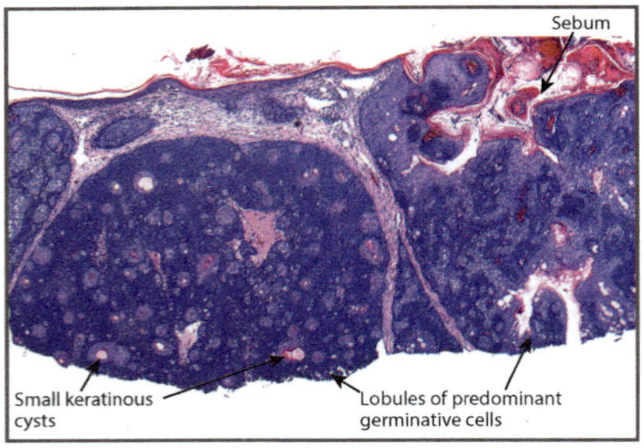

Figure 5.105 Sebaceoma: multinodular masses of smooth-contoured "bluish" lobules in the dermis composed mostly of germinative cells.

CUTANEOUS LYMPHOID NEOPLASMS

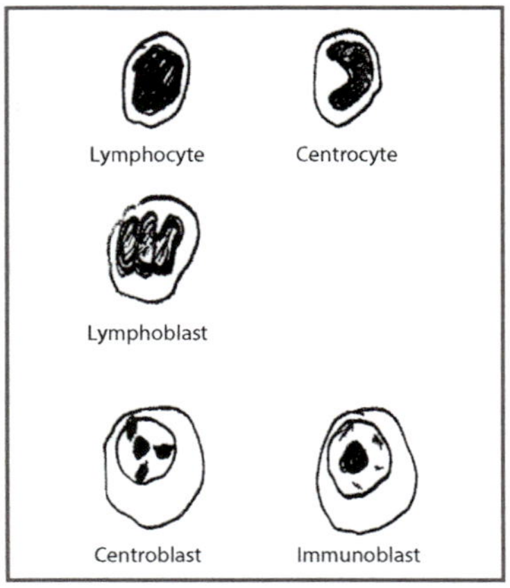

Figure 5.106 Lymphoid cells: a schematic presentation.

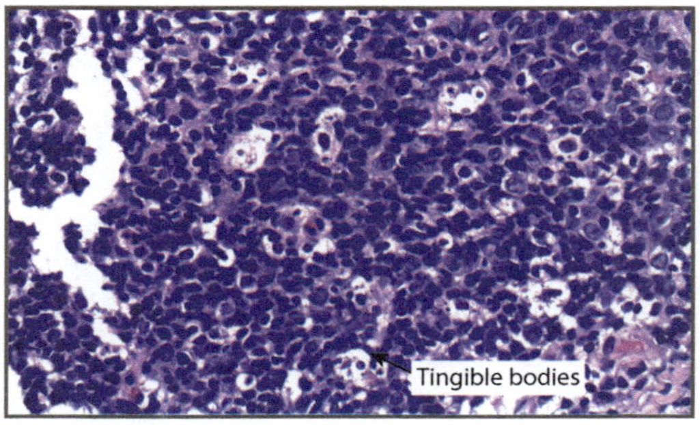

Figure 5.107 Apoptotic bodies within macrophages.

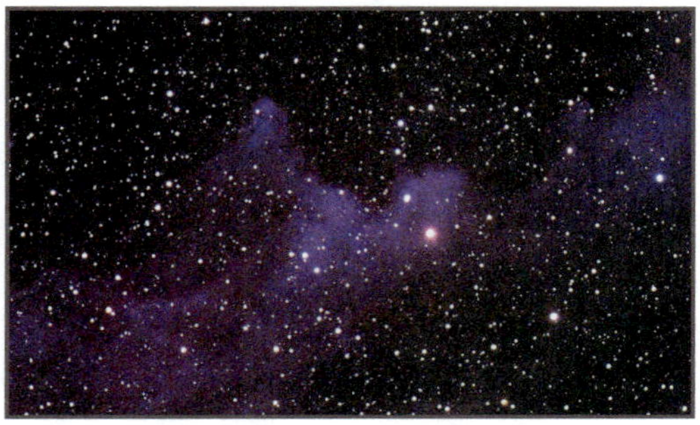

Photomnemonic 5.22 The apoptotic material in the germinal center resembles a starry sky.

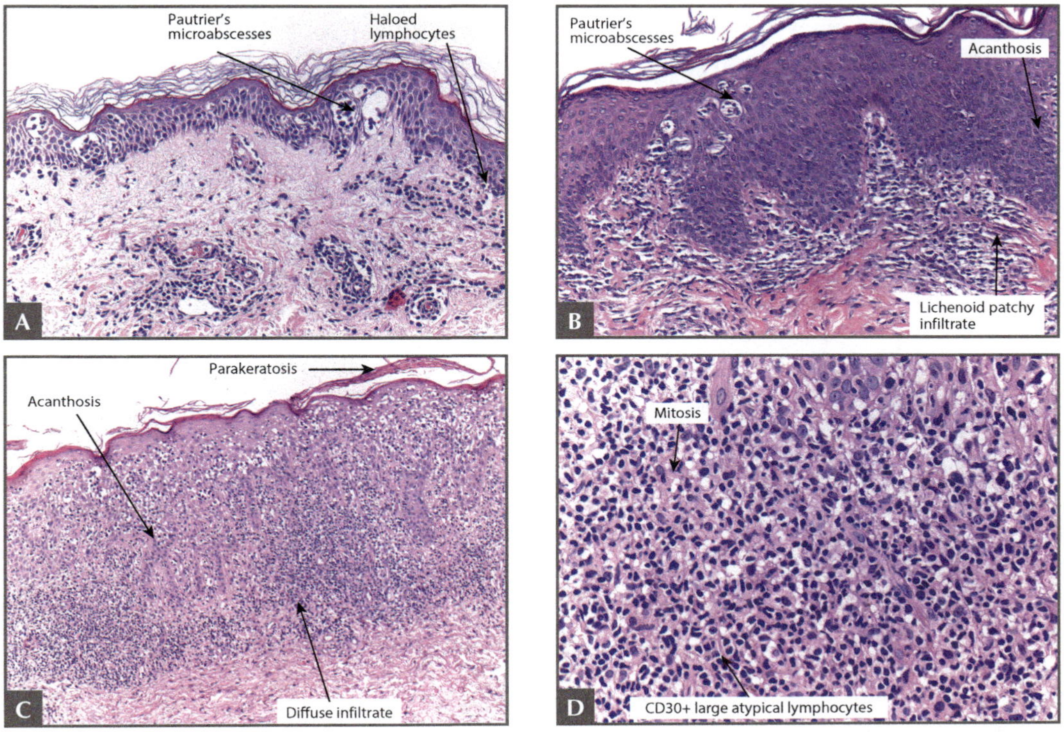

Figure 5.108 Mycosis fungoides (MF). **A** A patch stage. Note the individual haloed lymphocytes in the basal layer and the collections of same lymphocytes in Pautrier's microabscesses in the epidermis. **B** A plaque stage. Note the psoriasiform hyperplasia and the lichenoid patchy infiltrate which does not obscure the dermoepidermal junction. **C** A tumor stage, CD30+ transformation. There is diffuse dense infiltrate of atypical lymphoid cells in the dermis. **D** In the same case of MF, note the CD30+ blast-like cells and the mitoses.

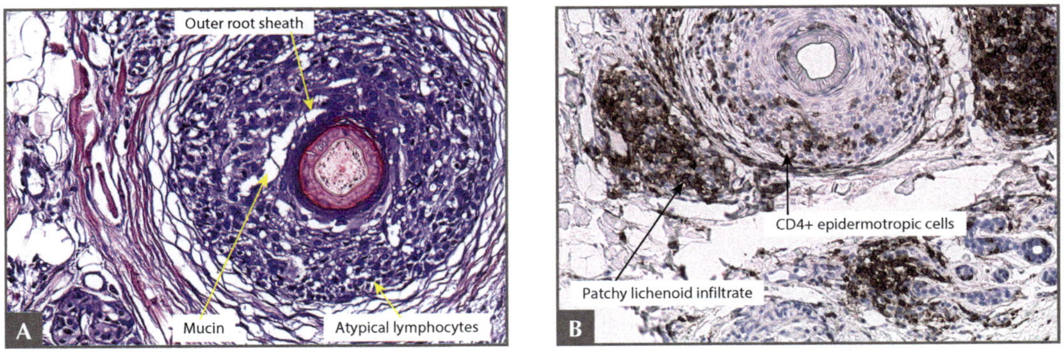

Figure 5.109 Mycosis fungoides. **A** A case of MF involving the scalp and presenting clinically with a non-scarring alopecia totalis-like pattern. Note the follicular epidermotropism in the outer root sheath and the mucin. **B** The same case shows the CD4+ follicular epidermotropism. Note also the patchy lichenoid perifollicular infiltrates.

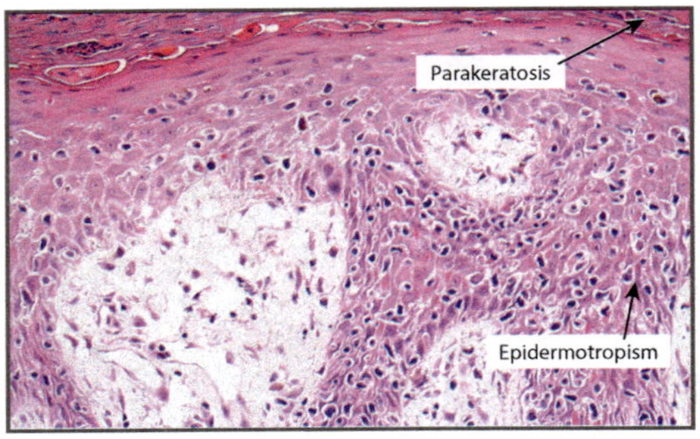

Figure 5.110 Pagetoid reticulosis. Note the haloed lymphocytes in the epidermis.

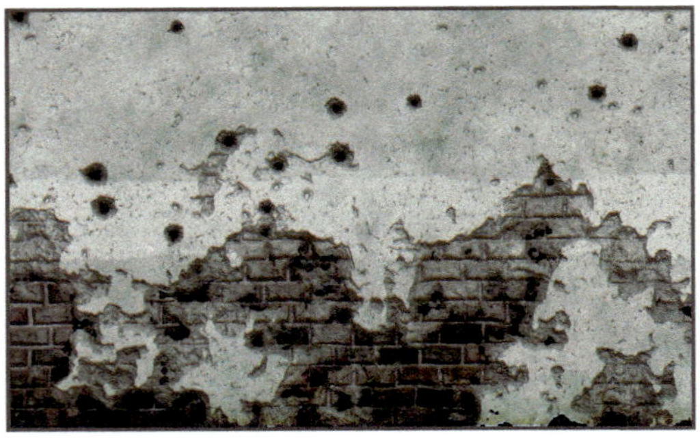

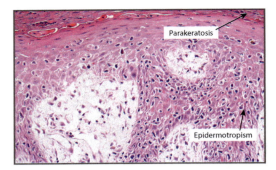

Photomnemonic 5.23 The pagetoid spread of atypical lymphocytes resembles a wall with bullet shots.

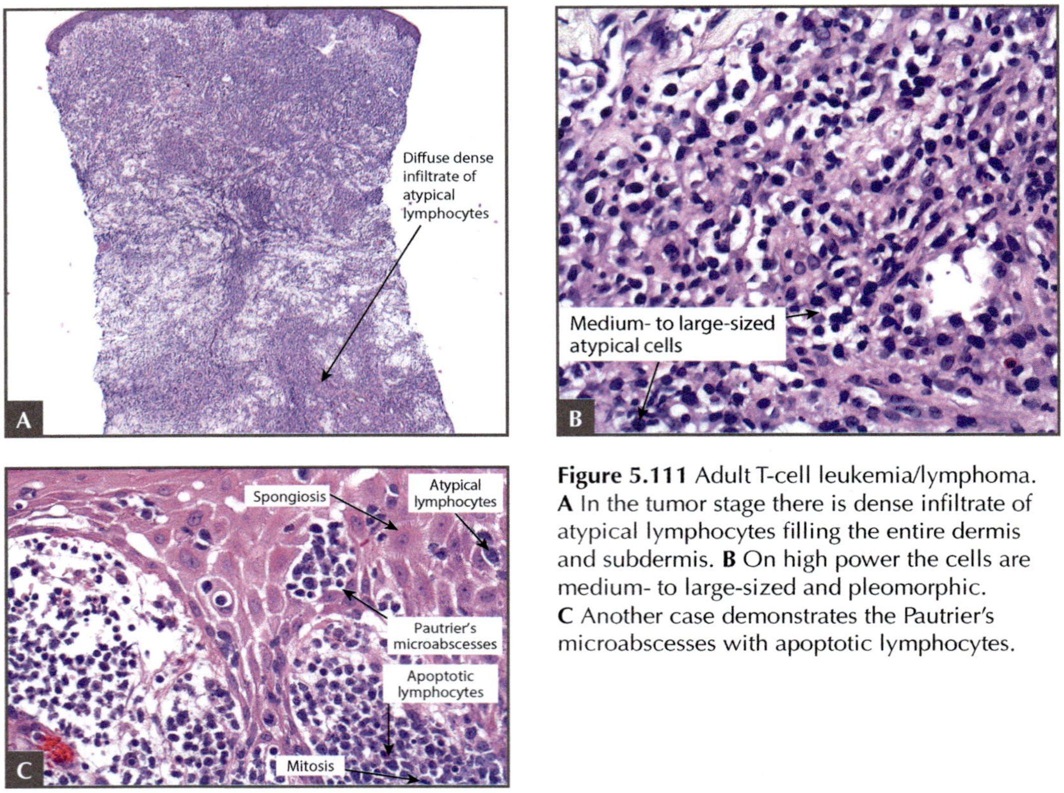

Figure 5.111 Adult T-cell leukemia/lymphoma. **A** In the tumor stage there is dense infiltrate of atypical lymphocytes filling the entire dermis and subdermis. **B** On high power the cells are medium- to large-sized and pleomorphic. **C** Another case demonstrates the Pautrier's microabscesses with apoptotic lymphocytes.

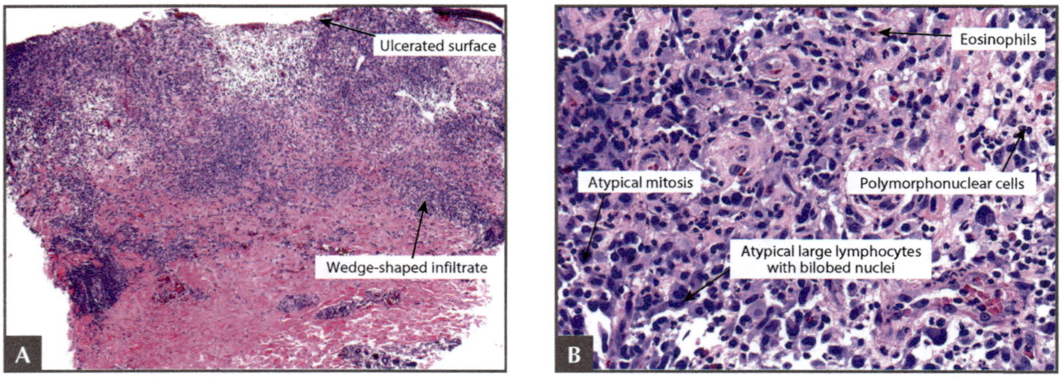

Figure 5.112 A, B Lymphomatoid papulosis, inflammatory/histiocytic type. **A** Note the wedge-shaped infiltrate in the dermis. **B** In inflammatory type the cells are large, pleomorphic, with ample cytoplasm and bilobed nuclei. Note the mixed infiltrate of inflammatory cells.

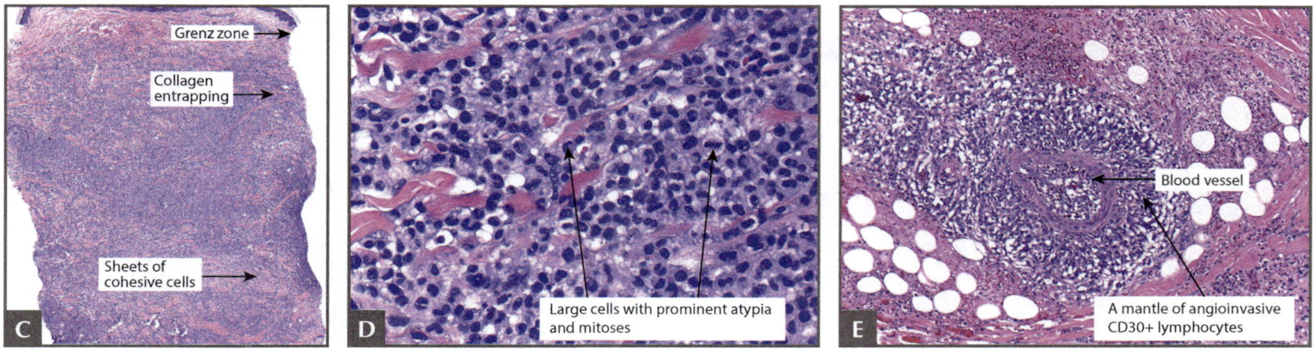

Figure 5.112 C, D Lymphomatoid papulosis, ALCL-like type. **C** Note the sheets of large atypical lymphocytes filling the entire dermis. **D** On high power the cells are large with bilobed nuclei (horseshoe-like) and show increased mitotic rate. **E** Lymphomatoid papulosis, angioinvasive type. Note large lymphocytes surrounding and invading the vessel wall.

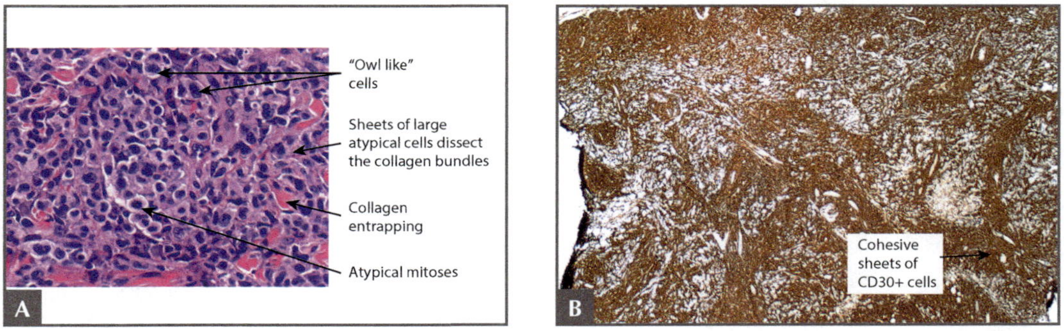

Figure 5.113 Anaplastic large cell lymphoma (ALCL). **A** The atypical cells are arranged in cohesive sheets and invade the subdermis. **B** Diffuse strong positivity for CD30.

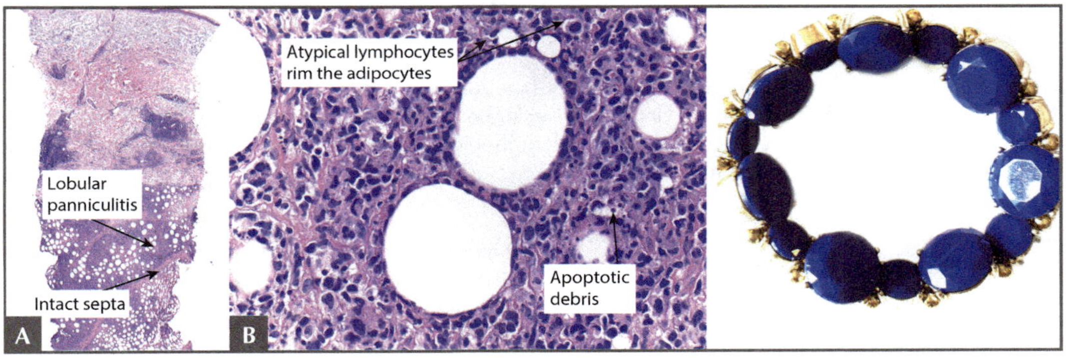

Figure 5.114 and Photomnemonic 5.24 Subcutaneous T-cell lymphoma. **A** Low power. **B** On high power the adipocytes show a rim of medium-sized atypical lymphocytes. The blue rim of atypical lymphocytes in subcutaneous T-cell lymphoma resembles a bracelet of blue stones.

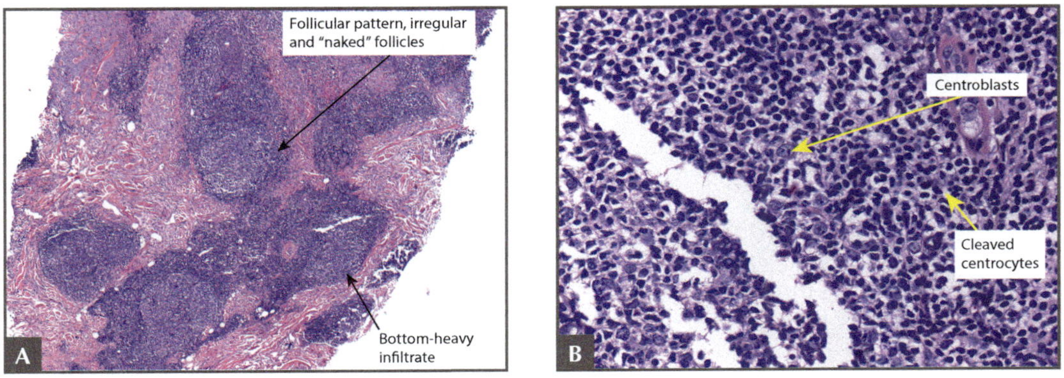

Figure 5.115 Primary cutaneous follicle center lymphoma (PCFCL). **A** Mixed follicular and diffuse pattern: the infiltrate involves the entire dermis and subdermis. **B** On high power: there is a mixture of centrocytes and centroblasts (see also Figure 5.106).

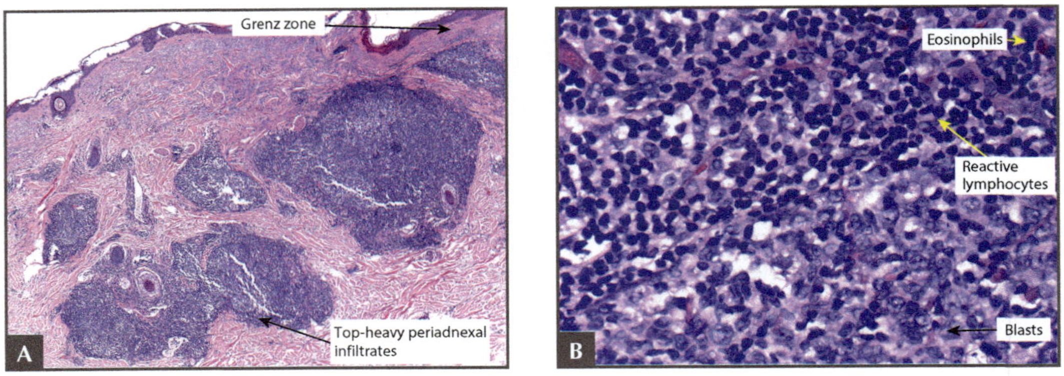

Figure 5.116 Primary cutaneous marginal zone lymphoma (PCMZL). **A** Nodular top-heavy infiltrate extends around sweat glands and hair follicles. **B** On high power: there are several blastoid cells admixed with reactive small to medium-sized lymphocytes and eosinophils.

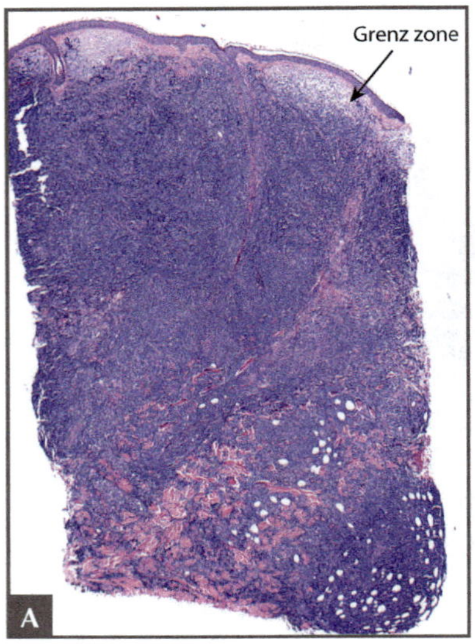

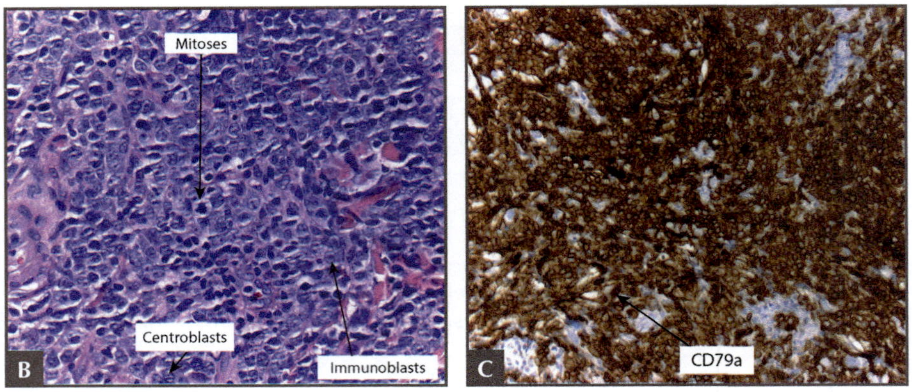

Figure 5.117 Primary cutaneous diffuse large B-cell lymphoma (DLBCL), leg type. **A** Note the dense blue infiltrate filling the entire specimen. **B** On high power the cells are large and atypical lymphocytes. **C** The cells are strongly positive for B-cell markers (CD79a).

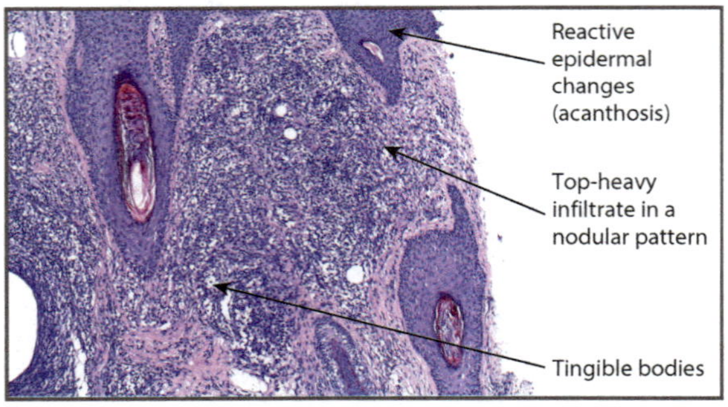

Figure 5.118 Lymphomatoid contact dermatitis. The infiltrate is nodular; no infiltration of the collagen bundles is noted.

NEURAL TUMORS

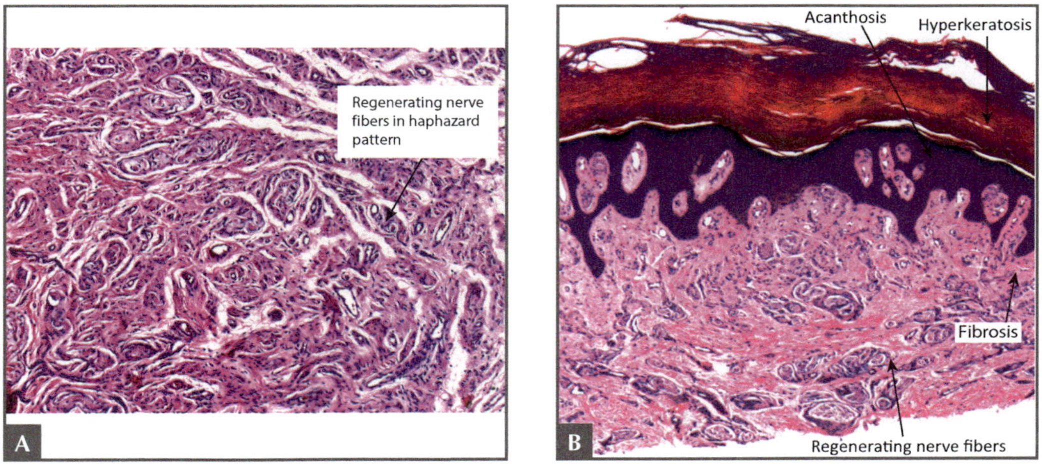

Figure 5.119 Acquired traumatic neuroma. **A** Note the haphazard fascicles of regenerating nerve fibers. **B** Rudimentary supernumerary digit is a variant of acquired traumatic neuroma. Note the acral location.

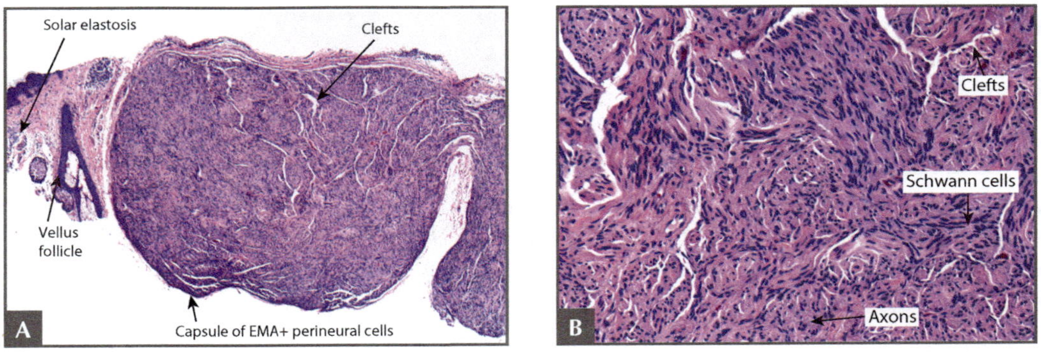

Figure 5.120 Palisaded encapsulated neuroma (PEN). **A** There are tightly interwoven fascicles with clefts among them. Note the absence of capsule at the surface. **B** PEN on high power shows the interlacing fascicles of axons (dots) and Schwann cells (spindled cells).

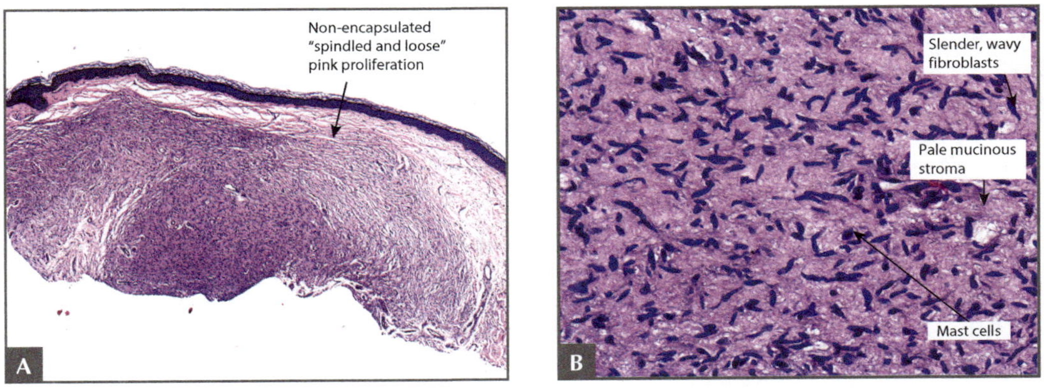

Figure 5.121 Extraneural neurofibroma (NF). **A** On low power. **B** On high power: note that the spindled cells have slender, wavy nuclei and there is an increased number of mast cells.

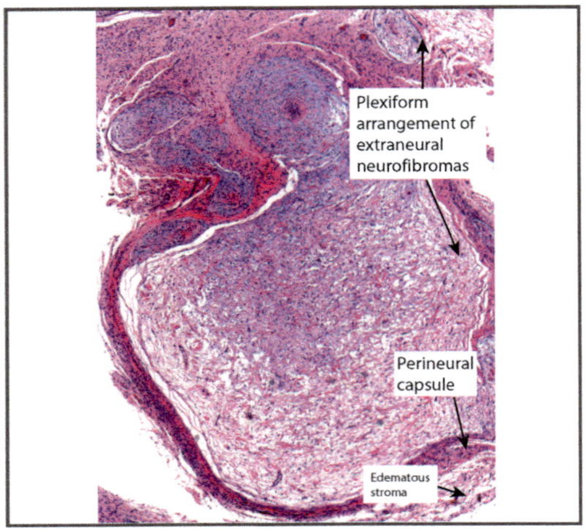

Figure 5.122 Intraneural (plexiform) NF: note the plexiform arrangement of encapsulated extraneural neurofibromas in a loose edematous stroma.

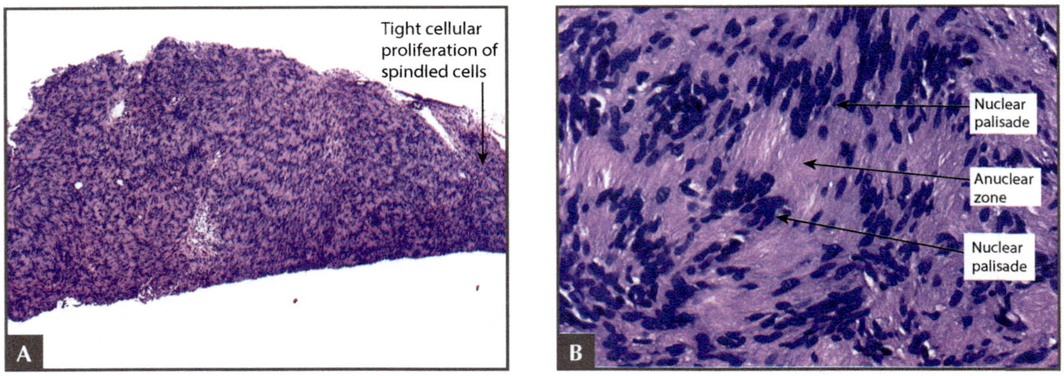

Figure 5.123 Schwannoma. **A** On low power: note the fascicular arrangement of spindled cells only and no clefts among the bundles (compare to Figure 5.120). **B** On high power: two nuclear palisades with the anuclear zone in the middle form the Verocay body.

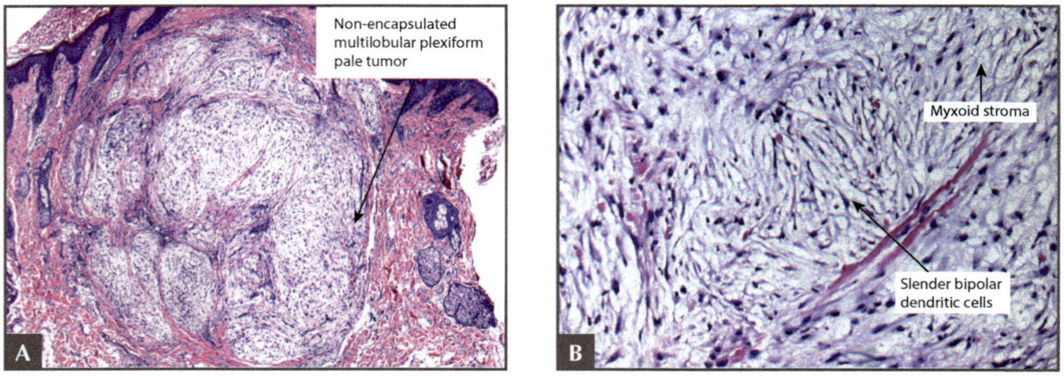

Figure 5.124 Nerve sheath myxoma (NSM). **A** The tumor is composed of bipolar/stellate immature cells embedded in a pale myxoid stroma. Note the plexiform arrangement. **B** On high power: note the bipolar cells.

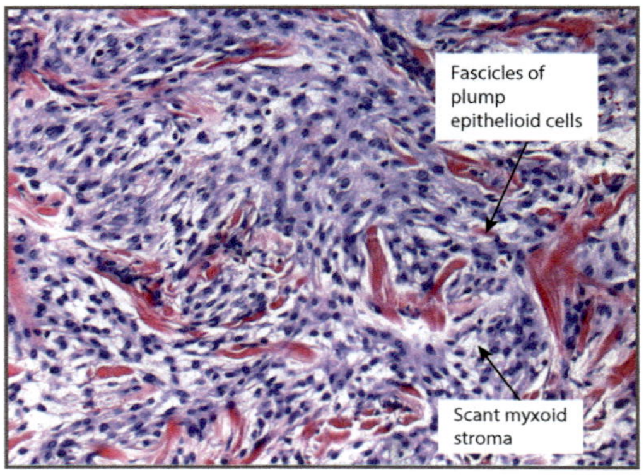

Figure 5.125 Cellular neurothekeoma. Note the fascicles of plump epithelioid cells in a scant myxoid stroma. The tumor may need to be distinguished from a melanocytic nevus.

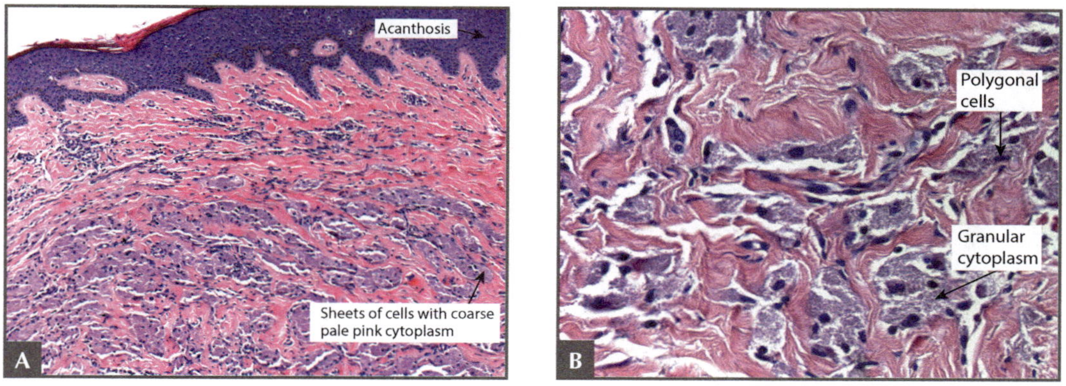

Figure 5.126 Granular cell tumor (GCT). **A** An ill-defined pale pink tumor infiltrates the collagen. **B** On high power the cells are polygonal and have an oval/round nucleus and pale granular cytoplasm.

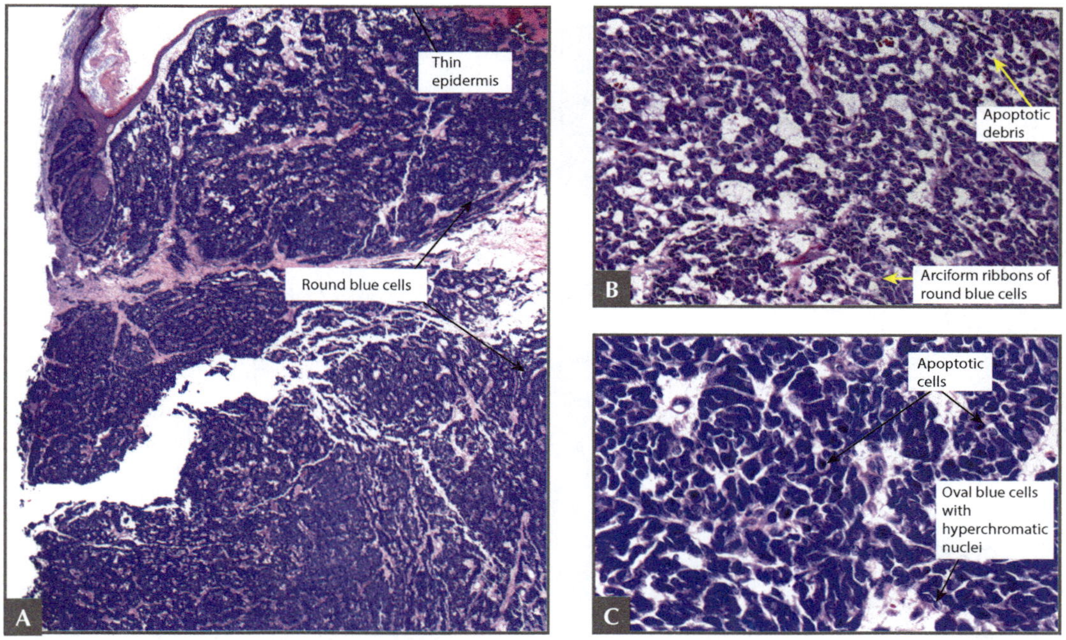

Figure 5.127 Merkel cell carcinoma (MCC). **A** A proliferation of round small blue cells organized in sheets occupies the entire specimen. **B** Note the trabecular pattern. **C** On high power the speckled chromatin is visible. There is also apoptotic debris among the blue cells.

CUTANEOUS METASTASES

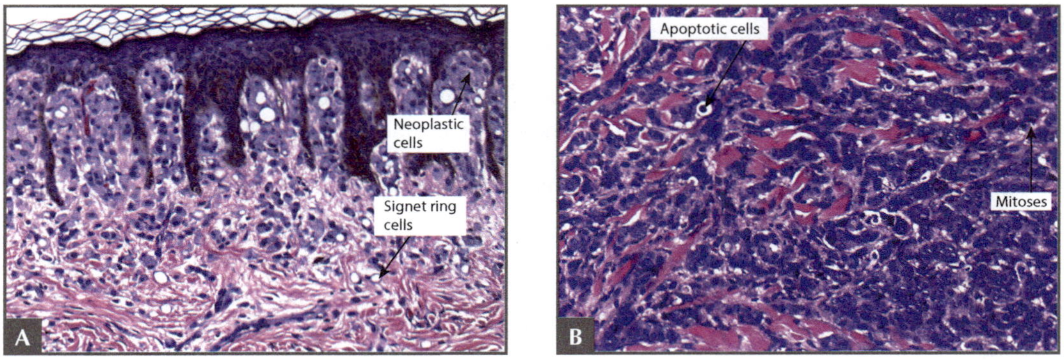

Figure 5.128 Metastatic breast carcinoma. **A** The papillary dermis is infiltrated by clusters of neoplastic cells with bluish granular, pale cytoplasm and peripheral nuclei. Some cells have a signet-ring appearance (central, cleared mucin-filled space compresses and marginalizes eccentric nucleus). **B** A different case demonstrates the infiltrative pattern in sheets and cords among the collagen bundles.

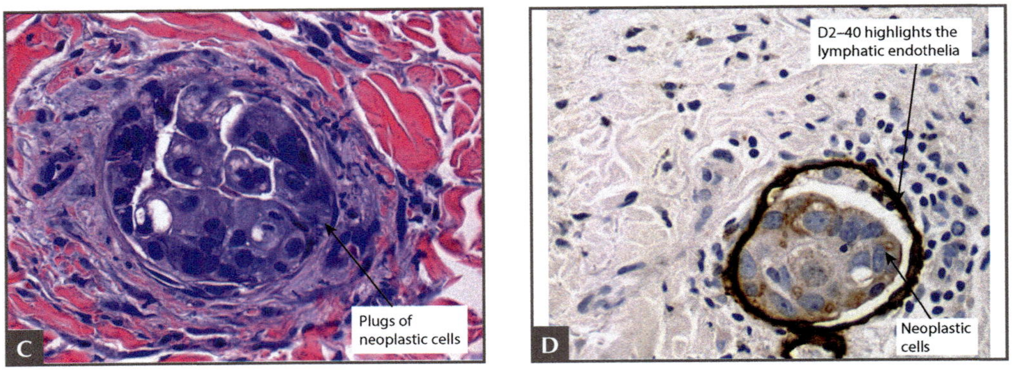

Figure 5.128 Metastatic breast carcinoma. **C** Note the malignant cells plugging the lymphatics in the dermis. **D** D2-40 highlights the lymphatic endothelia.

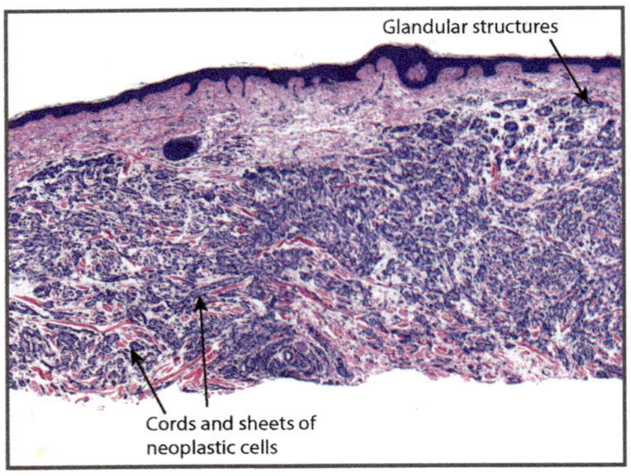

Figure 5.129 Metastatic prostate carcinoma. Cords, sheets, and glandular structures of undifferentiated atypical cells in the dermis.

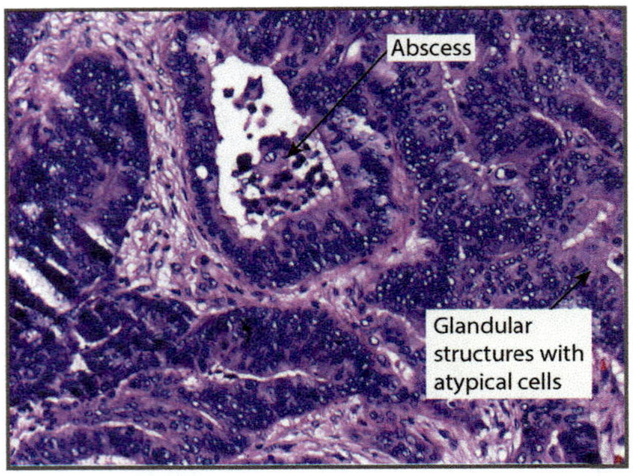

Figure 5.130 Metastatic colon carcinoma. Note the necrotic debris with abscess formation in the glandular lumina.

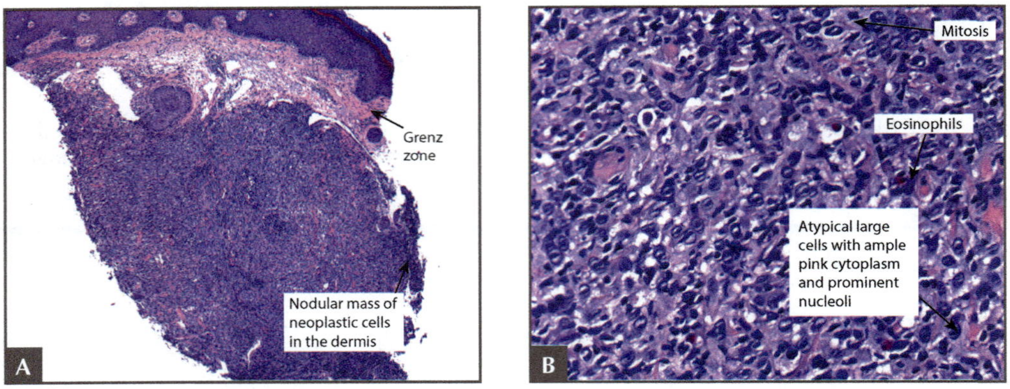

Figure 5.131 Metastatic squamous cell carcinoma (SCC) to skin. **A** Note the lack of connection to the epidermis. **B** On high power the cells show large angulated cells with ample pink cytoplasm and prominent nucleoli. Eosinophils can be identified in specimens particularly from head and neck squamous cell carcinomas (tumor-associated tissue eosinophilia, TATE).

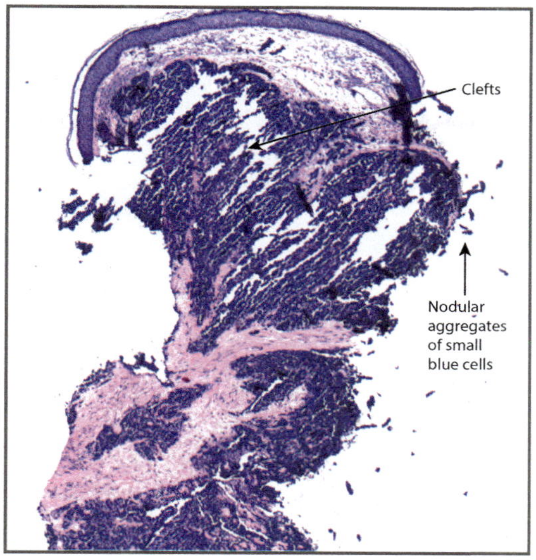

Figure 5.132 Metastatic small cell lung cancer. Note the striking resemblance to Merkel cell carcinoma. The small blue cells are organized in a nodular pattern in the entire dermis.

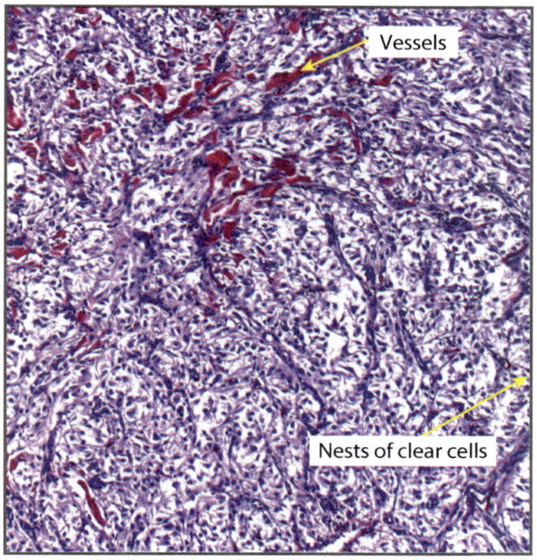

Figure 5.133 Metastatic renal cell carcinoma (RCC): the neoplastic cells have clear cytoplasm and are arranged in nests. Note the prominent vessels in a chicken-wire pattern.

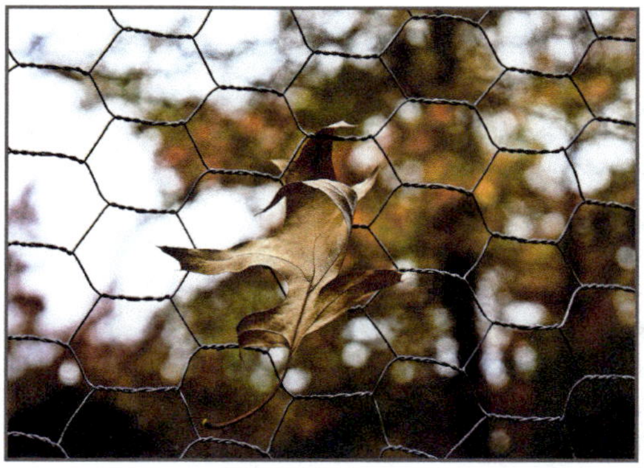

Photomnemonic 5.25 The vessels in RCC are organized in a chicken-wire pattern among the nests of neoplastic cells.

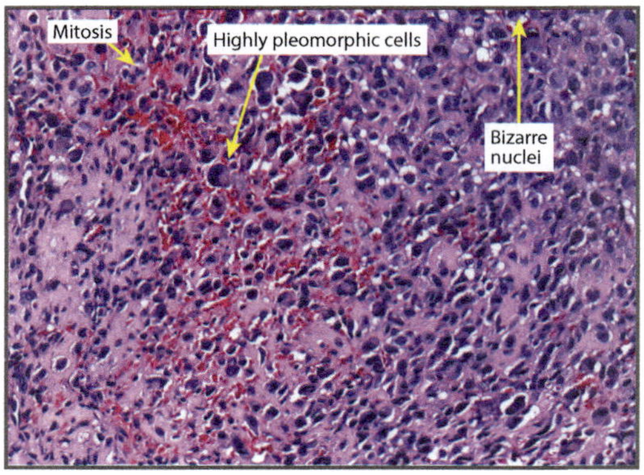

Figure 5.134 Undifferentiated pleomorphic sarcoma of the liver metastatic to skin: note the atypical infiltrate of cells with striking bizarre nuclei and atypical mitoses

SECTION III: "SPLIT SKIN": KEY PATHOLOGIC FINDINGS

6 Key pathologic findings for levels of the skin

Andrew Miner and Mariya Miteva

STRATUM CORNEUM

A. ORTHOKERATOSIS – normal, loose, "basket weave"

1. Normal skin
2. Acute dermatoses
   - Erythema multiforme
   - Stevens-Johnson syndrome
   - Acute spongiotic dermatitis

B. HYPERKERATOSIS – thickened stratum corneum *without* retained nuclei

Can be compact or loose (lamellar)

1. Compact hyperkeratosis
   - Lichen planus
   - Lichen simplex chronicus or prurigo nodularis
   - Acral skin
2. Lamellar hyperkeratosis
   - Seborrheic keratosis

C. PARAKERATOSIS – retention of nuclei within cells of the stratum corneum

1. Mound-like
   - Pityriasis rosea
   - Guttate psoriasis (often with neutrophils)
2. Confluent
   - Psoriasis vulgaris
3. Focal
   - Actinic keratosis
   - Subacute spongiotic dermatitis (often with serum: so-called "serum crust")
4. Rounded parakeratosis
   - Verruciform xanthoma
   - Premature keratinization
   - Atypical squamous proliferations (actinic keratosis, squamous cell carcinomas)
5. Checkerboard pattern –parakeratosis alternating with hyperkeratosis
   - Pityriasis rubra pilaris (often with follicular plugging)
   - Actinic keratosis (pink parakeratosis alternating with blue hyperkeratosis)
6. Cornoid lamella – 45° angle of parakeratosis with dyskeratotic cells underneath
   - Diagnostic of porokeratosis
7. "The sandwich model" – parakeratosis overlying normal lamellar stratum corneum overlying a granular layer
   - Dermatophyte infection

D. HOLES

- Normal eccrine gland ostia
- Area adjacent to scabies mite

E. RECOVERY SIGN – normal lamellar stratum corneum underlying parakeratosis or hyperkeratosis

Also called "last week's sign"
- Evidence of prior inflammation

F. NEUTROPHILS

- Candida (organisms perpendicular to epidermis)
- Tinea (organisms parallel to epidermis)
- Psoriasis
- Syphilis

G. RED BLOOD CELLS

- Talon noir
- Pityriasis rosea
- Pityriasis lichenoides

H. MELANIN

1. Acral nevi – regular columns in furrows
2. Acral melanoma – irregular columns

I. BUSY STRATUM CORNEUM

1. Parakeratosis, neutrophils and serum
   - Pityriasis lichenoides et variolis acuta (PLEVA)
   - Impetigenized spongiotic dermatitis
2. Parakeratosis and neutrophils only
   - Psoriasis (serum argues against psoriasis and favors PLEVA or spongiotic dermatitis)

EPIDERMIS

A. ABSENT EPIDERMIS

1. Erosion – partial absence of epidermis
   - Excoriation
   - Superficial acantholytic disease (keratinocytes falling apart):
     - Grover's disease
     - Pemphigus foliaceus
     - Darier's disease (with corps ronds, grains)
     - Bullous impetigo
     - Staphylococcal scalded skin syndrome
2. Ulcer – complete absence of epidermis
   - Excoriation
   - Underlying vascular compromise

B. SPACES

1. Spongiosis – spaces between cells with preserved desmosomal connections (versus acantholysis)
   - Eczematous processes (allergic contact dermatitis, nummular dermatitis)
2. Ballooning degeneration – extracellular edema in viral infections
3. Reticular degeneration – severe ballooning degeneration creating a net-like pattern in viral infections and contact dermatitis.
4. Spaces in the follicular epithelium
   - Spongiosis
   - Apocrine miliaria – inflammation in acrosyringium (intraepidermal portion of sweat duct)
   - Follicular mucinosis – mucin with/without folliculotropism of atypical lymphocytes
   - Acantholysis – cells falling apart
     - Pemphigus vulgaris often involves follicles

C. VACUOLAR DEGENERATION OF BASAL LAYER – in interface dermatides

Examples include:

- Discoid lupus erythematosus
- Dermatomyositis
- Erythema multiforme

D. ARTIFACTUAL VACUOLIZATION OF KERATINOCYTES

1. Frozen processing artifact – intracellular vacuoles in keratinocytes
2. Halos around lymphocytes
   - With spongiosis in spongiotic dermatitis
   - Without spongiosis in mycosis fungoides

E. ACANTHOLYSIS

1. Superficial acantholysis – cells falling apart in granular layer
   - Bullous impetigo (bacteria may be visible)
   - Staphylococcal scalded skin syndrome (NO bacteria seen – toxin-mediated)
   - Pemphigus foliaceus
2. Suprabasal epidermal acantholysis without dyskeratosis – cells falling apart above the basal layer without corps ronds and grains
   - Pemphigus vulgaris
3. Acantholysis with dyskeratosis (corps ronds and grains)
   - Darier's disease
   - Grover's disease (Darier's variant)
4. Acantholysis of dilapidated brick-wall pattern
   - Hailey-Hailey disease
   - Grover's disease (Hailey-Hailey variant)

F. SUPERFICIAL EPIDERMAL PALLOR AND VACUOLIZATION

1. Nutritional deficiencies
   - Pellagra
   - Glucagonoma syndrome
2. Liquid nitrogen therapy
3. Excoriation
4. Dermal vascular insult such as thrombotic vasculopathy

G. APOPTOSIS, NECROSIS, AND DYSKERATOSIS

1. Dyskeratotic cells – corps ronds and grains
   - Grover's disease
   - Darier's disease
   - Warty dyskeratoma
   - Acantholytic acanthoma

2. Apoptotic keratinocytes
   - Superficial apoptosis
     - Sunburn cells in phototoxic eruptions
   - Basal layer and/or acrosyringium apoptosis
     - Interface dermatitis
3. Satellite cell necrosis - apoptotic keratinocyte with an adjacent lymphocyte
   - Classic (but not specific) for graft-versus-host disease
4. Confluent necrosis
   - Intense interface dermatitis such as toxic epidermal necrolysis, grade IV GVHD, or bullous lichen planus

H. "FOREIGN" CELLS

1. With spongiosis
   - Lymphocytes (inconspicuous)
     - Spongiotic dermatitis
   - Neutrophils
     - Neutrophilic dermatoses such as Sweet's syndrome
     - Immunobullous diseases such as pemphigus
   - Eosinophils (eosinophilic spongiosis)
     - Bullous pemphigoid
     - Incontinentia pigmenti
     - Pemphigus vulgaris (especially the vegetans variant)
     - Pemphigus foliaceus
     - Spongiotic processes such as allergic contact dermatitis
   - Red blood cells
     - Pityriasis lichenoides
2. Without spongiosis
   - Lymphocytes (atypical): epidermotropism
     - Mycosis fungoides
   - Neutrophils
     - Subcorneal pustular dermatosis
     - IgA pemphigus
   - Pagetoid cells
     - Melanoma
     - Squamous cell carcinoma in situ
     - Intraepidermal sebaceous carcinoma
     - Pseudopagetoid melanocytes in tangentially cut sections (look for "holes of dermis" within the epidermis)
     - Paget's disease
     - Merkel cell carcinoma

I. ACANTHOSIS – THICKENING OF THE EPIDERMIS

1. Psoriasiform – long, regular acanthosis with thinning of suprapapillary plates (thin epidermis overlying elongated upward-reaching dermis)
   - Psoriasis
   - Syphilis
   - Tinea
2. Plump rete ridges with no suprapapillary thinning
   - Pityriasis rubra pilaris
3. Papillomatosis – undulations in the epidermis ranging from sharp, finger-like projections to broad, gradual changes in the epidermis
   - Sharp, finger-like projections
     - Stucco keratosis
     - Verruca filiformis
   - Broad, gradual undulations
     - Confluent and reticulated papillomatosis
     - Acanthosis nigricans
4. Pseudoepitheliomatous hyperplasia – pseudocarcinomatous changes sometimes including keratinocyte enlargement, squamous eddies, and keratin pearls
   - Reactive
     - Prurigo nodularis
     - Hypertrophic lichen planus
     - Hypertrophic discoid lupus erythematosus
   - Infections
     - Blastomycosis
     - Coccidioidomycosis
     - Chromoblastomycosis
     - Blastomycosis-like pyoderma (staphylococcal infection)

J. PERFORATING DERMATOSES

See Chapter 4, Table 4.9

K. ATROPHY

1. With collagen homogenization
   - Lichen sclerosis et atrophicus
2. With normal collagen
   - Goltz syndrome
   - Anetoderma

DERMIS

A. SPACES

1. Cysts
2. Dermal fillers
3. Artifact
4. Edema
   - Urticaria – intravascular neutrophils
   - Arthropod bite reaction – superficial and deep with eosinophils
   - Sweet's syndrome – neutrophils and leukocytoclasia without vasculitis
   - Polymorphous light eruption – lymphocytes
   - Pernio (aka chilblains) – superficial and deep lymphocytes on acral skin
5. Separation epidermis/dermis
   - Cell-poor subepidermal blisters
     - Artifact overlying scar

    - Porphyria cutanea tarda
    - Epidermolysis bullosa acquisita
    - Cell-poor bullous pemphigoid
  - Cell-rich subepidermal blisters
    - Bullous pemphigoid (eosinophils)
    - Dermatitis herpetiformis (neutrophils and eosinophils)
    - IgA pemphigus (neutrophils)
6. Lymphatics – endothelial lining, no blood cells in the lumen
  - Lymphangioma
  - Lymphedema
7. Mucin deposition
  - Mucocele
  - Focal mucinosis
  - Pretibial myxedema
8. Foamy cells in the dermis (xanthoma)
  - Xanthelasma – eyelid skin with vellus hairs, foamy histiocytes
  - Eruptive xanthoma – foamy histiocytes with extracellular lipid and admixed acute and chronic inflammation
  - Tuberous xanthoma – nodular aggregates of foamy cells without inflammatory cells
9. Pale infiltrates in the dermis
  - Granulomas
    - Tuberculoid – admixed prominent inflammation +/– necrobiosis
      - Tuberculosis
      - Leprosy
      - Lupus miliaris disseminatus faciei
    - Sarcoidal – epithelioid round granulomas with only sparse surrounding inflammation and NO necrobiosis
      - Sarcoidosis
      - Beryllium
      - Zirconium
    - Necrobiotic – altered collagen with histiocytes and often other inflammatory cells
      - Granuloma annulare
      - Necrobiosis lipoidica – layers of altered collagen alternating with layers of inflammatory cells
      - Necrobiotic xanthogranuloma – cholesterol clefts, altered collagen, associated IgG kappa monoclonality
  - Tumors
    - Clear cell squamous cell carcinoma
    - Balloon cell nevus/melanoma
    - Clear cell sarcoma
    - Renal cell carcinoma

B. FOREIGN BODIES

1. Crystals
  - Keratin – fine filaments of keratin often present within clefts
  - Cholesterol – needle-like clefts seen in embolic diseases, necrobiotic xanthogranuloma, or post-steroid panniculitis
  - Urate – seen in gout; foamy "feathery" altered collagen surrounding clefts
2. Calcium – purple material
3. Bone – osteoma cutis with pink bone and osteocytes

C. BAND-LIKE INFILTRATE

1. Lymphocytes
  - Lichenoid dermatoses
  - Lichenoid tumor reactions (benign lichenoid keratosis)
2. Neutrophils
  - With edema
    - Neutrophilic dermatoses such as Sweet's syndrome
3. Plasma cells
  - Zoon's balanitis
  - Syphilis
4. Eosinophils
  - Lichenoid drug eruption
5. Pigment incontinence
  - Non-specific finding seen in lichenoid dermatoses, dysplastic nevi, and postinflammatory hyperpigmentation among other entities

D. PAPILLARY DERMIS

1. Expanded
  - Lichenoid dermatitis
  - Urticaria pigmentosa
  - Mycosis fungoides
  - Pigmented purpura
2. Spared (Grenz zone)
  - Cutaneous B-cell lymphoma
  - Lepromatous leprosy
  - Granuloma faciale

E. CONNECTIVE TISSUE ABNORMALITIES

1. Sclerosis
  - Morphea
  - Lichen sclerosus et atrophicus
  - Scleromyxedema
2. Fibrosis
  - Scar
  - Nephrogenic systemic fibrosis
3. Necrobiosis of collagen
  - Granuloma annulare
  - Rheumatoid nodule
  - Necrobiosis lipoidica
  - Necrobiotic xanthogranuloma
4. Red collagen (flame figure)
  - Wells' syndrome
  - Any entity with numerous eosinophils (arthropod bite reaction, parasitic reaction)

5. Hypotrophic/absent elastic tissue
   - Cutis laxa
   - Scar
   - Anetoderma – may be primary or secondary
   - Mid-dermal elastolysis
   - Solar elastosis – basophilic alteration of collagen

F. INFLAMMATORY INFILTRATES

1. Superficial – often non-specific finding on its own
   - Urticaria (neutrophils and/or eosinophils)
   - Drug eruption
   - Viral exanthems
2. Superficial and deep
   - Arthropod bite reaction
   - Lichen striatus (perieccrine inflammation)
   - Discoid or tumid lupus (increased mucin)
3. Wedge-shaped
   - Pityriasis lichenoides
   - Inflammatory cells along nerves
     - Leprosy

G. "BUSY DERMIS" PATTERN

1. Necrobiosis lipoidica
2. Granuloma annulare
3. Early Kaposi's sarcoma
4. Folliculitis

H. VASCULAR ABNORMALITIES

1. Vasculitis
   - Size of vessel involved and inflammatory infiltrate are key to diagnosis.
   - Incidental vasculitis under ulcers common and not necessarily pathologic.
2. Hemorrhage – extravasated red blood cells with minimal inflammation
   - Traumatic
   - Actinic purpura
3. Thrombi – fibrin plugs without significant inflammation
   - Coagulopathies
   - Cryoglobulinema
   - Degos disease
   - Deep fungal infections (*Aspergillus*)
   - Angiolipoma

I. PILOSEBACEOUS AND SWEAT GLAND ABNORMALITIES

1. Follicular plugging
   - Keratosis pilaris
   - Discoid lupus erythematosus
   - Pityriasis rubra pilaris
2. Adnexotropism of inflammatory cells
   - Lichen planopilaris
   - Discoid lupus erythematosus
3. Adnexotropism of neoplastic cells
   - With lymphocytes and mucin – folliculotropic mycosis fungoides
   - Atypical squamous cells – squamous cell carcinoma in situ
   - Atypical melanocytes – melanoma in situ
4. Tumors with vellus follicles
   - Accessory tragus – preauricular papule, often with cartilage
   - Hair follicle nevus – papule with vellus follicles but without cartilage (may be variant of accessory tragus)
   - Preauricular pit – invagination with vellus hairs
   - Trichofolliculoma – many vellus follicles feeding a central "mother follicle"
5. Eosinophils around sweat coils and ducts – arthropod bite reaction
6. Lymphocytes around sweat coils
   - Perniosis
   - Lupus erythematosus (tumid lupus)
7. Neutrophils around sweat coils (neutrophilic hidradenitis)
8. Black granules around sweat coils: argyria

J. FOREIGN SUBSTANCES

1. Banana bodies – ochronosis
2. Black granules around sweat coils – argyria
3. Superficial dermal yellow–brown granules – hydroxychloroquine, amiodarone, and omeprazole have all been described with this pattern
4. Red granules on fluorescent microscopy – clofazimine

SUBDERMIS

A. LIPOATROPHY – lost or diminished subcutaneous fat (shrunken lobules, shrunken adipocytes, increased number of vessels)

1. Primary
2. Secondary (usually due to inflammation and intralesional steroid therapy)

B. EMPTY SPACES

1. Cysts of different size with crystals – dermal fillers
2. Needle-like clefts
   - Without inflammation
     - Sclerema neonatorum
   - With inflammation
     - Subcutaneous fat necrosis of the newborn
     - Post-steroid panniculitis

C. INFLAMMATION

See Chapter 3, Panniculitis

1. Septal
   - Erythema nodosum – Miescher's granulomas
   - Morphea profunda

2. Lobular
    - Erythema induratum – prominent vasculitis with associated panniculitis
    - Alpha-1 antitrypsin – neutrophils
    - Pancreatic panniculitis – saponification with nuclear dust and ghost cells
    - Subcutaneous panniculitis-like T-cell lymphoma – lymphocytes rimming adipocytes (classic but not entirely specific sign)
    - Infection – suppurative, granulomatous, or eosinophilic depending on etiology
    - Hyalinization of the fat (systemic lupus erythematosus)
    - Honeycomb pattern in neoplasms (dermatofibrosarcoma protuberans)

FASCIA

A. EOSINOPHILIC FASCIITIS

Eosinophils sometimes prominent, but inflammatory cells typically present

B. SCLERODERMA/MORPHEA

Thickened fascia of eosinophilic fasciitis without the inflammation; typically overlying sclerotic collagen present

C. NODULAR FASCIITIS

Randomly arranged spindle cells with mitoses, inflammatory cells, and extravasated red cells